Imaging of Bone Tumors in Shoulder and Elbow

Xiaoguang Cheng • Yongbin Su
Mingqian Huang

Imaging of Bone Tumors in Shoulder and Elbow

中国协和医科大学出版社
Peking Union Medical College Press

Springer

Xiaoguang Cheng
Department of Radiology
Beijing Jishuitan Hospital
Beijing
China

Yongbin Su
Department of Radiology
Beijing Jishuitan Hospital
Beijing
China

Mingqian Huang
Department of Diagnostic
Molecular and Interventional Radiology
Mount Sinai Health System
New York, NY
USA

ISBN 978-981-33-6149-2 ISBN 978-981-33-6150-8 (eBook)
https://doi.org/10.1007/978-981-33-6150-8
Jointly published with Peking Union Medical College Press

This Springer imprint is published by the registered company Springer Nature Singapore Pte Ltd.
The registered company address is: 152 Beach Road, #21-01/04 Gateway East, Singapore 189721, Singapore

Foreword

Beijing Jishuitan Hospital has a long history and experience in the diagnosis and treatment of various orthopedic diseases. Despite this abundant experience, the diagnosis of bone tumors remains difficult because of the low morbidity of this condition. Professor Song Xian-wen, known as the father of Chinese bone tumors, recalled the establishment of the Chinese bone tumor treatment team in the 1970s and said that "After we had done a lot of clinical work and treated hundreds of orthopaedic patients, we found the complexity of bone tumors… the diagnosing of bone tumors needed the combination of clinical, radiological test and pathological result…." The diagnosis of bone tumors is difficult because bone tumors are a type of orthopedic diseases and also have imaging features that are common to other orthopedic diseases such as congenital abnormalities and degenerative bone disease. Furthermore, there are similarities between bone tumors and metabolic bone diseases, and even between the different subtypes of bone tumors.

The World Health Organization's classification system for bone tumors has undergone a transition from being based on histoembryology to histogenesis. The introduction of bone tumor "radiomics" has also further revealed the complexity of bone tumors. The complexity of bone tumors necessitates a combination of clinical, radiological, and pathological findings for accurate diagnosis.

One point that requires special emphasis is that even though some people think that pathological diagnosis is the "gold standard" in combination diagnosis, imaging is actually more reliable than pathology for diagnosing some types of bone tumors. Therefore, in general, we believe that imaging should be the basis for the final diagnosis of bone tumors.

The study of bone tumors requires strong integration of theories and practice. These theories are only fully assimilated after continuous practice. Thus, the importance of practice is endorsed by many famous professors in Beijing Jishuitan Hospital. Professor Song Xian-wen from the Department of Bone Tumors and Professor Wang Yun-zhao from the Department of Radiology had done a lot of work in determining the correlations between histology and radiology.

I recall Professor Wang Yun-zhao holding an imaging meeting in a small room that was about 6 m^2; this meeting was so popular that most of the doctors had to listen from outside the room. This tradition of discussing imaging and the thirst for practical knowledge drive us all. The good news is that this tradition has been inherited by the Department of Radiology in Beijing

Jishuitan Hospital. The writing of this book is the cumulative product of continuous practice and imaging meetings that have been held over the past several decades.

This book contains high-quality images, which will increase the ability of clinicians to use imaging to diagnose bone tumors. I believe that there are at least two important benefits to be gained from this book. The first one is the provision of examples of typical radiological findings of bone tumors, which can be consulted as needed. The second one is the description of the analysis process used in bone tumor imaging diagnosis. This describes a real practice that can help the reader to train, verify, and improve his or her diagnostic skills and finally become a "master of bone tumor imaging diagnosis."

In conclusion, this book is a crystallization of collective wisdom that contains rich content and detailed information that is both scientific and practical. This book provides doctors and students with a valuable reference related to bone tumors, which is important in increasing the ability of clinicians to use imaging to diagnose bone tumors.

I am pleased to write the foreword for this book and hope that its publication aids in the development of bone tumor radiology in China.

November 1, 2020

Niu Xiaohui
Department of Orthopaedic Oncology Surgery
Beijing Jishuitan Hospital
Beijing, China

Preface

The correct diagnosis of bone tumor and tumor-like lesions is challenging due to their low prevalence, lack of features, and the variety of bone tumors. The close teamwork of orthopedist, radiologist, and pathologist is the key to meeting this challenge.

The Bone Tumor Department of Beijing Jishuitan Hospital, founded in 1984, was the first center to specialize in bone tumor treatment in China and is well regarded both in China and abroad. Professor Wang Yun-zhao, the most famous musculoskeletal radiologist in China, established the Department of Radiology and performed extensive radiology–pathology correlation studies on bone tumors. He was very good at the diagnosis of bone tumors and accumulated a rich database of case studies. Fellows from all over China participated in the bone tumor training course in the department every year. However, we found a lack of books about bone tumors, particularly books with a case-based approach. Therefore, a few years ago we started to collect this series of bone tumors, with carefully selected cases that included comprehensive X-ray, CT, and MRI studies. We present the cases as in the way of the morning roundtable discussion at Jishuitan Hospital, pointing out the key features of each case.

One of the features of this book is that we document the real roundtable discussion of cases in our department. Usually, a young radiologist presents the case with medical history, then the residents or fellows read the images and propose possible differential diagnosis, followed by the attending radiologist, pros and cons of the opinion of the residents, then one of the most experienced professors, Xiaoguang Cheng, presents his opinion on the case. Finally, the pathological finding is presented and carefully correlated with the radiological findings to find the pros and cons of the diagnosis. In some cases, if the pathological finding was inconsistent with radiology or orthopedics, then the case was sent to the pathology department with a request for a review. Finally, the treatment and follow-up of the patients by the orthopedist is an important part of the discussion. This book exemplifies the close teamwork required between radiologists, orthopedists, and pathologists.

We greatly appreciate the hard work of graduates and fellows in sorting out the cases and documentation. The publication of this first edition of *Imaging of Bone Tumors in Shoulder and Elbow* would not have been possible without the help of the Peking Union Medical College Press and Lei Nan in particular.

Beijing, China — Xiaoguang Cheng
New York, NY, USA — Mingqian Huang
Beijing, China — Yongbin Su
November 18, 2020

Contents

List of Authors and Contributors

Authors

Xiaoguang Cheng Department of Radiology, Beijing Jishuitan Hospital, Beijing, People's Republic of China

Health Science Center, Peking University, Beijing, People's Republic of China

Mingqian Huang Department of Diagnostic, Molecular and Interventional Radiology, Mount Sinai Health System, New York, NY, USA

Yongbin Su Department of Radiology, Beijing Jishuitan Hospital, Beijing, People's Republic of China

Contributors

Wei Cai Department of Radiology, Beijing Jishuitan Hospital, Beijing, People's Republic of China

Ling Chen Department of MRI, Heping Hospital Affiliated to Changzhi Medical College, Shanxi, People's Republic of China

Xiang-Shu Chen Department of Radiology, Beijing Jishuitan Hospital, Beijing, People's Republic of China

Ke-Bin Cheng Department of Radiology, Beijing Jishuitan Hospital, Beijing, People's Republic of China

Yi Ding Department of Pathology, Beijing Jishuitan Hospital, Beijing, People's Republic of China

Qiang-Qiang Feng Department of Radiology, Beijing Jishuitan Hospital, Beijing, People's Republic of China

Li-Hua Gong Department of Pathology, Beijing Jishuitan Hospital, Beijing, People's Republic of China

Xiang Gu Department of Radiology, Beijing Jishuitan Hospital, Beijing, People's Republic of China

Zhe Guo Department of Radiology, Beijing Jishuitan Hospital, Beijing, People's Republic of China

Xue Hou Department of Radiology, Beijing Jishuitan Hospital, Beijing, People's Republic of China

Wen Jiang Department of Radiology, Beijing Jishuitan Hospital, Beijing, People's Republic of China

Dong-Ming Li Department of Radiology, Sichuan Provincial Orthopedics Hospital, Sichuan, People's Republic of China

Kai Li Department of Radiology, Beijing Jishuitan Hospital, Beijing, People's Republic of China

Na Li Department of Radiology, Beijing Jishuitan Hospital, Beijing, People's Republic of China

Xin-Min Li Department of Radiology, Beijing Jishuitan Hospital, Beijing, People's Republic of China

Xin-Tong Li Department of Radiology, Beijing Jishuitan Hospital, Beijing, People's Republic of China

Bao-Yue Liu Department of Pathology Beijing Jishuitan Hospital, Beijing, People's Republic of China

Wei-Feng Liu Department of Orthopaedic Oncology, Beijing Jishuitan Hospital, Beijing, People's Republic of China

Yan-Dong Liu Department of Radiology, Beijing Jishuitan Hospital, Beijing, People's Republic of China

Lu-Xin Lou Department of Radiology, Beijing Jishuitan Hospital, Beijing, People's Republic of China

Ning Ma Department of Radiology, Beijing Hepingli Hospital, Beijing, People's Republic of China

Yi-Min Ma Department of Radiology, Beijing Jishuitan Hospital, Beijing, People's Republic of China

Shu-Qin Meng Department of Pathology, Beijing Jishuitan Hospital, Beijing, People's Republic of China

Peng-Ying Niu Department of Radiology, People's Hospital of Ningxia Hui Autonomous Region, Ningxia, People's Republic of China

Cheng-Ming Pu Department of Radiology, Traditional Chinese Medicine Hospital of Yunyang County, Chongqing, People's Republic of China

Zhan-Hua Qian Department of Radiology, Beijing Jishuitan Hospital, Beijing, People's Republic of China

Tao Qin Department of Radiology, Qinghuangdao Workers' Hospital, Hebei, People's Republic of China

Chen Wang Department of Radiology, Beijing Jishuitan Hospital, Beijing, People's Republic of China

Jun Wang Department of Radiology, Taihe County People's Hospital, Anhui, People's Republic of China

Ling Wang Department of Radiology, Beijing Jishuitan Hospital, Beijing, People's Republic of China

Song-Ming Wang Department of Radiology, Beijing Hepingli Hospital, Beijing, People's Republic of China

Tao Wang Department of Orthopaedic Oncology, Beijing Jishuitan Hospital, Beijing, People's Republic of China

Hai-Rong Xu Department of Orthopaedic Oncology, Beijing Jishuitan Hospital, Beijing, People's Republic of China

Li Xu Department of Radiology, Beijing Jishuitan Hospital, Beijing, People's Republic of China

Xiao-Min Xu Department of Radiology, Beijing Jishuitan Hospital, Beijing, People's Republic of China

Dong Yan Department of Radiology, Beijing Jishuitan Hospital, Beijing, People's Republic of China

Ruo-Pei Yang Department of Magnetic Resonance Imaging, Xi'an Honghui Hospital, Xi'an, People's Republic of China

De-Qiu Ye Department of Radiology, Quanzhou First Hospital, Fujian, People's Republic of China

Hong-Zhi Yin Department of Radiology, Gucheng County Hospital, Hebei, People's Republic of China

Hui-Li Zhan Department of Radiology, Beijing Jishuitan Hospital, Beijing, People's Republic of China

Hong-Hong Zhang Department of Radiology, The First Hospital of Fangshan District, Beijing, People's Republic of China

Jing Zhang Department of Radiology, Beijing Jishuitan Hospital, Beijing, People's Republic of China

Xiao-Yu Zhang Department of Radiology, General Hospital of Ningxia Medical University, Ningxia, People's Republic of China

Zi-Kun Zong Department of Radiology, Integrated Traditional Chinese and Western Medicine Hospital of Tongzhou District, Beijing, People's Republic of China

Part I

Shoulder

1 Giant Cell Tumor of Bone: Case 1

1.1 Medical History

The patient is a 26-year-old male. He experienced pain around the proximal left humerus from vibration when riding a bike. Outside radiographs showed pathological fracture with subsequent fine needle biopsy. He reported a history of right shoulder arthroplasty for the right proximal humeral giant cell tumor about 7 years ago.

1.2 Physical Examination

Swelling around the left shoulder without point tenderness. Scar tissues noted around the right shoulder.

1.3 Imaging Findings

1.3.1 Radiograph

X. Cheng et al., *Imaging of Bone Tumors in Shoulder and Elbow*,
https://doi.org/10.1007/978-981-33-6150-8_1

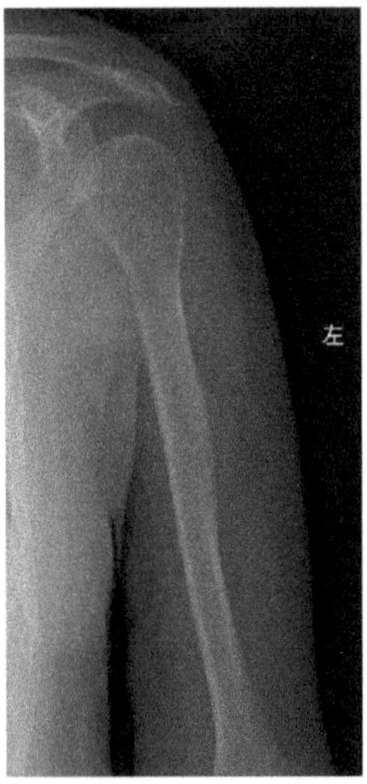

Fig. 1.1 Frontal view of the left shoulder

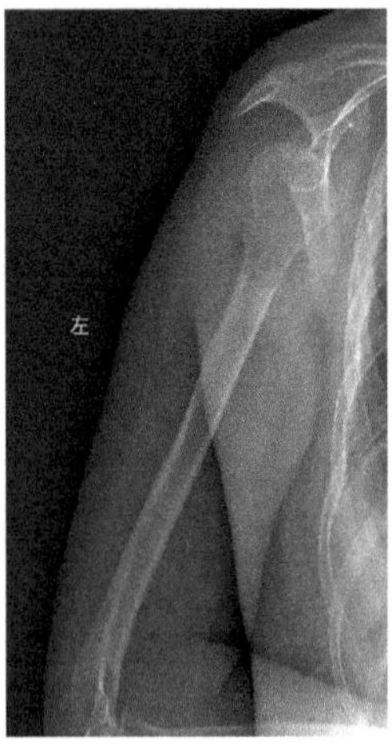

Fig. 1.2 Lateral view of the left shoulder

Radiographs of the left shoulder demonstrate lytic bony destructive changes of the right proximal humerus with cortical break. There is no peripheral sclerosis or periosteal reaction noted.

1.3.2 CT Imaging

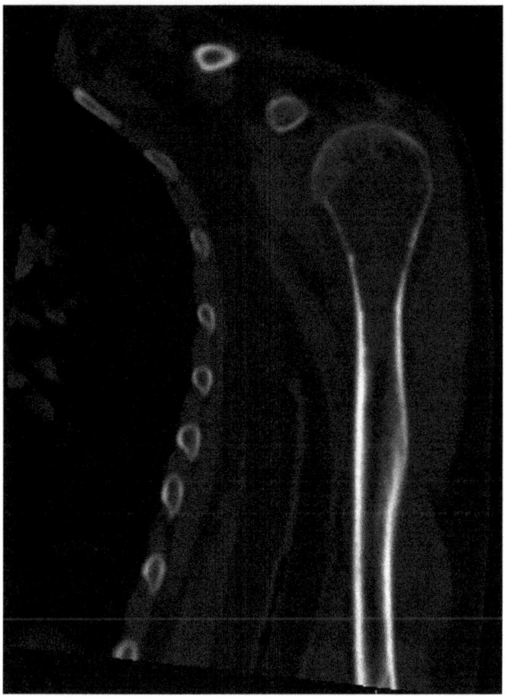

Fig. 1.3 Coronal CT image of the left shoulder in bone window

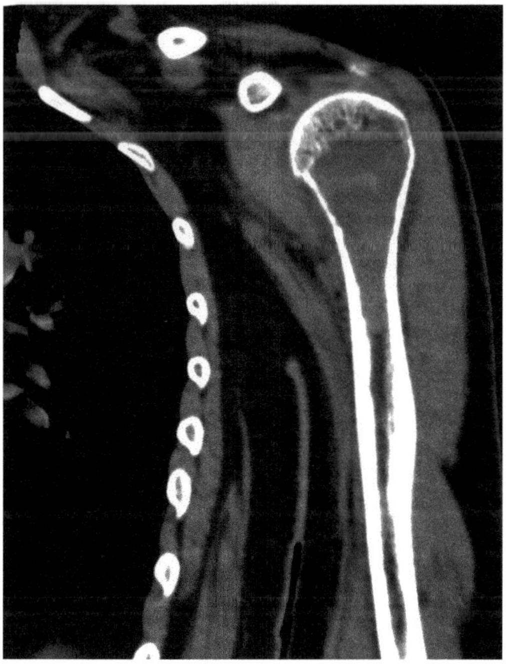

Fig. 1.4 Coronal CT image of the left shoulder in soft tissue window

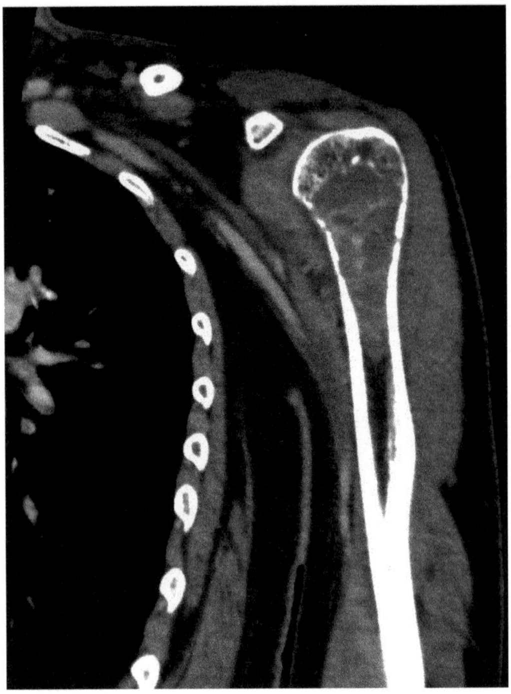

Fig. 1.5 Coronal post-contrast CT image of the left shoulder in soft tissue window

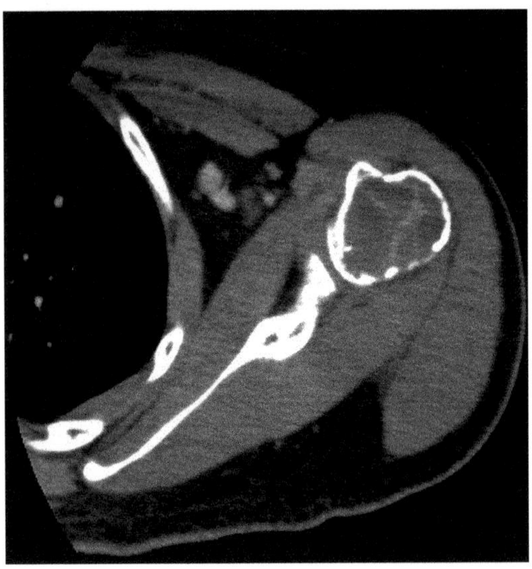

Fig. 1.6 Axial post-contrast CT image of the left shoulder in soft tissue window

CT images of the left shoulder demonstrate the lytic bony destructive changes at the proximal left humerus. The lesion is slightly expansile, with cortical break. The long axis of the lesion is parallel to the long axis of the humerus. Internal septations are noted with enhancement.

1.3.3 MR Imaging

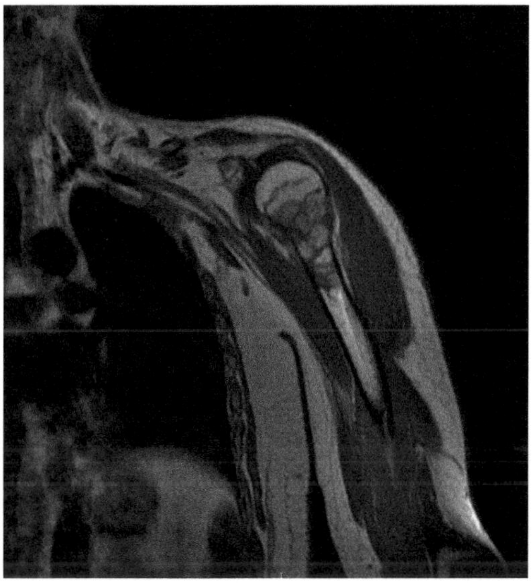

Fig. 1.7 Coronal T1-weighted MR image of left shoulder

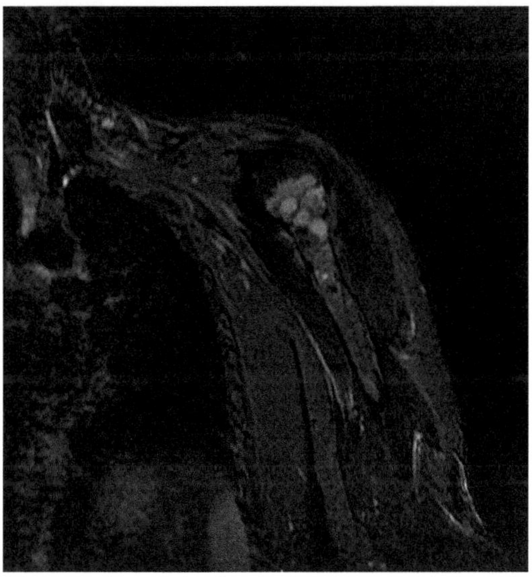

Fig. 1.8 Coronal fat-suppressed T2-weighted MR image of left shoulder

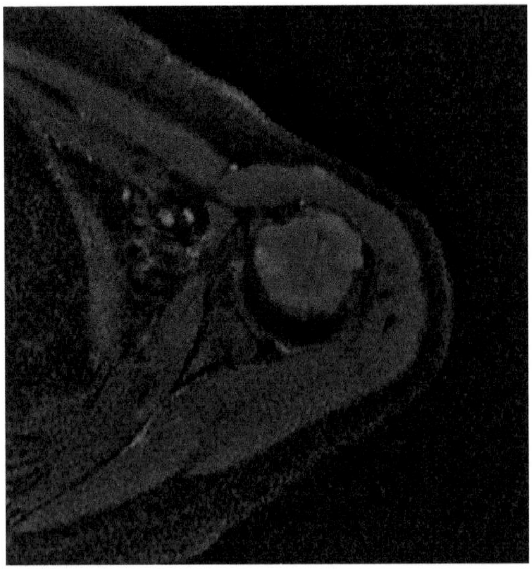

Fig. 1.9 Axial post-contrast fat-suppressed T1-weighted MR image of the left shoulder

MR images of the left shoulder demonstrate the mildly expansile lesion in the proximal left humerus. The lesion shows a heterogeneous signal with hemorrhage, internal septations, and multiple fluid–fluid levels. There are cystic and solid components within the lesion and enhancements are noted in the solid portion.

1.4 Description and Discussion from Residents

The patient is a young male. He has a past medical history of giant cell tumor of the bone and outside radiographs showed pathological fracture. Our radiographs demonstrate lytic bony destructive changes with clear margin and cortical break. The lesion appears mildly expansile with some matrix within. There is no peripheral sclerosis or periosteal reaction. Fracture cannot be adequately excluded based on radiographs alone. The lesion on CT images is again noted to be mildly expansile and located around the metaphysis with cortical break and internal septations. No sclerosis is seen and enhancements around the septations are noted. Septations and multiple fluid–fluid levels are noted on the MRI images. There are cystic and solid components within the lesion with enhancement along the solid portion. Based on history, age, the differential diagnoses include: (A) Giant cell tumor with secondary aneurismal bone cyst (ABC), favored. However, the following features argue against giant cell tumor: (1) lesion is not at end of the bone, with no asymmetrical expansion; (2) very mild enhancement of the solid component; (3) lesion's long axis parallels along the humerus. (B) Fibrous lesion with secondary ABC.

1.5 Analysis and Comments from Professor Xiaoguang Cheng

Young male presents with prior history of giant cell tumor of the right humerus and current history of trauma. Radiographs show destructive changes around the left proximal humerus with underlying normal bone mineralization and suspected pathological fracture on the lateral view. CT images show the lesion at metaphysis with heterogeneous densities and suggestion of cystic component, and enhancement along the septations. MR images show fluid–fluid levels and enhancement at the solid portion of the lesion. The bones around the shoulder joint show normal mineralization. Given the past medical history, first, we need to correlate with laboratory testing (blood phosphatase level, calcium level, and parathyroid level) to exclude brown tumors from hyperparathyroidism. Multicentric giant cell tumor of bone is very rare. When thinking about multicentric giant cell tumor of bone, hyperparathyroidism should be excluded first. Please pay attention to the MR signal within the lesion, check to see if there is internal hemorrhage or heterogeneous enhancement. Overall, the differential diagnoses are: (1) Hyperparathyroidism; (2) ABC.

1.6 Diagnosis

Giant cell tumor of bone with secondary ABC (Multicentric giant cell tumor of bone).

Suggested Reading

Dhillon MS, Prasad P. Multicentric giant cell tumour of bone. Acta Orthop Belg. 2007;73(3):289–99.

Hoch B, Inwards C, Sundaram M, et al. Multicentric giant cell tumor of bone. Clinicopathologic analysis of thirty cases. J Bone Joint Surg Am. 2006;88(9):1998–2008.

Simple Bone Cyst: Case 2

2

2.1 Medical History

The patient is a 17-year-old male. He was found to have a pathologic fracture of the right humerus after a fall 5 years ago. Follow-up studies showed enlargement of the lesion.

2.2 Physical Examination

Point tenderness around the proximal right humerus.

2.3 Imaging Findings

2.3.1 Radiograph

X. Cheng et al., *Imaging of Bone Tumors in Shoulder and Elbow*,
https://doi.org/10.1007/978-981-33-6150-8_2

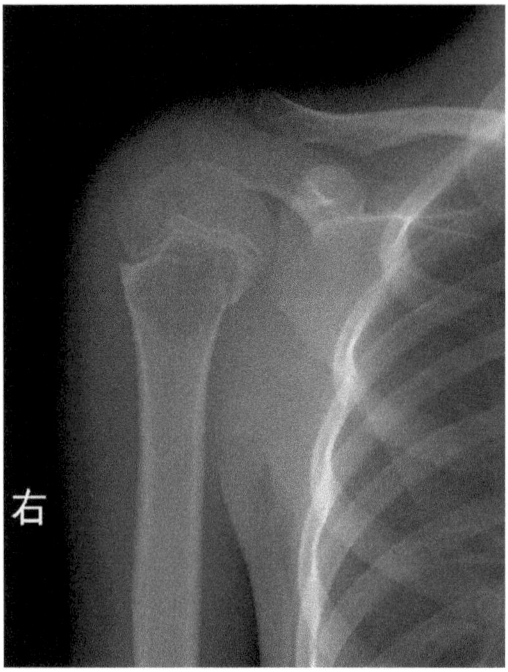

Fig. 2.1 Frontal view of the right humerus (2013)

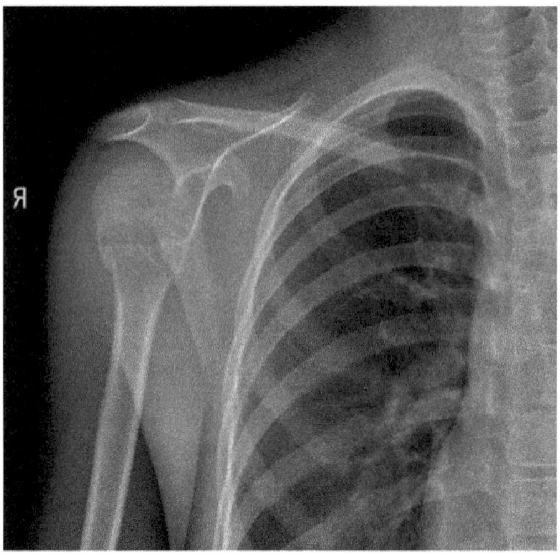

Fig. 2.2 Lateral view of the right humerus (2013)

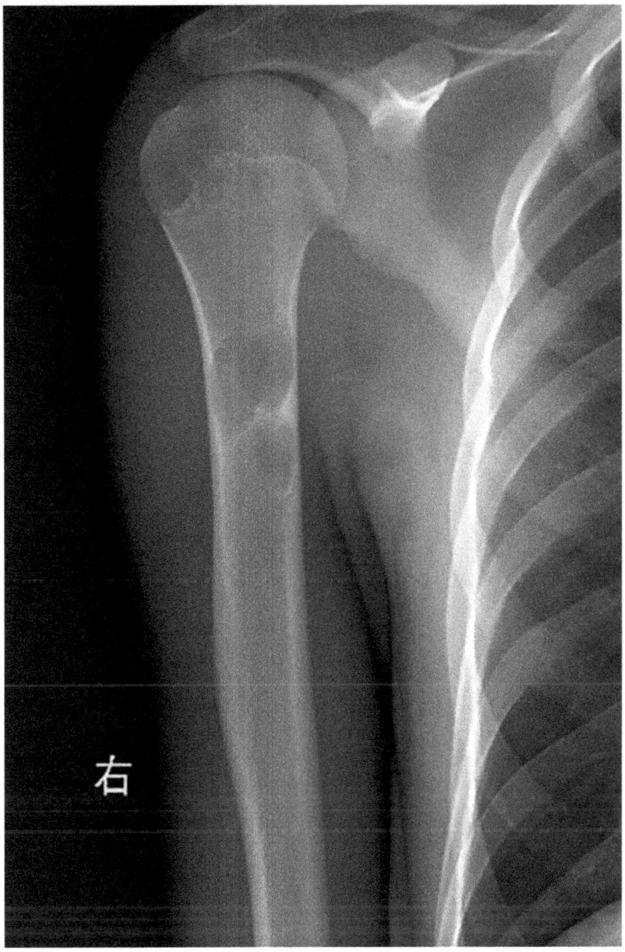

Fig. 2.3 Frontal view of the right humerus (2018)

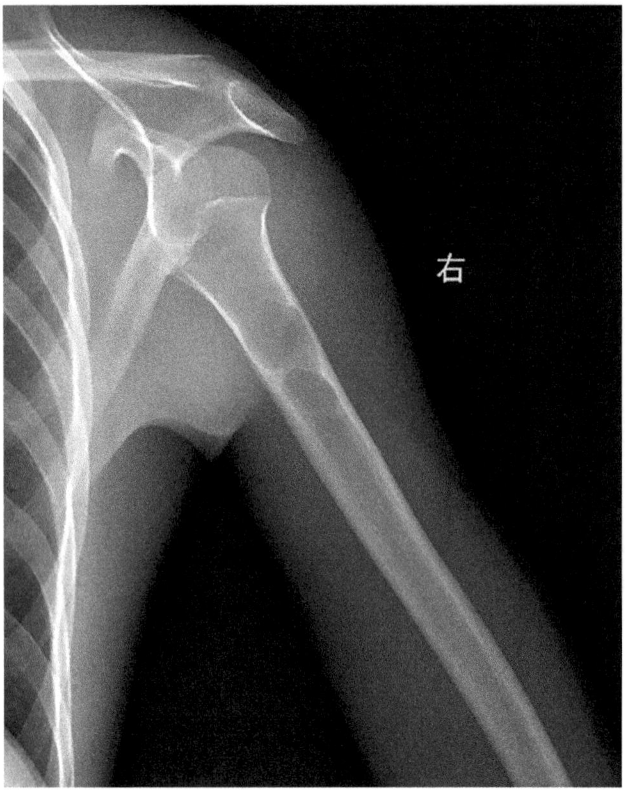

Fig. 2.4 Lateral view of the right humerus (2018)

Radiographs of the right humerus demonstrate a lucent, well-circumscribed lesion at the proximal right humerus with thinning of the cortex and associated pathologic fracture. There is internal septation. No periosteal reaction is noted.

2.3.2 CT Imaging

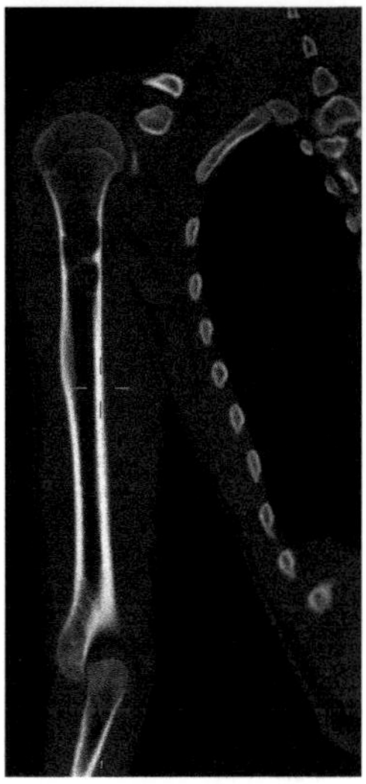

Fig. 2.5 Coronal CT image of the right humerus in bone window (2018)

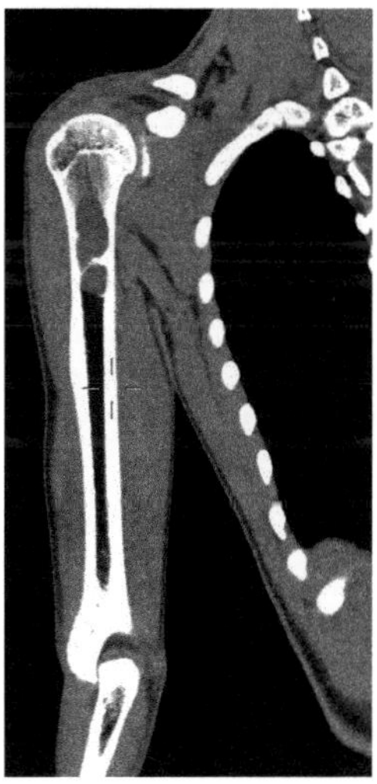

Fig. 2.6 Coronal CT image of the right humerus in soft tissue window (2018)

CT images of the right humerus demonstrate the intramedullary lesion at the proximal humerus with a clear margin and internal septation. The lesion shows relatively homogenous density with the long axis parallel to the bone. There is no clear enhancement.

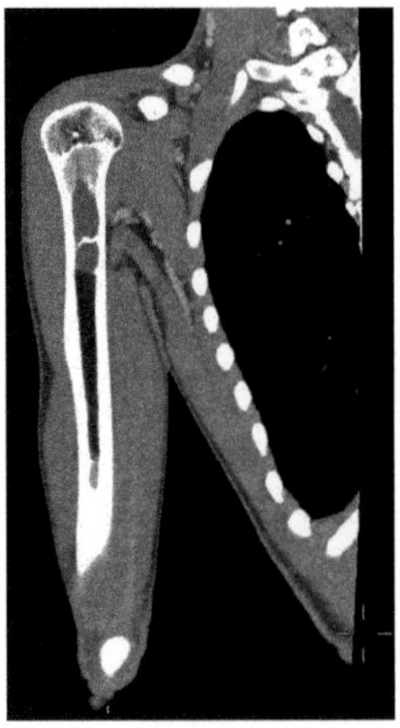

Fig. 2.7 Coronal post-contrast CT image of the right humerus in soft tissue window (2018)

2.4 Description and Discussion from Residents

The patient is an adolescent male. The radiographs from 2013 demonstrate expansile lesion around the metaphysis of the right humerus with cortical destruction with pathologic fracture and internal septation. In the follow-up study from 2018, the lesion is noted expanding along the long axis of the diaphysis with increasing internal septations, most suggestive of benign fibrous lesion, such as non-ossifying fibroma. CT images demonstrate some patchy ground-glass density in the intramedullary cavity, raising concern for fibrous dysplasia. However, the appearance of the lesion extending to the diaphysis from metaphysis with age is more suggestive of simple bone cyst. Usually, there are not many internal septations within the bone cyst.

2.5 Analysis and Comments from Professor Xiaoguang Cheng

Young male presents with metaphyseal lesion with clear margin, most likely benign. Pathological fracture is noted. On the lateral view, there is a linear high density within the lesion, raising concern for fallen fragments. On the 5-year follow-up study, the lesion extends to the diaphysis, consistent with the pattern of a simple bone cyst. CT images demonstrate the intramedullary lesion with mild expansion and homogenous density and internal septation without significant enhancement, all suggestive of simple bone cyst. Non-ossifying fibroma usually originates around the cortex, asymmetrical, affects the intramedullary cavity later, and with enhancement, not consistent with the current case, should not be considered in the differential diagnosis.

2.6 Diagnosis

Simple bone cyst.

Suggested Reading

Mascard E, Gomez-Brouchet A, Lambot K. Bone cysts: unicameral and aneurysmal bone cyst. Orthop Traumatol Surg Res. 2015;101(1 Suppl):S119–27.

Rosenblatt J, Koder A. Understanding unicameral and aneurysmal bone cysts. Pediatr Rev. 2019;40(2):51–9.

Sullivan RJ, Meyer JS, Dormans JP, et al. Diagnosing aneurysmal and unicameral bone cysts with magnetic resonance imaging. Clin Orthop Relat Res. 1999;366:186–90.

3 Osteochondroma: Case 3

3.1 Medical History

The patient is a 5-year-old boy. He presented with a left shoulder mass without pain or fever.

3.2 Physical Examination

Palpable 2.5 cm × 3 cm lesion along the left proximal humerus medially with suggestion of an attached pedicle. The lesion feels hard, with clear margin, non-mobile, and without point tenderness.

3.3 Imaging Findings

3.3.1 Radiograph

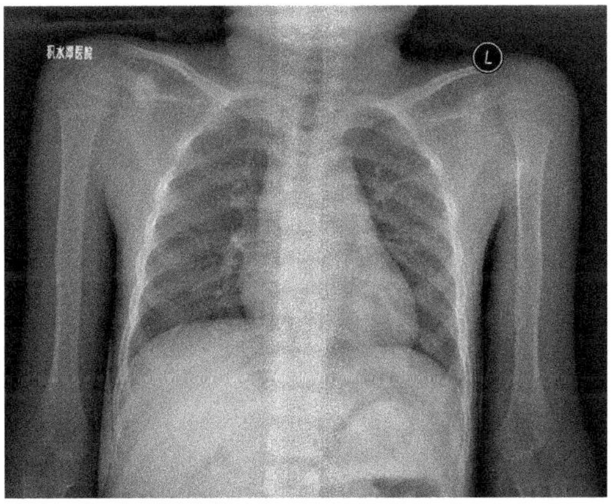

Fig. 3.1 Frontal view of both humeri

X. Cheng et al., *Imaging of Bone Tumors in Shoulder and Elbow*,
https://doi.org/10.1007/978-981-33-6150-8_3

Radiograph of both humeri demonstrates an exostosis along the proximal left humerus medially.

3.3.2 CT Imaging

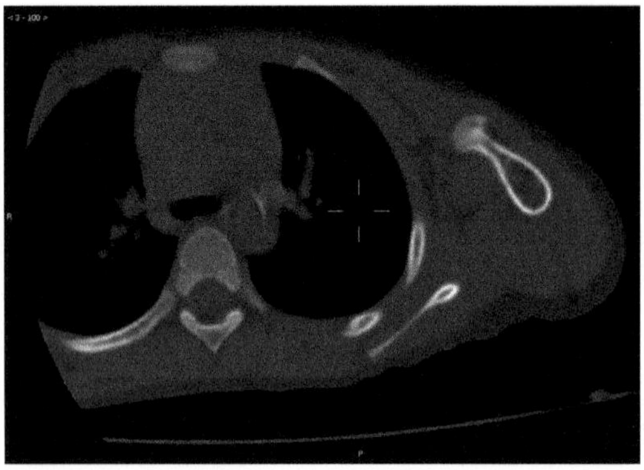

Fig. 3.2 Axial CT image of the left shoulder in bone window

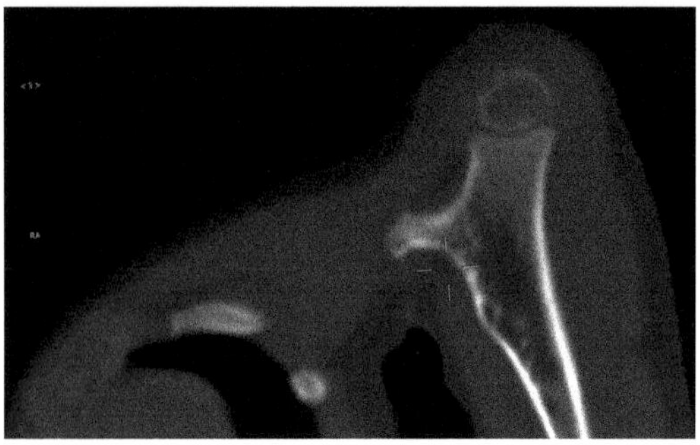

Fig. 3.3 Coronal CT image of the left shoulder in bone window

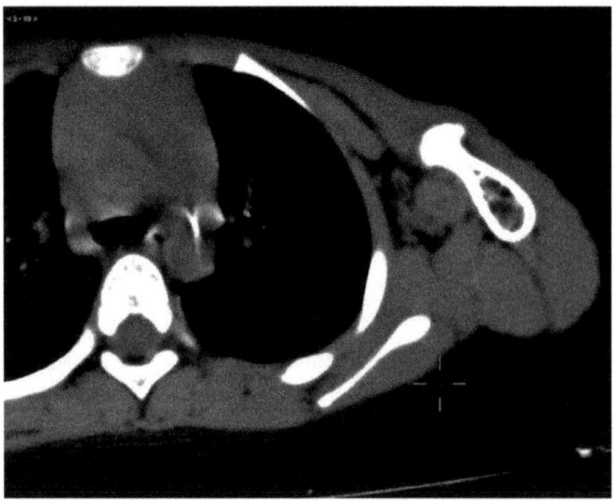

Fig. 3.4 Axial CT image of the left shoulder in soft tissue window

CT images of the left shoulder demonstrate a bony exostosis along the left proximal humeral metaphysis with medullary continuity.

3.4 Description and Discussion from Residents

The patient is a boy. The radiograph demonstrates an exostosis at the left proximal humerus medially. On the CT scan, there is a stalk attached to the lesion and the lesion demonstrates medullary continuity, consistent with classic pedunculated osteochondroma. Patient with osteochondroma usually is asymptomatic and the lesion likely to be an incidental finding. The management is to leave it alone. If the patient is older with symptoms, concern for malignant transformation is raised. Then, MRI is indicated to evaluate the thickness of the cartilaginous cap. It would be concerning for malignant transformation if the thickness is more than 2 cm.

3.5 Analysis and Comments from Professor Xiaoguang Cheng

The radiograph does not demonstrate the detail of the lesion, just as bony density along the medial aspect of the left proximal humerus. CT images demonstrate the medullary continuity of the exostosis, classic for osteochondroma. There is no other differential diagnosis. Medullary continuity and cortical continuity must be present for the diagnosis. MRI is also helpful for the evaluation of the intramedullary fat.

3.6 Diagnosis

Osteochondroma.

Suggested Reading

Bernard SA, Murphey MD, Flemming DJ, et al. Improved differentiation of benign osteochondromas from secondary chondrosarcomas with standardized measurement of cartilage cap at CT and MR imaging. Radiology. 2010;255(3):857–65.

Murphey MD, Choi JJ, Kransdorf MJ, et al. Imaging of osteochondroma: variants and complications with radiologic-pathologic correlation. Radiographics. 2000;20(5):1407–34.

4 Multiple Osteochondromas: Case 4

4.1 Medical History

The patient is a 3-year-old boy. He presented with multiple masses around the right shoulder.

4.2 Physical Examination

Palpable mass around the right shoulder, hard with clear margin and non-mobile. There is no point tenderness.

4.3 Imaging Findings

4.3.1 Radiograph

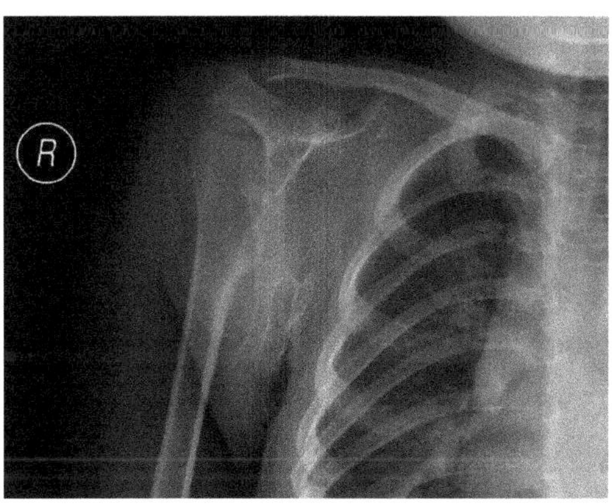

Fig. 4.1 Frontal view of the right scapula

X. Cheng et al., *Imaging of Bone Tumors in Shoulder and Elbow*,
https://doi.org/10.1007/978-981-33-6150-8_4

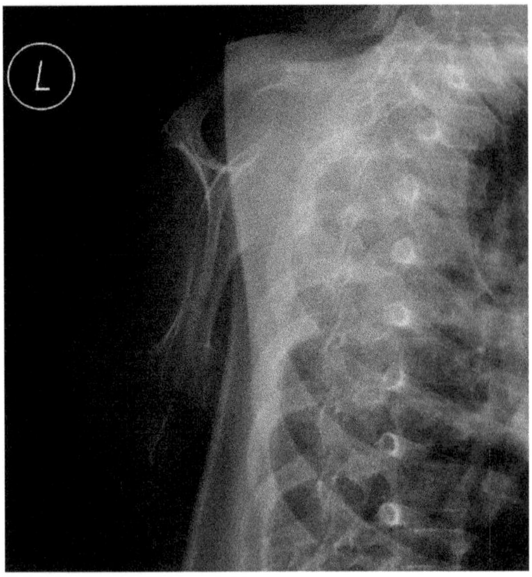

Fig. 4.2 Lateral view of the right scapula

Radiographs of the right scapula demonstrate multiple bony exostosis around the right scapula, involving the scapula spine and body.

4.3.2 CT Imaging

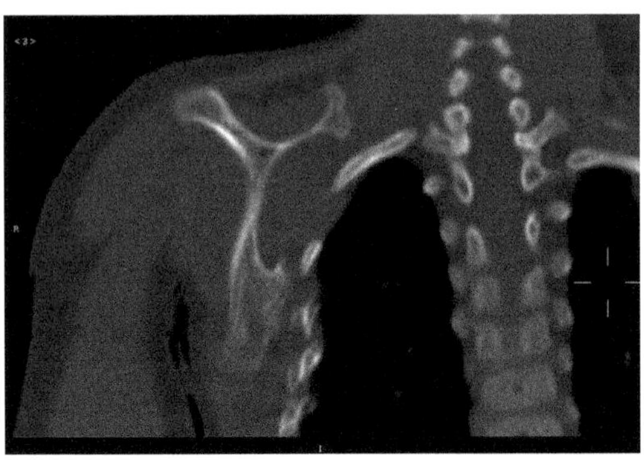

Fig. 4.3 Coronal CT image of the right scapula in bone window

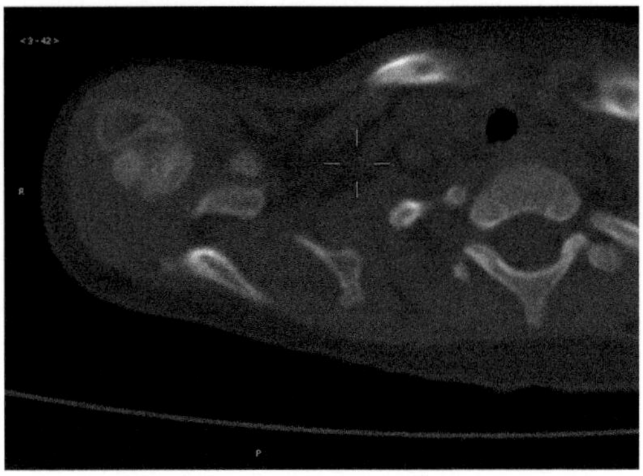

Fig. 4.4 Axial CT image of the right scapula in bone window

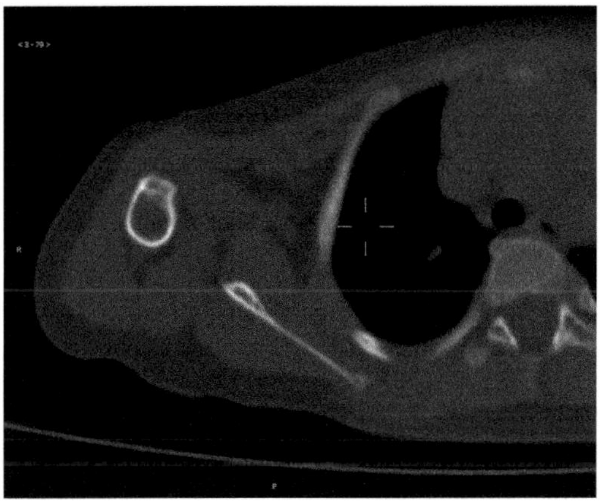

Fig. 4.5 Axial CT image of the right scapula in bone window

CT images of the right scapula demonstrate multiple bony exostosis along the right scapula. The lesions demonstrate medullary continuity with broad base and cortical continuity. There is an irregular shape of the lesion but with a clear margin.

4.4 Description and Discussion from Residents

The patient is a boy. The radiographs demonstrate multiple bony exostosis around the right scapula body and spine with cortical and medullary continuity. The lesions are well-circumscribed without associated periosteal reaction. There is also cortical irregularity around the right humeral metaphysis. CT scan shows the same findings as on radiographs. This is most consistent with multiple osteochondromas given the patient's age and imaging findings.

4.5 Analysis and Comments from Professor Xiaoguang Cheng

The patient is a young boy and asymptomatic. Radiographs demonstrate multiple bony exostosis around the scapula body and spine with cortical and medullary continuity. Additionally, there is cortical irregularity around the right proximal humeral metaphysis. The finding along the right proximal humerus is subtle and can easily be missed. Cartilaginous cap can be seen on this CT scan. This is consistent with multiple osteochondromas given the patient's age and typical imaging findings.

4.6 Diagnosis

Multiple osteochondromas.

Suggested Reading

D'Arienzo A, Andreani L, Sacchetti F, et al. Hereditary multiple exostoses: current insights. Orthop Res Rev. 2019;11:199–211.

Murphey MD, Choi JJ, Kransdorf MJ, et al. Imaging of osteochondroma: variants and complications with radiologic-pathologic correlation. Radiographics. 2000;20(5):1407–34.

5 Hemangioma: Case 5

5.1 Medical History

The patient is a 42-year-old female. She presented with left shoulder discomfort for 10 years and worsened in the last half-year with radiation to the left upper extremity.

5.2 Physical Examination

There is a deep palpable mass in the medial aspect of the left shoulder posteriorly.

5.3 Imaging Findings

5.3.1 Radiograph

X. Cheng et al., *Imaging of Bone Tumors in Shoulder and Elbow*,
https://doi.org/10.1007/978-981-33-6150-8_5

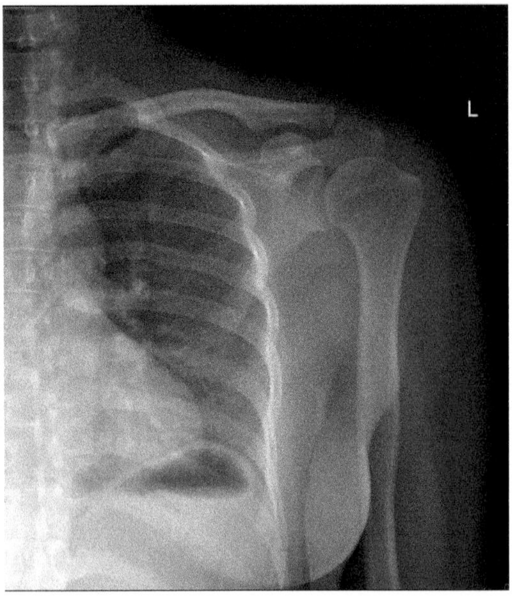

Fig. 5.1 Frontal view of the left shoulder

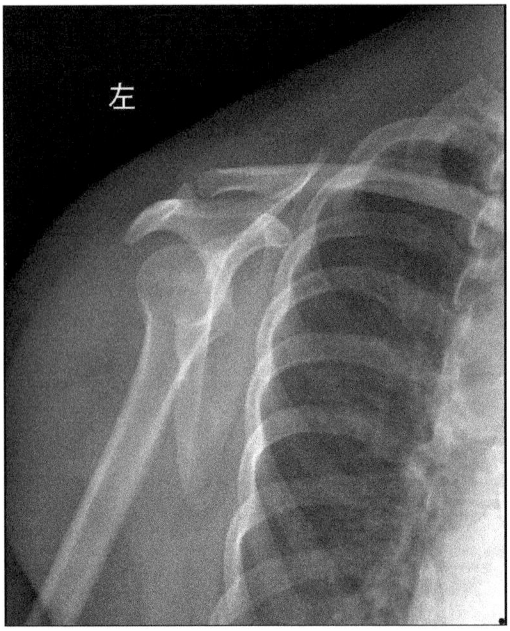

Fig. 5.2 Lateral view of the left shoulder

Radiographs of the left shoulder demonstrate no cortical irregularity and unremarkable soft tissue

5.3.2 MR Imaging

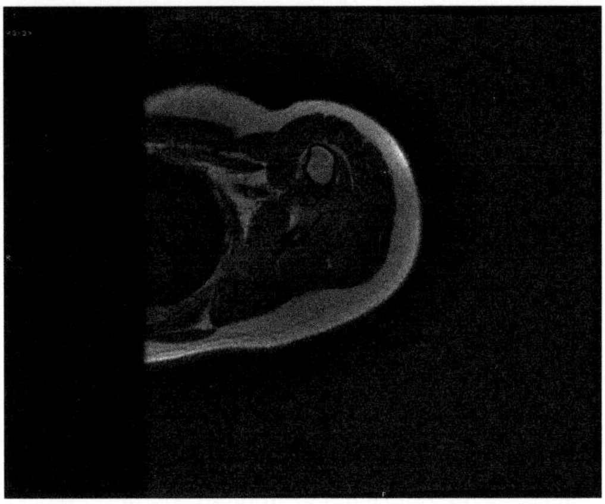

Fig. 5.3 Axial T1-weighted MR image of the left shoulder

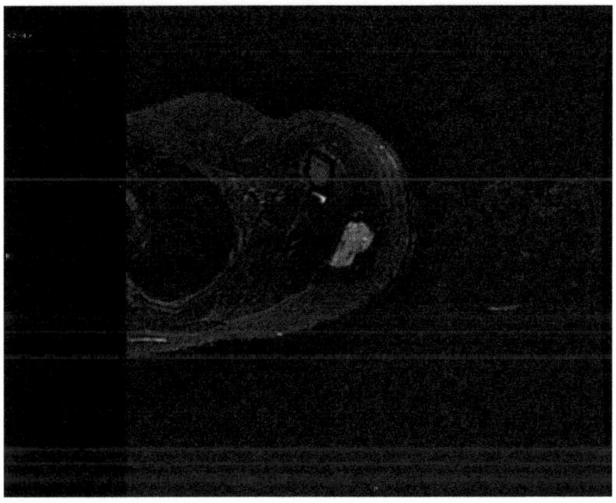

Fig. 5.4 Axial fat-suppressed T2-weighted MR image of the left shoulder

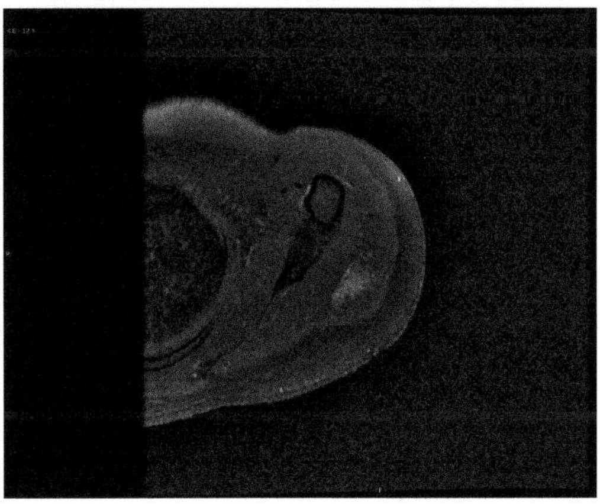

Fig. 5.5 Axial post-contrast fat-suppressed T1-weighted MR image of the left shoulder

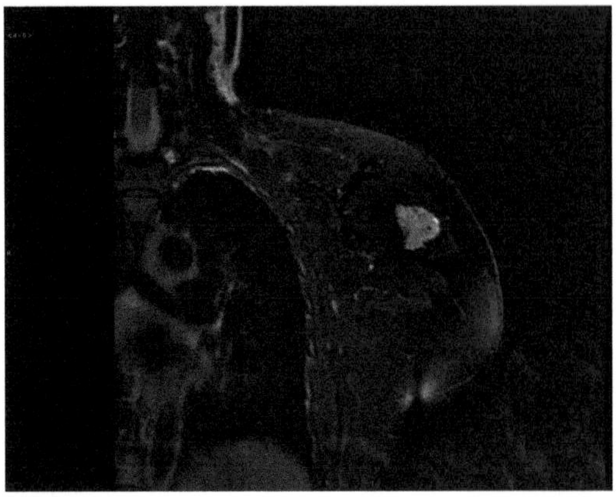

Fig. 5.6 Coronal fat-suppressed T2-weighted MR image of the left shoulder

MR images of the left shoulder demonstrate a soft tissue mass in the posterior left deltoid muscle with iso-intense T1 and hyper-intense T2 signal and internal punctuate low signal. There is enhancement after contrast administration.

5.4 Description and Discussion from Residents

The patient is a middle-aged female. Radiographs show no abnormality in the bone or soft tissue. MR images of the left shoulder demonstrate lesion within the left deltoid muscle with T1 iso-intense signal and hyper-intense T2 signal with irregular. There are punctate low T2 signals on fat-suppressed sequences, which could be flow voids. Avid enhancement is noted. The above constellation of findings is most suggestive of hemangioma.

5.5 Analysis and Comments from Professor Xiaoguang Cheng

The patient is a middle-aged female with a prolonged history. No abnormal findings are noted on the radiographs. MRI of the left shoulder demonstrates a lesion in the posterior left deltoid muscle with internal iso-intense T1 and hyper-intense T2 signal and irregular margin and no capsule. There is an internal high T1 signal. Fat-suppressed sequences can be used to differentiate fat from hemorrhage. The internal punctuate low signals on fat-suppressed sequences may represent flow voids. CT can be performed to exclude subtle calcifications. There is an avid enhancement of the lesion. The above features are most suggestive of hemangioma. Soft tissue mass within the muscle tends to be malignant, except for hemangioma. Characteristics of hemangioma: (1) internal heterogeneous signal, containing fat; (2) no capsule.

5.6 Diagnosis

Hemangioma.

Suggested Reading

Cohen EK, Kressel HY, Perosio T, et al. MR imaging of soft-tissue hemangiomas: correlation with pathologic findings. AJR Am J Roentgenol. 1988;150(5):1079–81.

Walker EA, Salesky JS, Fenton ME. Magnetic resonance imaging of malignant soft tissue neoplasms in the adult. Radiol Clin North Am. 2011;49(6):1219–34, vi

6 Desmoid-Type Fibromatosis (Recurrence): Case 6

6.1 Medical History

The patient is a 25-year-old male. He presented with a painful mass around the right shoulder for a month, with a history of soft tissue mass resection in this region 4 years ago.

6.2 Physical Examination

There is a protuberance at the right deltoid region posteriorly, measuring about 18 cm × 6 cm, hard with point tenderness.

6.3 Imaging Findings

6.3.1 MR Imaging

X. Cheng et al., *Imaging of Bone Tumors in Shoulder and Elbow*,
https://doi.org/10.1007/978-981-33-6150-8_6

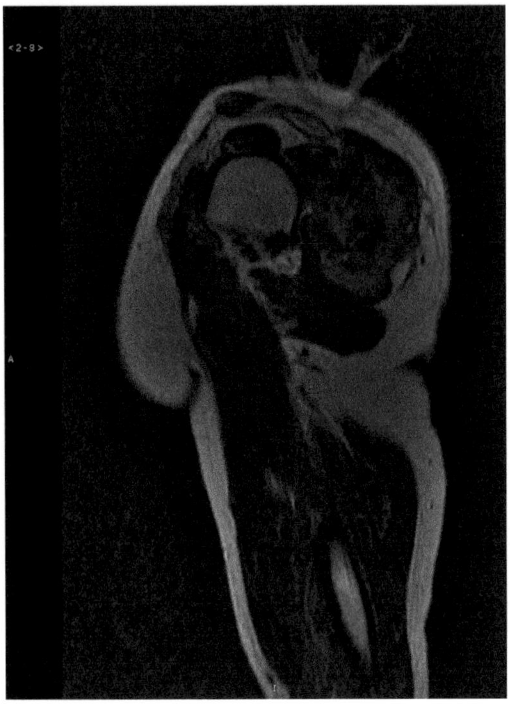

Fig. 6.1 Sagittal T1-weighted MR image of the right shoulder

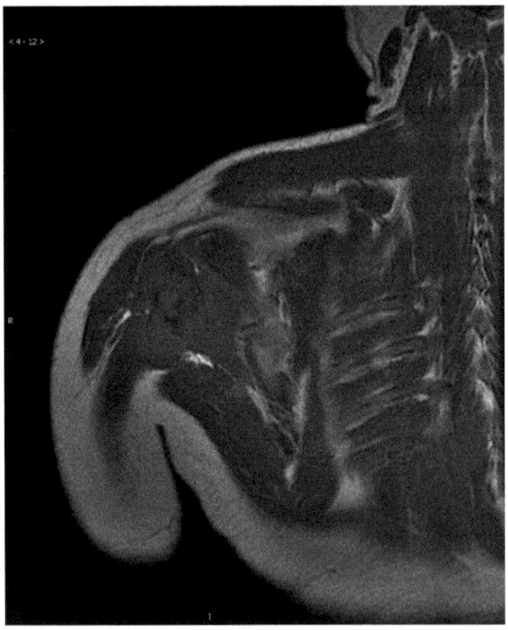

Fig. 6.2 Coronal T1-weighted MR image of the right shoulder

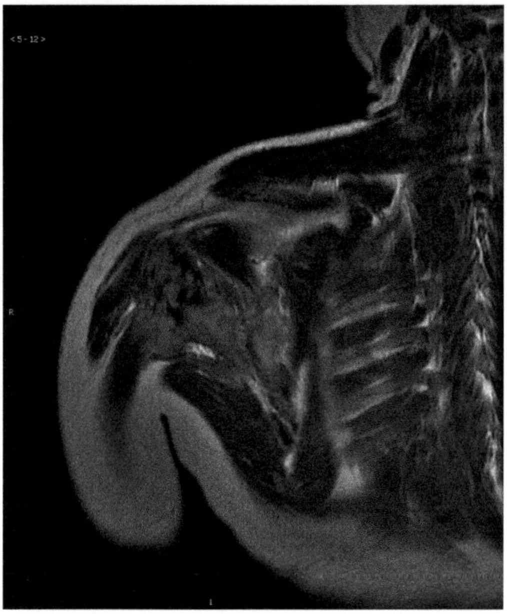

Fig. 6.3 Coronal T2-weighted MR image of the right shoulder

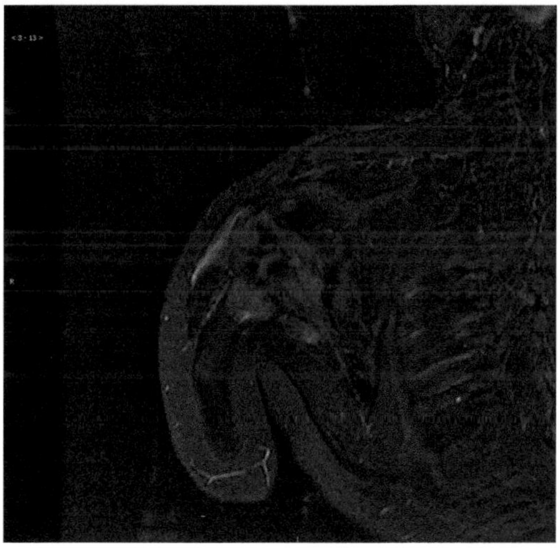

Fig. 6.4 Coronal fat-suppressed T2-weighted MR image of the right shoulder

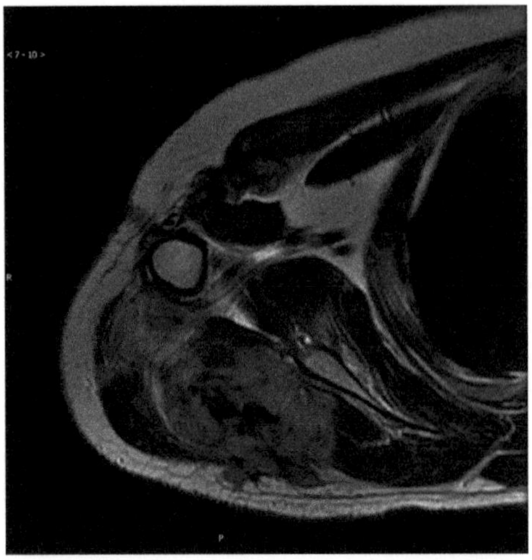

Fig. 6.5 Axial T2-weighted MR image of the right shoulder

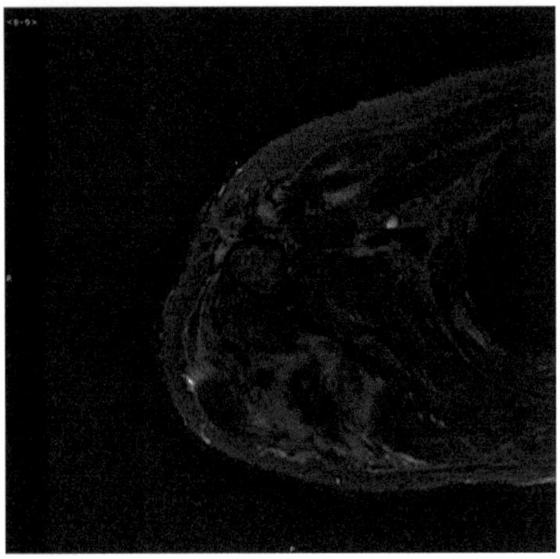

Fig. 6.6 Axial fat-suppressed T2-weighted MR image of the right shoulder

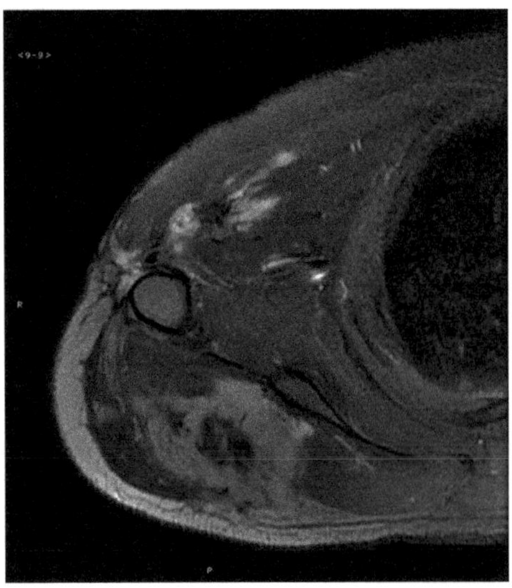

Fig. 6.7 Axial post-contrast fat-suppressed T1-weighted MR image of the right shoulder

MR images of the right shoulder demonstrate a soft tissue mass in the infraspinatus muscle with internal heterogeneous signal and patch low T2 signal with irregular margin and heterogeneous enhancement.

6.4 Description and Discussion from Residents

The patient is a young male. On MR images, there are heterogeneous T1 and T2 signals within the mass in the infraspinatus muscle. On the fat-suppressed sequences, there is a high T2 signal. The internal patchy low signal in the lesion likely represents fibrous tissue. This could be confirmed by radiograph and CT scan to exclude the possibility of calcification. There is an irregular margin of the lesion. After contrast administration, there is peripheral enhancement and non-enhancement centrally of the low signal region. Combined with clinical history, the top consideration is a recurrence of desmoid-type fibromatosis.

6.5 Analysis and Comments from Professor Xiaoguang Cheng

The patient is a young male with a history of soft tissue mass resection 4 years ago. MRI scan shows a solid mass with heterogeneous signal within the right infraspinatus muscle with irregular margin. The low signal component in the lesion likely represents fibrous tissues. The lesion appears to be predominantly posterior in location and the anterior abnormal signal likely related to postoperative changes. This is most likely a desmoid-type fibromatosis recurrence given the patient's clinical history and the high recurrence rate of desmoid-type fibromatosis. Characteristics of desmoid-type fibromatosis: (1) no clear margin, benign histologically, though very difficult for total resection; (2) fibrous tissue predominant with internal fibrous scar as multiple linear low signal bands on T2-weighted images.

6.6 Diagnosis

Desmoid-type fibromatosis (recurrence).

Suggested Reading

Otero S, Moskovic EC, Strauss DC, et al. Desmoid-type fibromatosis. Clin Radiol. 2015;70(9):1038–45.

Robbin MR, Murphey MD, Temple HT, et al. Imaging of musculoskeletal fibromatosis. Radiographics. 2001;21(3):585–600.

Desmoid-Type Fibromatosis: Case 7

7

7.1 Medical History

The patient is a 15-year-old boy. He presented with a right axillary mass for 1 year.

7.2 Physical Examination

There is a palpable deep mass at the right axillary region, about 4 cm × 3 cm with clear margin, smooth, rubbery, and nonmobile without point tenderness.

7.3 Imaging Findings

7.3.1 MR Imaging

X. Cheng et al., *Imaging of Bone Tumors in Shoulder and Elbow*,
https://doi.org/10.1007/978-981-33-6150-8_7

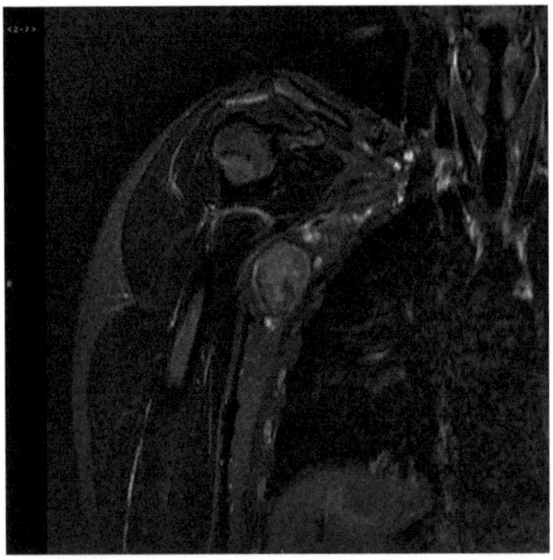

Fig. 7.1 Coronal fat-suppressed T2-weighted MR image of the right shoulder

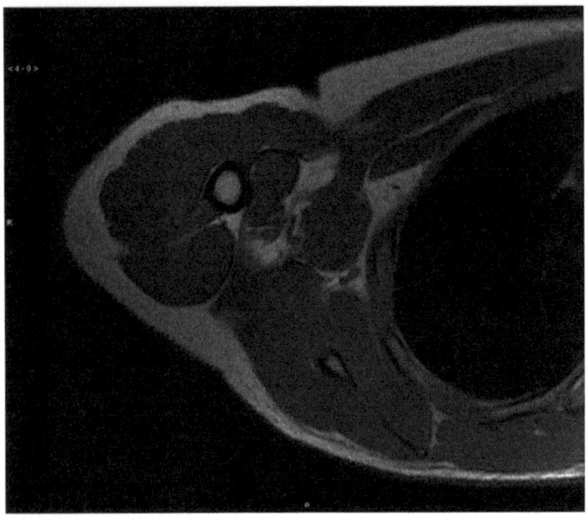

Fig. 7.2 Axial T1-weighted MR image of the right shoulder

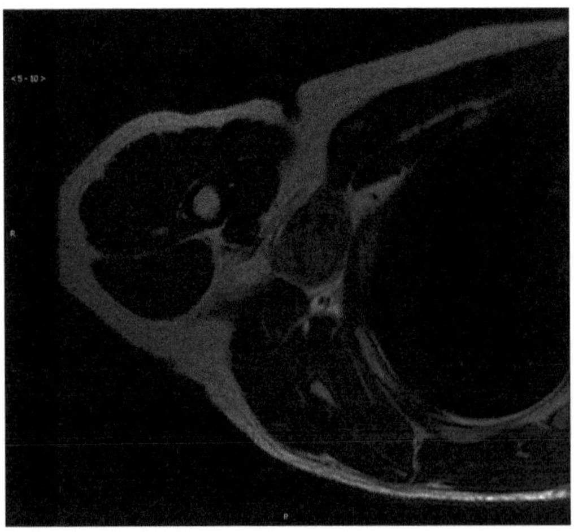

Fig. 7.3 Axial T2-weighted MR image of the right shoulder

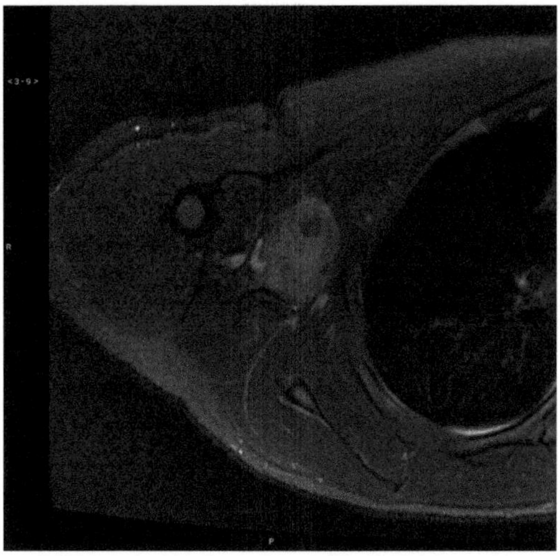

Fig. 7.4 Axial fat-suppressed T2-weighted MR image of the right shoulder

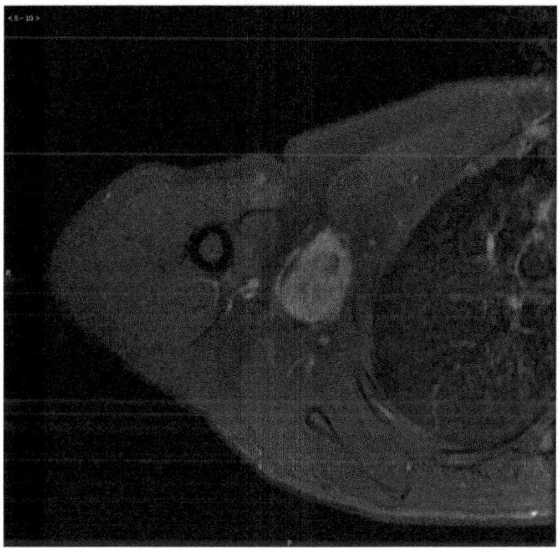

Fig. 7.5 Axial post-contrast fat-suppressed T1-weighted MR image of the right shoulder

MR images demonstrate a space-occupying lesion at the right axillary region, oval in shape with iso-intense T1 signal and heterogeneous T2 signal and enhancement.

7.4 Description and Discussion from Residents

The patient is an adolescent male. On MR images, there is a space-occupying lesion in the right axillary region, along the chest wall. The lesion demonstrates iso-intense signal on T1-weighted image, mild high signal with internal patchy, and linear low signals on T2-weighted image. The lesion is well-circumscribed without lobulated morphology. There is enhancement after contrast administration, but no enhancement along the patchy and linear low signal areas in the lesion. This is most likely a desmoid-type fibromatosis, given the location. When diagnosing desmoid-type fibromatosis, sometimes emphasis is better placed on location or region of involvement than imaging features. A soft tissue lesion with an internal low T2 signal along the anterior, lateral chest wall, around the scapula or in gluteal region, favors desmoid-type fibromatosis. The imaging features of desmoid-type fibromatosis could be extensive, such as clear margin or not, central or peripheral low T2 signal of the lesion. Nerve sheath tumor with commonly seen central low signal should be included in the differential diagnosis.

7.5 Analysis and Comments from Professor Xiaoguang Cheng

The patient is an adolescent male. The lesion locates at the right axillary region, the differential diagnosis should include: enlarged lymph nodes, tumor from the brachial plexus. On the MR images, the lesion is along the right chest wall with a clear margin and surrounded by fatty tissue. This is most suggestive of a benign or low-grade malignant tumor. Low signal is noted within the lesion on T2-weighted images, but no corresponding low T1 signal, unlikely to be calcification. Mild high signal on T2-weighted images; myxoid component can be excluded. Rather homogenous enhancement after contrast administration is noted. Given the location of the lesion and imaging features, lymphadenopathy or nerve sheath tumor can be excluded; this is most likely a desmoid-type fibromatosis. Location is important in narrowing down a differential diagnosis for soft tissue tumors. Identification of lesions along the neurovascular bundle or originate intramuscularly can be very helpful for diagnosis.

7.6 Diagnosis

Desmoid-type fibromatosis.

Suggested Reading

Otero S, Moskovic EC, Strauss DC, et al. Desmoid-type fibromatosis. Clin Radiol. 2015;70(9):1038–45.

Robbin MR, Murphey MD, Temple HT, et al. Imaging of musculoskeletal fibromatosis. Radiographics. 2001;21(3):585–600.

8 Giant Cell Tumor of Bone: Case 8

8.1 Medical History

The patient is a 21-year-old female. She presented with left shoulder pain for 6 months and exacerbated with decreased range of motion after a recent fall 6 days ago.

8.2 Physical Examination

Focal swelling of the left shoulder with obvious point tenderness and decreased range of motion.

8.3 Imaging Findings

8.3.1 Radiograph

X. Cheng et al., *Imaging of Bone Tumors in Shoulder and Elbow*,
https://doi.org/10.1007/978-981-33-6150-8_8

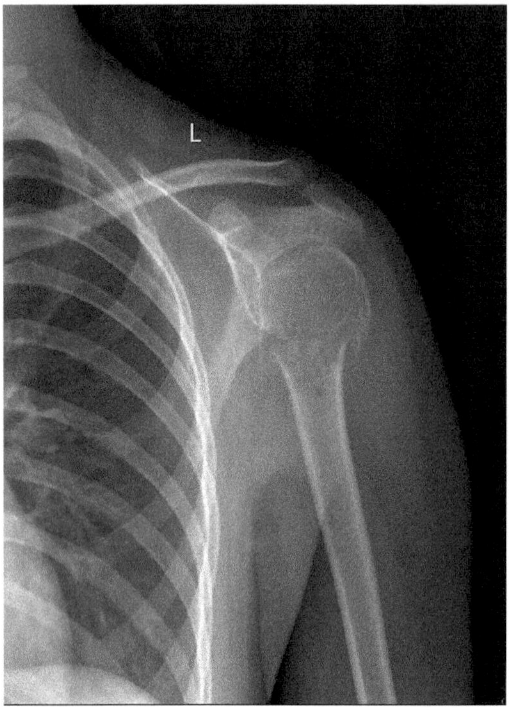

Fig. 8.1 Frontal view of the left shoulder

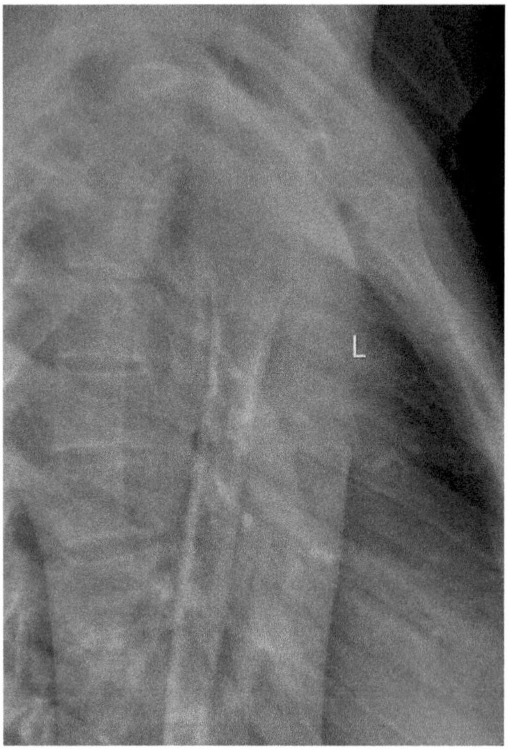

Fig. 8.2 Lateral view of the left shoulder

Radiographs of the left shoulder demonstrate a lytic lesion at the proximal humerus with cortical destruction and associated pathological fracture through the surgical neck.

8.3.2 CT Imaging

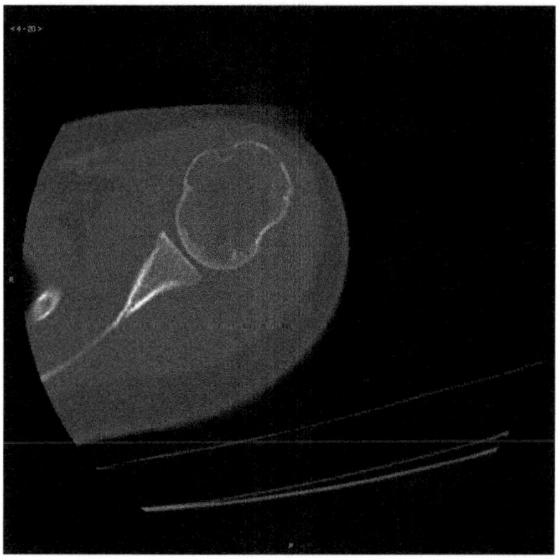

Fig. 8.3 Axial CT image of the left shoulder in bone window

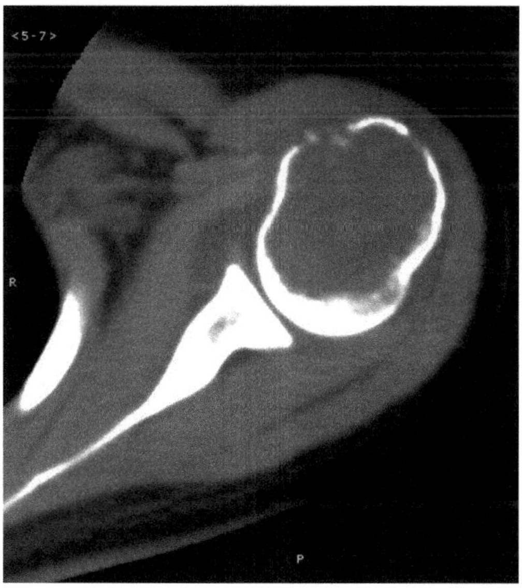

Fig. 8.4 Axial CT image of the left shoulder in soft tissue window

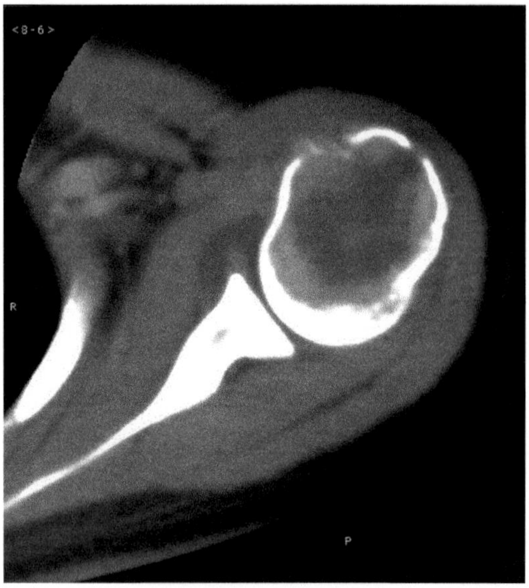

Fig. 8.5 Axial post-contrast CT image of the left shoulder in soft tissue window

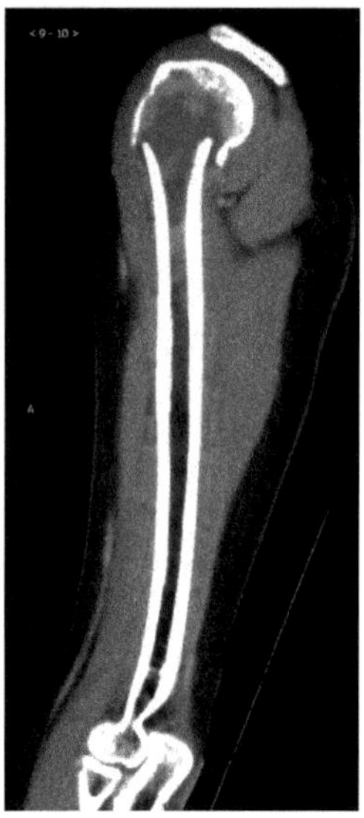

Fig. 8.6 Sagittal post-contrast CT image of the left shoulder in soft tissue window

CT images of the left shoulder demonstrate left proximal humeral lytic, expansile lesion with destruction of the cortex and associated pathological fracture. After contrast administration, there is avid enhancement in the solid component of the lesion and surrounding soft tissue swelling.

8.4 Description and Discussion from Residents

The patient is a young female. Radiographs show left proximal humeral lytic bony destructive lesion with thinning of the cortex and associated pathological fracture. Given the patient's age, area of involvement, this is most likely a giant cell tumor. Associated pathological fracture complicates the diagnosis. CT images again demonstrate the expansile bony destruction and enhancement, again most suggestive of giant cell tumor. Humeral head, greater and lesser tuberosities can all be considered as epiphysis. Thus, proximal humeral giant cell tumor can affect the humeral head along the articular surface or greater tuberosity with less involvement of the humeral head articular surface. Nowadays, most experts believe that giant cell tumor originates from the metaphysis side along the closed physis, so tends to extend along the diaphysis. This is more common in lesions at the proximal humerus. Differential diagnosis includes chondroblastoma. Pathologic fracture is present in the current case, causing surrounding soft tissue edema, joint effusion, but no thickening of the synovium and no secondary inflammatory changes commonly seen with chondroblastoma. Additionally, there is no internal calcification, not consistent with chondroblastoma. Chondroblastoma tends to occur around the humeral epiphysis, so could be excluded. Benign fibrous histiocytoma of bone can behave similarly to giant cell tumor on imaging, however, rare, would not consider it here. If the patient is older, a metastatic lesion would be in the differential diagnosis. Regardless of age, brown tumor from hyperparathyroidism should be considered. However, hyperparathyroidism tends to involve the diaphysis more.

8.5 Analysis and Comments from Professor Xiaoguang Cheng

Radiographs demonstrate the proximal humeral lesion with pathological fracture and irregular margin. There are heterogeneous densities of the lesion on the soft tissue window of the CT scan without calcification and with joint effusion. Heterogeneous enhancement after contrast with focal area of avid enhancement is noted. The above constellation of findings is consistent with giant cell tumor. Given the location of the lesion, the enhancement pattern, chondroblastoma can be excluded. Osteopenia is usually present in patients with brown tumor from hyperparathyroidism, not present in the current case, and can be excluded.

8.6 Diagnosis

Giant cell tumor of bone.

Suggested Reading

Chakarun CJ, Forrester DM, Gottsegen CJ, et al. Giant cell tumor of bone: review, mimics, and new developments in treatment. Radiographics. 2013;33(1):197–211.

Murphey MD, Nomikos GC, Flemming DJ, et al. Imaging of giant cell tumor and giant cell reparative granuloma of bone: radiologic-pathologic correlation. Radiographics. 2001;21(5):1283–309.

9 Chondrosarcoma: Case 9

9.1 Medical History

The patient is an 83-year-old male. He presented with pain in the right upper arm with swelling, deformity, and restricted range of motion after a fall 45 days ago.

9.2 Physical Examination

Deformity of the right humerus with point tenderness and palpable mass, nonmobile.

9.3 Imaging Findings

9.3.1 Radiograph

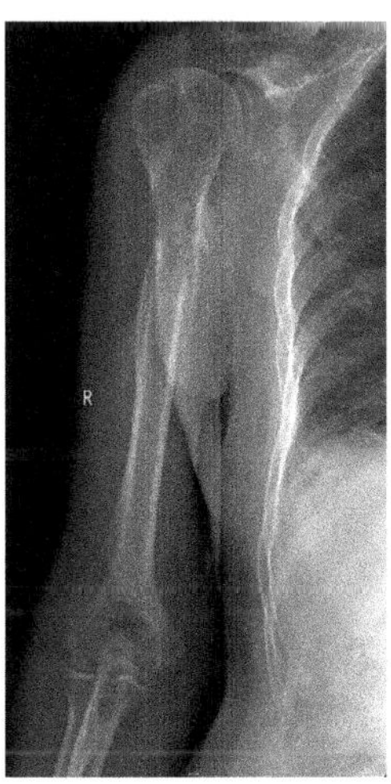

Fig. 9.1 Frontal view of the right humerus

X. Cheng et al., *Imaging of Bone Tumors in Shoulder and Elbow*,
https://doi.org/10.1007/978-981-33-6150-8_9

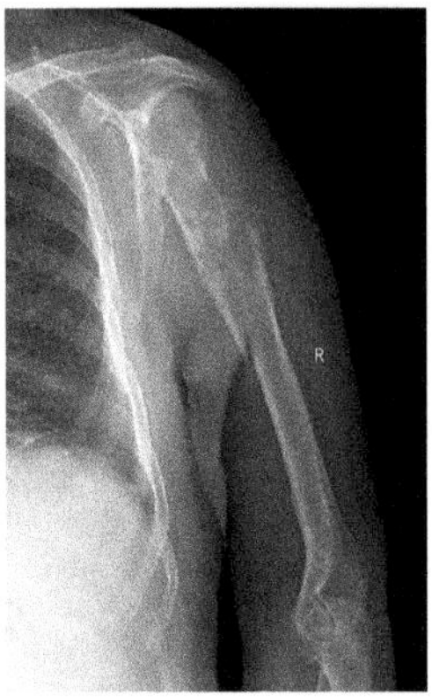

Fig. 9.2 Lateral view of the right humerus

Radiographs of the right humerus demonstrate bony destruction along the proximal one-third of the right humerus and associated pathological fracture. There is an irregular margin with internal heterogeneous densities.

9.3.2 CT Imaging

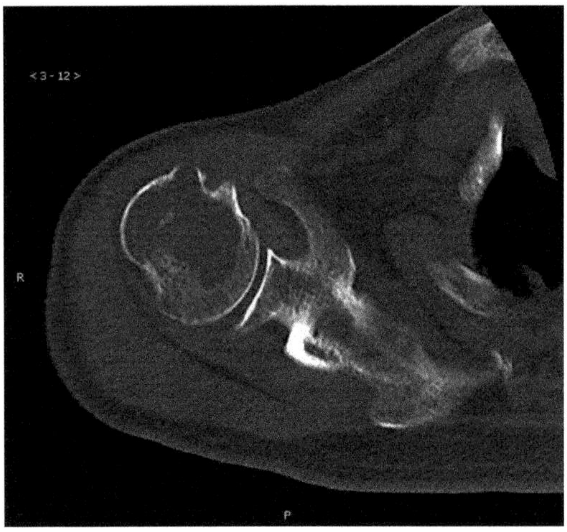

Fig. 9.3 Axial CT image of the right shoulder in bone window

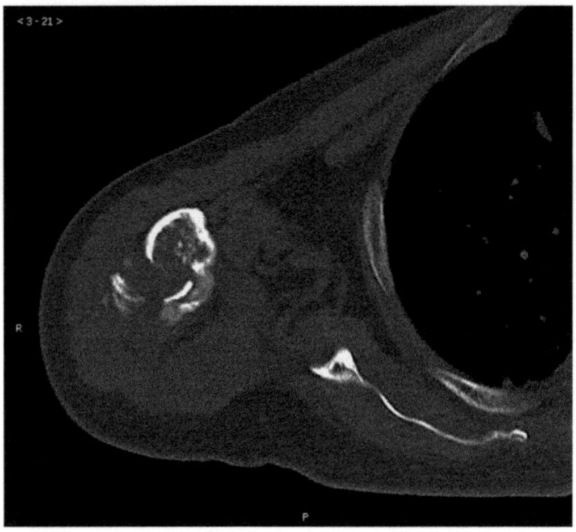

Fig. 9.4 Axial CT image of the right shoulder in bone window

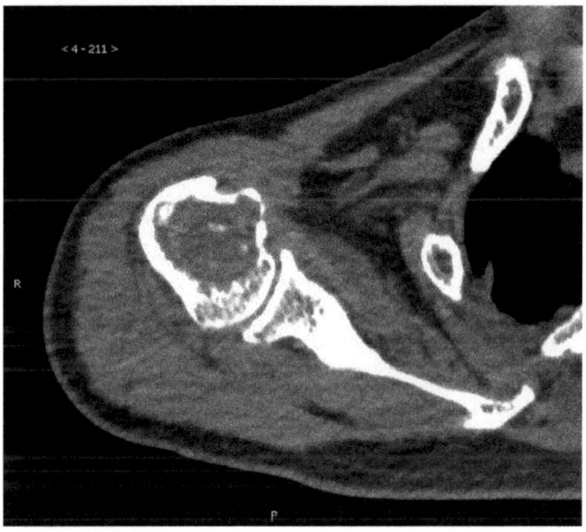

Fig. 9.5 Axial CT image of the right shoulder in soft tissue window

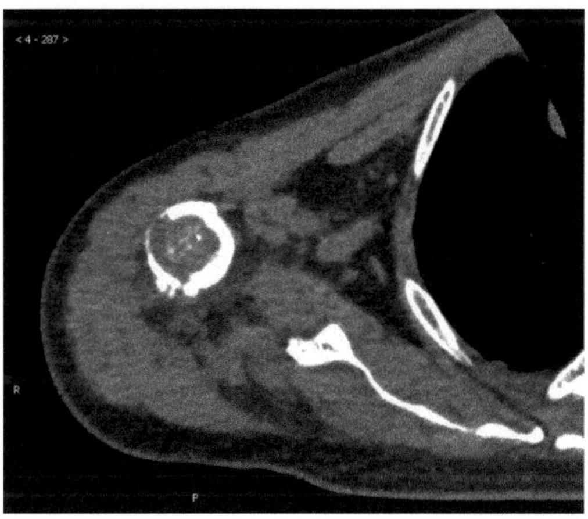

Fig. 9.6 Axial CT image of the right shoulder in soft tissue window

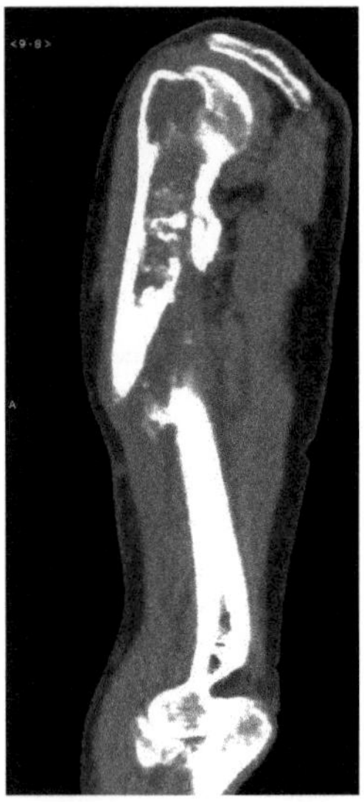

Fig. 9.7 Sagittal CT image of the right shoulder in soft tissue window

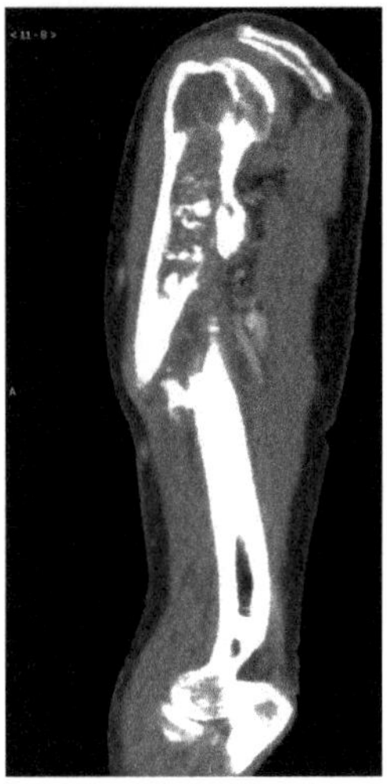

Fig. 9.8 Sagittal post-contrast CT image of the right shoulder in soft tissue window

CT images of the right humerus demonstrate osseous destruction of the proximal one-third of the right humerus with pathological fracture. There are multiple intramedullary calcifications and destruction of the cortex.

9.3.3 MR Imaging

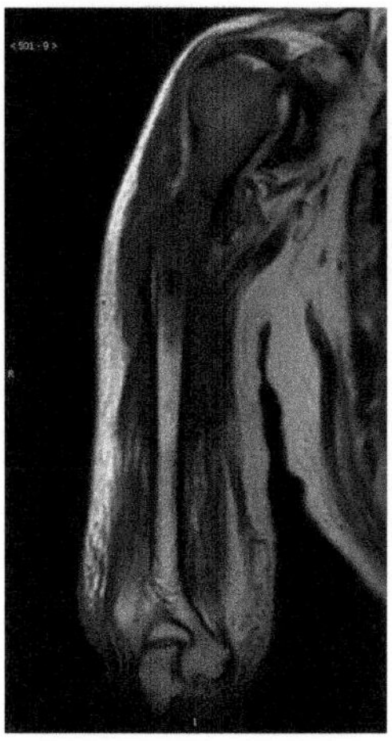

Fig. 9.9 Coronal T1-weighted MR image of the right shoulder

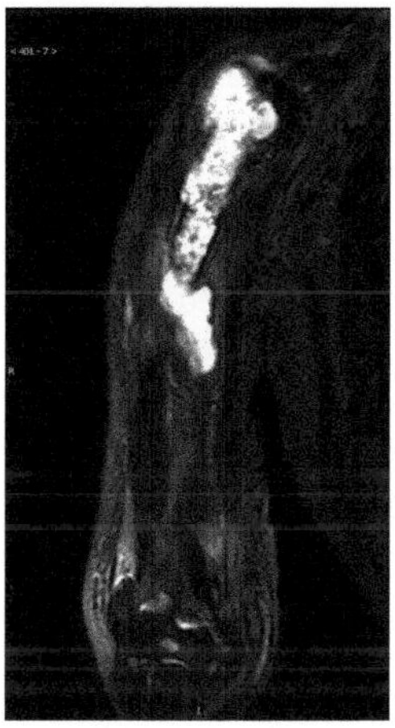

Fig. 9.10 Coronal fat-suppressed T2-weighted MR image of the right shoulder

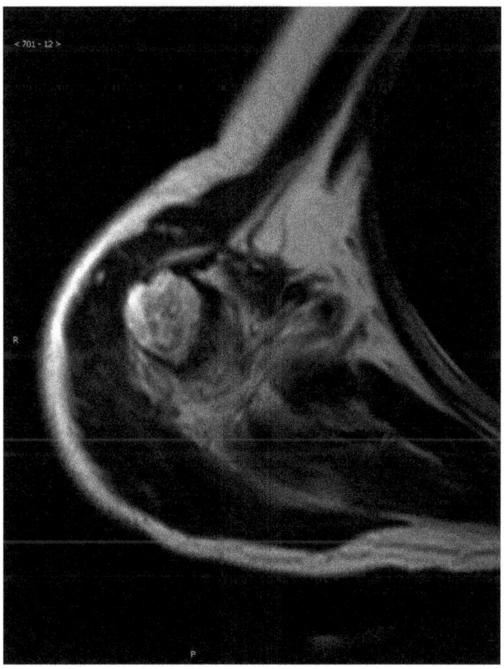

Fig. 9.11 Axial T2-weighted MR image of the right shoulder

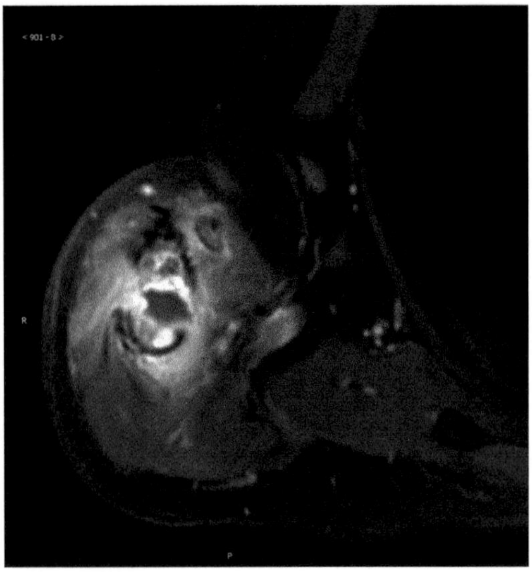

Fig. 9.12 Axial post-contrast fat-suppressed T1-weighted MR image of the right shoulder

MR images of the right shoulder demonstrate heterogeneous high T2 signal in the lesion and heterogeneous enhancement. Nodular enhancement is noted around the peripheral of the lesion.

9.4 Description and Discussion from Residents

The patient is an older male. Radiographs demonstrate right proximal humeral bony destruction with mild expansile appearances of the humeral head and patchy high densities around the diaphysis, with thinning of the cortex and pathological fracture, most suggestive of permeative aggressive bony changes. It is important to point out that with pathological fracture, the patchy high densities within the lesion could be fracture fragments or hemorrhage, not calcified matrix. CT images show multiple calcifications along the long axis of the humerus within the lesion and involvement of the cortex but no soft tissue component beyond the cortex. Part of the lesion demonstrates lobular contour without much permeative bony changes. On the post-contrast images, there is almost no enhancement in the lesion. All these features are consistent with chondrosarcoma. When diagnosing primary malignant tumor in elderly patients, metastatic lesion must be excluded. On MRI, there is a heterogeneous high T2 signal within the lesion, signaling fluid, but not excluding hemorrhage. Enhancement is noted at the inferior portion of the lesion, probably from callus formation of the pathological fracture. Nodular enhancement at the proximal portion of the lesion is consistent with chondrosarcoma. Overall, the lesion is most consistent with chondrosarcoma.

9.5 Analysis and Comments from Professor Xiaoguang Cheng

The patient is an older male. Radiographs show pathological fracture along the inferior portion of the lesion with some callus formation, indicating the subacute nature of the injury. The lesion is rather large with internal patchy high densities. On the CT images, the margin is relatively clear with patchy calcification, combined with pathological fracture, organizing hematoma with periosteal reaction; and no clear enhancement. On MR images, chondroid matrix and calcifications are noted in the lesion with peripheral lace-like enhancement of the proximal portion of the lesion. The changes of the inferior portion of the lesion are likely due to the pathological fracture. Overall, this is most consistent with chondrosarcoma, and given the patient's advanced age, metastatic lesion should be excluded.

9.6 Diagnosis

Chondrosarcoma.

Suggested Reading

Douis H, Saifuddin A. The imaging of cartilaginous bone tumours. II. Chondrosarcoma. Skeletal Radiol. 2013;42(5):611–26.

Murphey MD, Walker EA, Wilson AJ, et al. From the archives of the AFIP: imaging of primary chondrosarcoma: radiologic-pathologic correlation. Radiographics. 2003;23(5):1245–78.

Varma DG, Ayala AG, Carrasco CH, et al. Chondrosarcoma: MR imaging with pathologic correlation. Radiographics. 1992;12(4):687–704.

Chondrosarcoma: Case 10

10

10.1 Medical History

The patient is a 51-year-old male. He presented with pain at the right shoulder for 10 months, with spontaneous resolution.

10.2 Physical Examination

Point tenderness of the right scapula in the outer lateral aspect with increased temperature of the skin.

10.3 Imaging Findings

10.3.1 Radiograph

X. Cheng et al., *Imaging of Bone Tumors in Shoulder and Elbow*,
https://doi.org/10.1007/978-981-33-6150-8_10

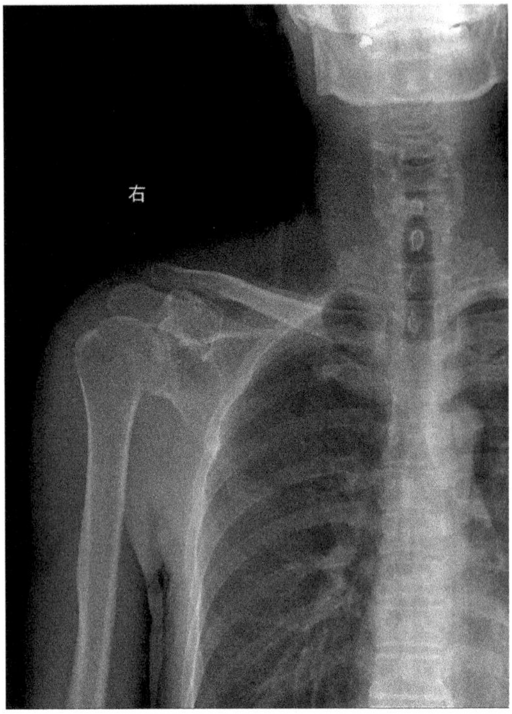

Fig. 10.1 Frontal view of the right scapula

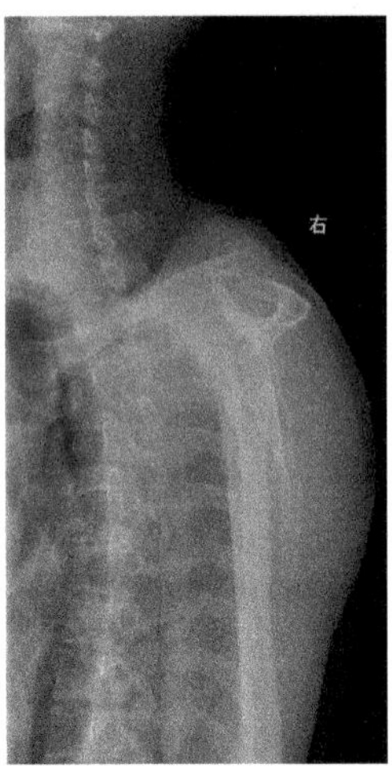

Fig. 10.2 Lateral view of the right scapula

Radiographs of the right scapula demonstrate lytic osseous destruction, involving around the scapula spine and coracoid process with expansile appearances and peripheral sclerosis.

10.3.2 CT Imaging

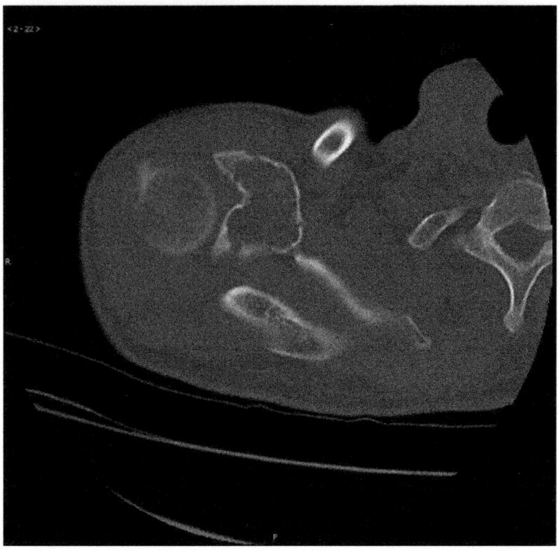

Fig. 10.3 Axial CT image of the right shoulder in bone window

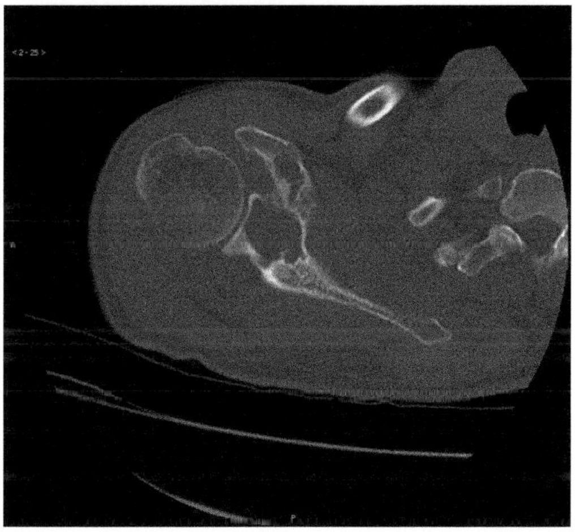

Fig. 10.4 Axial CT image of the right shoulder in bone window

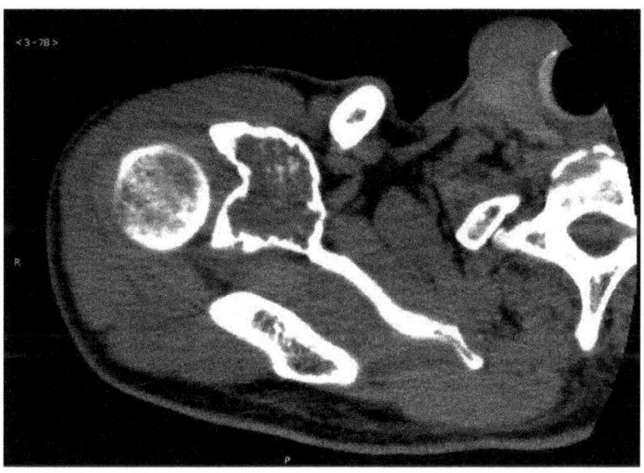

Fig. 10.5 Axial CT image of the right shoulder in soft tissue window

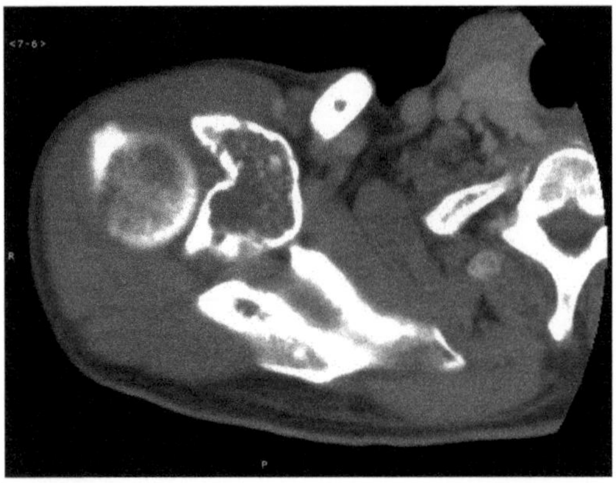

Fig. 10.6 Axial CT post-contrast image of the right shoulder in soft tissue window

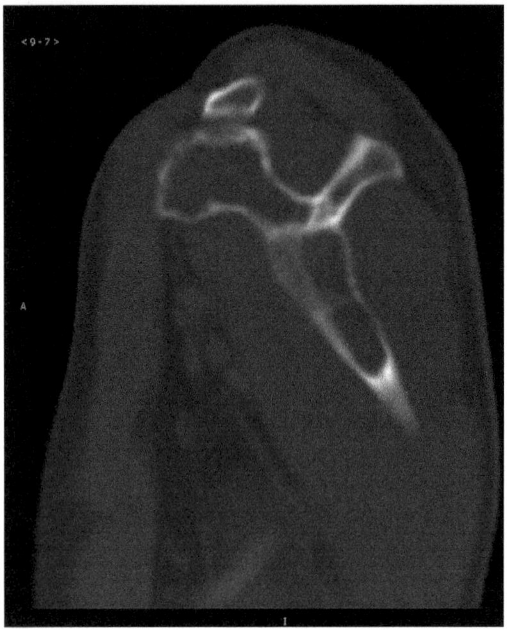

Fig. 10.7 Sagittal CT image of the right shoulder in bone window

CT images of the right shoulder demonstrate the well-circumscribed lesion with cortical disruption and internal scattered calcifications. There is mild inhomogeneous enhancement.

10.3.3 MR Imaging

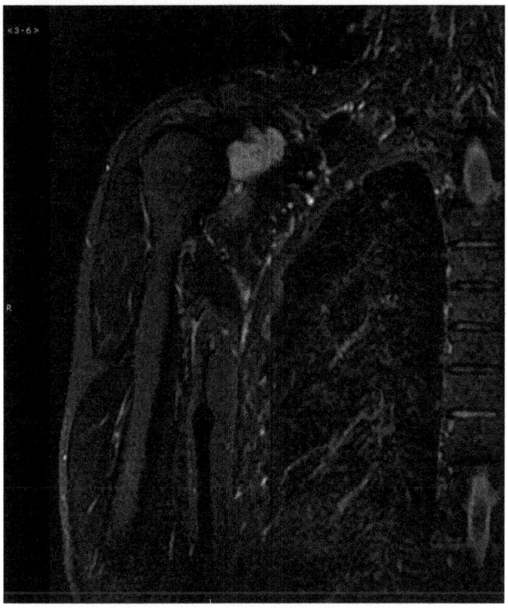

Fig. 10.8 Coronal fat-suppressed T2-weighted MR image of the right shoulder

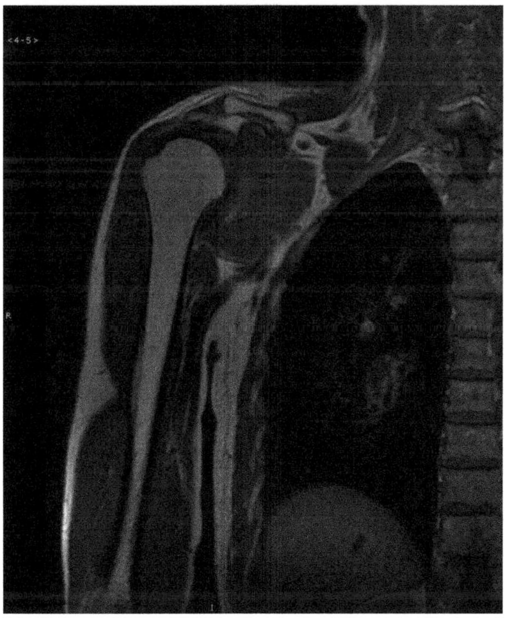

Fig. 10.9 Coronal T1-weighted MR image of the right shoulder

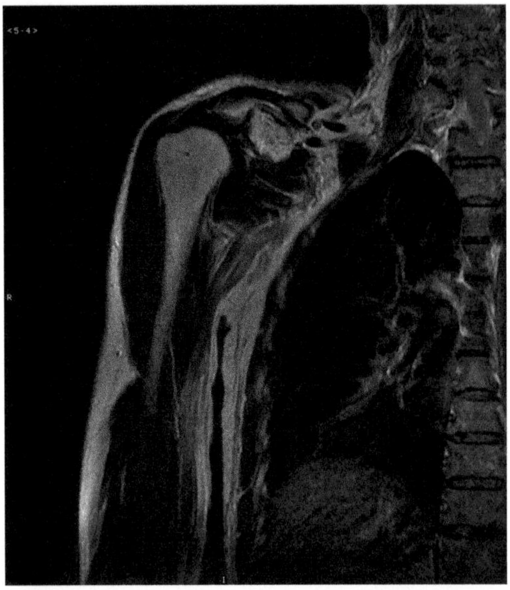

Fig. 10.10 Coronal T2-weighted MR image of the right shoulder

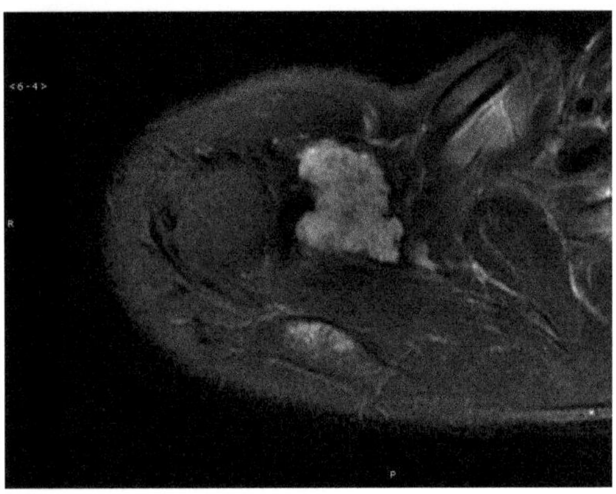

Fig. 10.11 Axial fat-suppressed T2-weighted MR image of the right shoulder

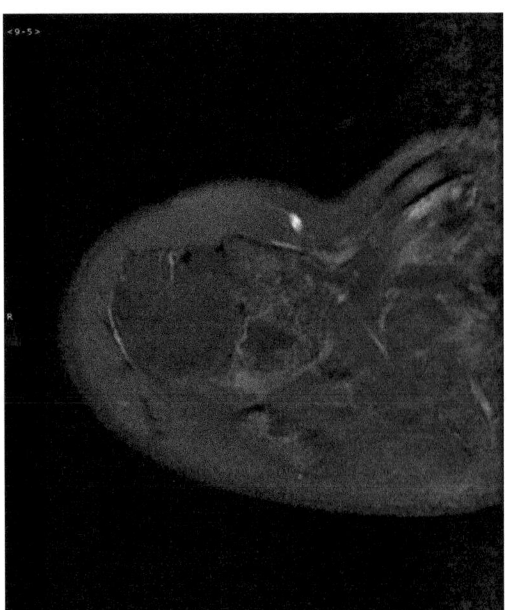

Fig. 10.12 Axial post-contrast fat-suppressed T1-weighted MR image of the right shoulder

MR images of the right shoulder demonstrate heterogeneous high T2 signal and iso-intense T1 signal of the lesion with peripheral enhancement.

10.4 Description and Discussion from Residents

Radiographs demonstrate the lesion involves the scapula spine and coracoid process with lytic osseous destruction and mild peripheral sclerosis. The lesion is well-circumscribed with internal heterogeneous densities and small septations. There is no destruction of the glenoid articular surface or adjacent soft tissue swelling. CT images again demonstrate the well-circumscribed lesion with peripheral sclerosis and some cortical disruption; internal scattered calcifications and mild heterogeneous enhancement. The lesion demonstrates a heterogeneous high T2 signal and iso-intense T1 signal. The T2 signal characteristics are consistent with chondroid matrix. Low signal of calcifications and peripheral enhancement with lobular contour represent a pattern seen in chondrosarcoma. Scapula and pelvis are common locations for chondrosarcoma. Overall, this is most suggestive of chondrosarcoma.

10.5 Analysis and Comments from Professor Xiaoguang Cheng

Radiographs show a clear margin of the lesion. CT images demonstrate expansile lesion with lytic osseous destruction and internal scattered calcifications with mild enhancement. MR images show lobular enhancement. This is consistent with a chondrogenic tumor. If in short tubular bone, this would be enchondroma. In other locations, with the above findings, the top consideration is chondrosarcoma and metastatic lesion should be included in the differential diagnosis.

10.6 Diagnosis

Chondrosarcoma.

Suggested Reading

Douis H, Saifuddin A. The imaging of cartilaginous bone tumours. II. Chondrosarcoma. Skeletal Radiol. 2013;42(5):611–26.

Murphey MD, Walker EA, Wilson AJ, et al. From the archives of the AFIP: imaging of primary chondrosarcoma: radiologic-pathologic correlation. Radiographics. 2003;23(5):1245–78.

Varma DG, Ayala AG, Carrasco CH, et al. Chondrosarcoma: MR imaging with pathologic correlation. Radiographics. 1992;12(4):687–704.

Osteomyelitis: Case 11

11

11.1 Medical History

The patient is an 11-year-old girl. She presented with redness and swelling of her right upper arm with pain. She had fever and elevated CRP and ESR.

11.2 Physical Examination

Point tenderness of the right upper arm with restricted range of motion of the right shoulder.

11.3 Imaging Findings

11.3.1 Radiograph

X. Cheng et al., *Imaging of Bone Tumors in Shoulder and Elbow*,
https://doi.org/10.1007/978-981-33-6150-8_11

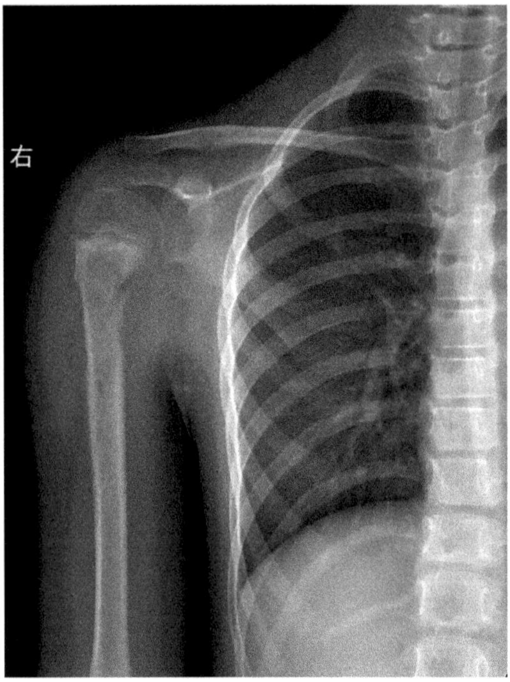

Fig. 11.1 Frontal view of the right shoulder

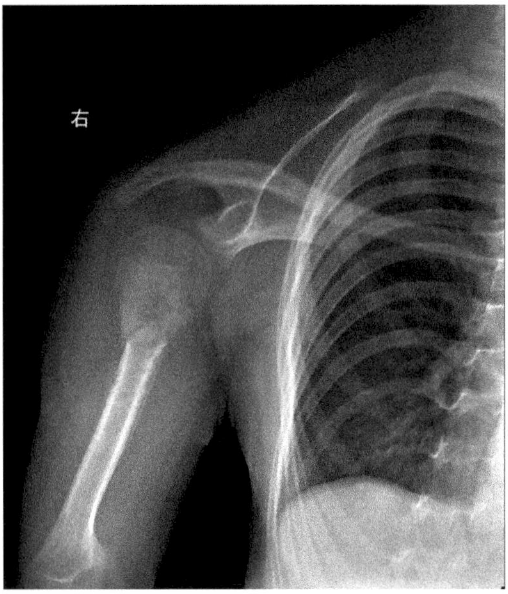

Fig. 11.2 Lateral view of the right shoulder

Radiographs of the right shoulder demonstrate bony destruction of the right proximal humerus with interrupted periosteal reaction. There is associated secondary pathological fracture.

11.3.2 CT Imaging

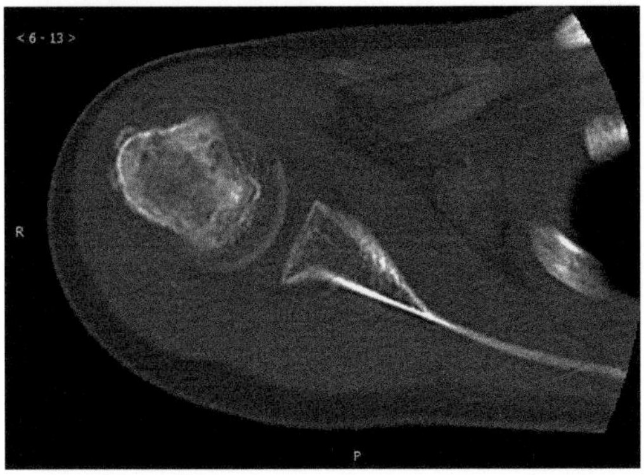

Fig. 11.3 Axial CT image of the right shoulder in bone window

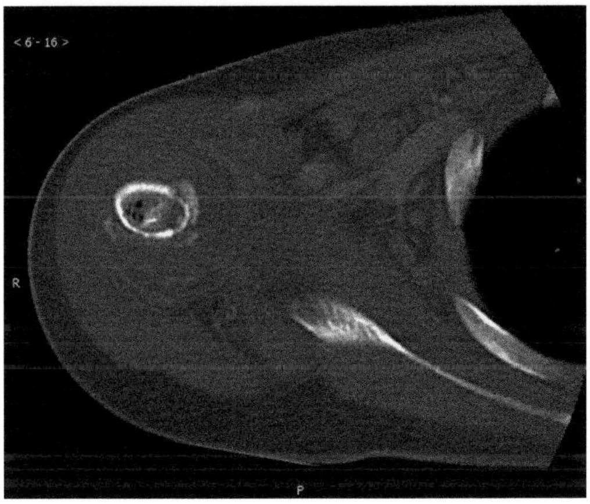

Fig. 11.4 Axial CT image of the right shoulder in bone window

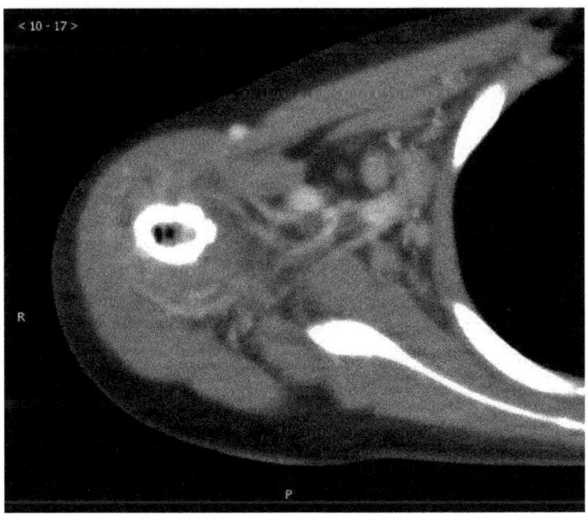

Fig. 11.5 Axial post-contrast CT image of the right shoulder in soft tissue window

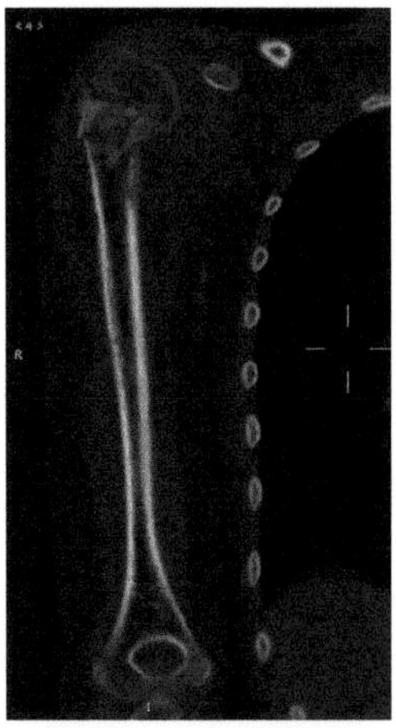

Fig. 11.6 Coronal CT image of the right shoulder in bone window

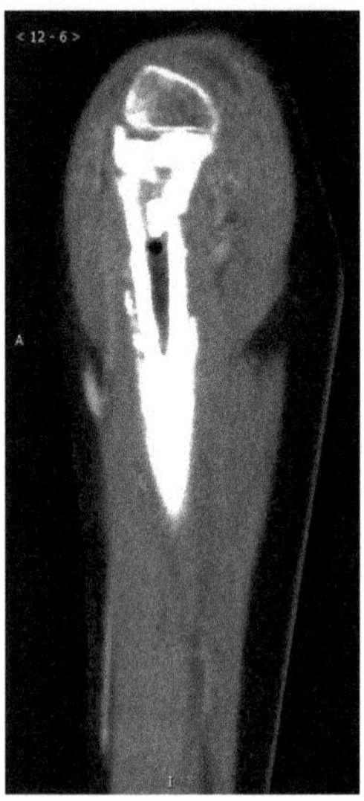

Fig. 11.7 Sagittal post-contrast CT image of the right shoulder in soft tissue window

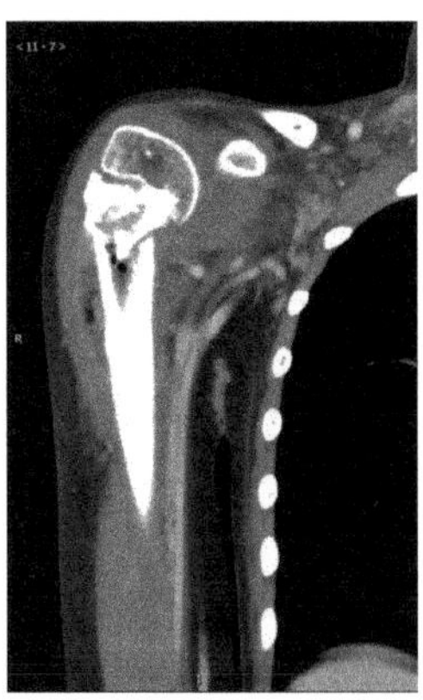

Fig. 11.8 Coronal post-contrast CT image of the right shoulder in soft tissue window

CT images of the right shoulder demonstrate bony destruction of the proximal humerus with cortical break and periosteal reaction. There is fluid like low density in the adjacent soft tissue with peripheral enhancement. Air is noted in the intramedullary cavity. Pathological fracture is seen.

11.4 Description and Discussion from Residents

The patient presents with pain, redness with swelling, and elevated inflammatory markers. Radiographs demonstrate right proximal humeral bone destruction with pathologic fracture. On the lateral view, there is an interruption of the periosteal reaction around the pathologic fracture with destruction around the medullary cavity. On the CT scan, there is proximal humeral bone destruction with cortical disruption in a permeative pattern, with clear periosteal reaction and adjacent air–fluid level in the soft tissue, most consistent with osteomyelitis.

11.5 Analysis and Comments from Professor Xiaoguang Cheng

The clinical presentation is most suggestive of an inflammatory process. Right proximal humeral bone destruction with inhomogeneous densities in the intramedullary cavity is demonstrated on radiographs. On the CT images, there is air noted in the intramedullary cavity and adjacent soft tissue, typical of infection.

11.6 Diagnosis

Osteomyelitis (with pathologic fracture).

Suggested Reading

Beaman FD, von Herrmann PF, Kransdorf MJ, et al. ACR appropriateness Criteria® suspected osteomyelitis, septic arthritis, or soft tissue infection (excluding spine and diabetic foot). J Am Coll Radiol. 2017 May;14(5S):S326–37.

Oudjhane K, Azouz EM. Imaging of osteomyelitis in children. Radiol Clin N Am. 2001 Mar;39(2):251–66.

Saigal G, Azouz EM, Abdenour G. Imaging of osteomyelitis with special reference to children. Semin Musculoskelet Radiol. 2004 Sep;8(3):255–65.

Bony Metastatic Lesion (Liver Cancer): Case 12

12

12.1 Medical History

The patient is a 65-year-old male. He presented with right shoulder pain, discomfort for a year, worsened by activity with restriction for 7 months.

12.2 Physical Examination

Not done.

12.3 Imaging Findings

12.3.1 Radiograph

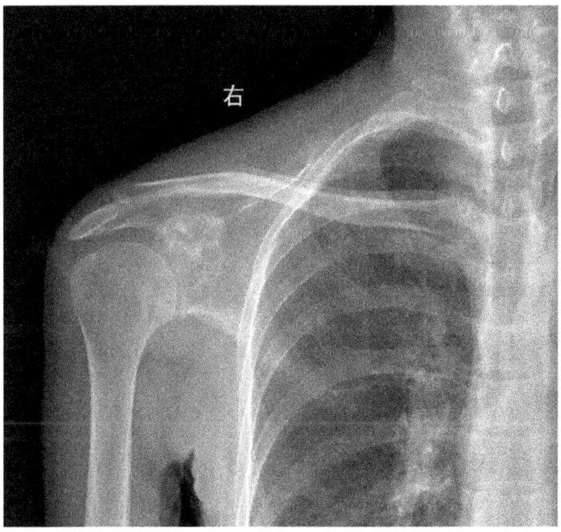

Fig. 12.1 Frontal view of the right scapula

X. Cheng et al., *Imaging of Bone Tumors in Shoulder and Elbow*,
https://doi.org/10.1007/978-981-33-6150-8_12

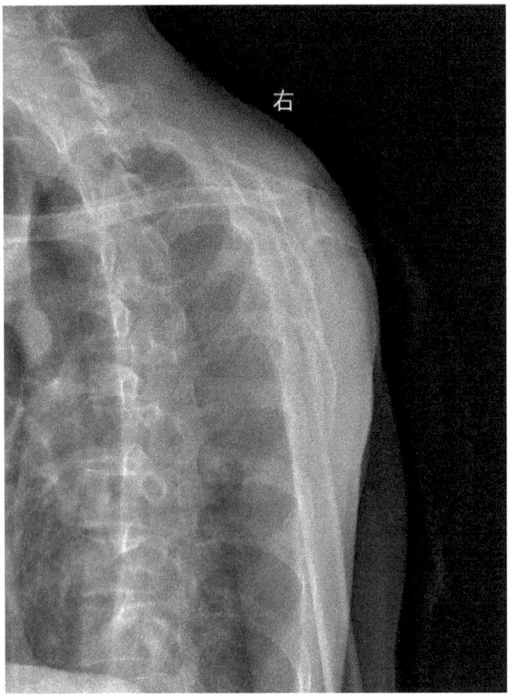

Fig. 12.2 Lateral view of the right scapula

Radiographs of the right scapula demonstrate expansile bony destruction around the scapula spine and coracoid process with internal heterogeneous densities.

12.3.2 CT Imaging

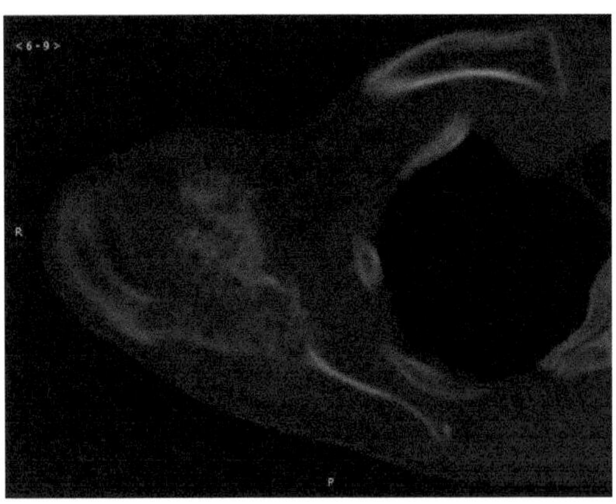

Fig. 12.3 Axial CT image of the right shoulder in bone window

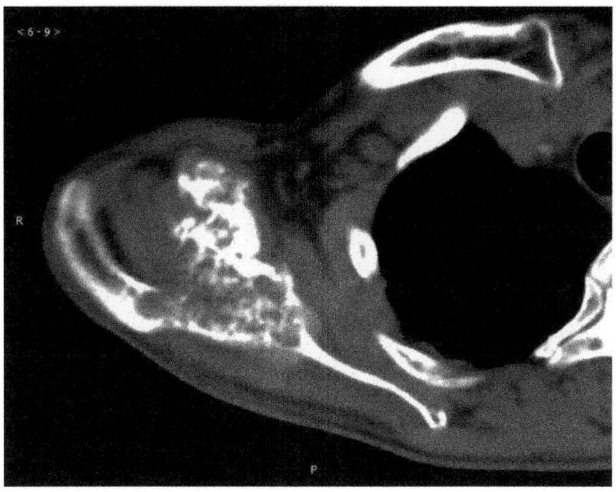

Fig. 12.4 Axial CT image of the right shoulder in soft tissue window

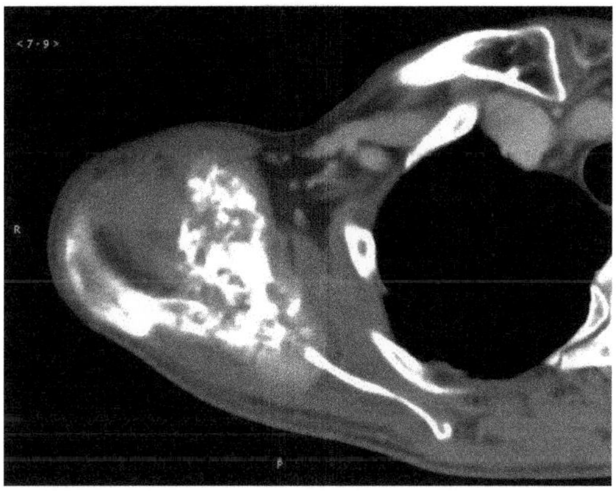

Fig. 12.5 Axial post-contrast CT image of the right shoulder in soft tissue window

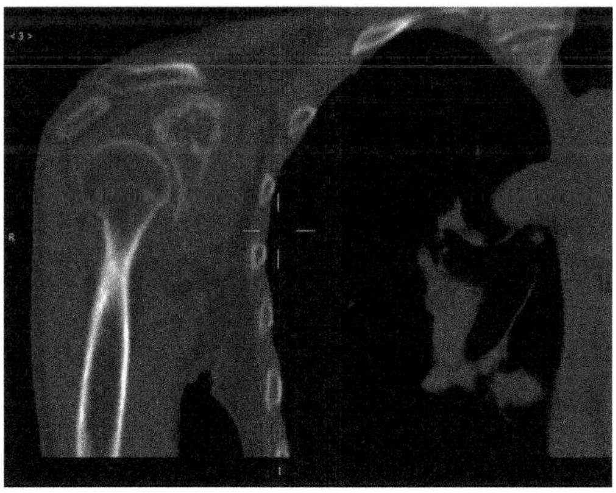

Fig. 12.6 Coronal CT image of the right shoulder in bone window

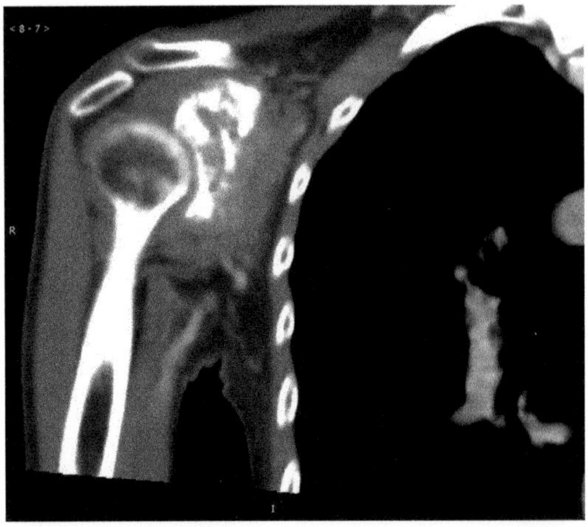

Fig. 12.7 Coronal post-contrast CT image of the right shoulder in soft tissue window

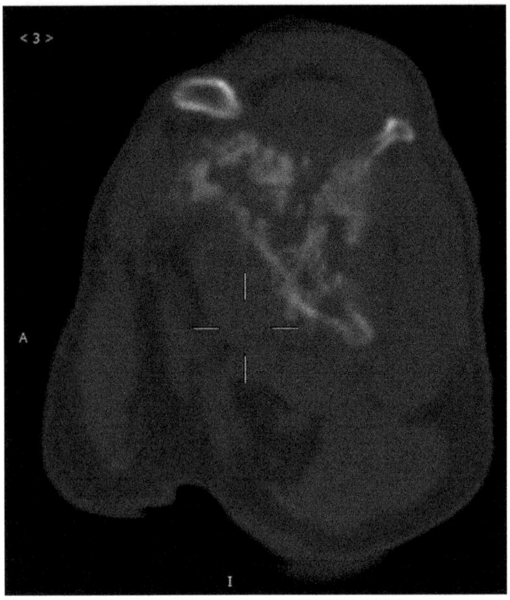

Fig. 12.8 Sagittal CT image of the right shoulder in bone window

CT images of the right shoulder demonstrate extensive bony destruction with mixed sclerotic and lytic appearances of the scapula and no clear margin. There is cortical disruption with adjacent soft tissue nodule and avid enhancement.

12.4 Description and Discussion from Residents

The patient is an older male. Radiographs demonstrate bony destruction around the right scapula spine, body, and coracoid process. There are mild expansile appearances with internal heterogeneous densities and no definite adjacent soft tissue mass. On the CT scan, the lesion demonstrates an ill-defined margin with extensive bony destruction in a mixed pattern, causing cortical disruption and associated soft tissue mass with avid enhancement. Given the patient's age, the first consideration would be a metastatic lesion. This is most consistent with a highly aggressive lesion. Most chondrosarcoma is usually not highly aggressive on imaging, so not at the top of the differential diagnosis.

12.5 Analysis and Comments from Professor Xiaoguang Cheng

Images demonstrate a mixed pattern of osseous destruction of the right scapula spine, body, and coracoid process with avid enhancement. Chondrosarcoma can be excluded based on the imaging findings. Given patient is an older male, the metastatic lesion is at the top of differential diagnosis. Metastatic lesions from liver cancer, thyroid cancer, and renal cell carcinoma all can have the above findings. Differential diagnosis should include osteosarcoma.

12.6 Diagnosis

Bony metastatic lesion (Liver cancer).

Suggested Reading

Roberts CC, Daffner RH, Weissman BN, et al. ACR appropriateness criteria on metastatic bone disease. J Am Coll Radiol. 2010 Jun;7(6):400–9.

Velloni F, Ramalho M, AlObaidy M, et al. Bone metastases of hepatocellular carcinoma: appearance on MRI using a standard abdominal protocol. AJR Am J Roentgenol. 2016 May;206(5):1003–12.

13 Bony Metastatic Lesion (Renal Clear Cell Carcinoma): Case 13

13.1 Medical History

The patient is a 78-year-old male. He presented with right shoulder pain for 8 months.

13.2 Physical Examination

Mild swelling around the right shoulder with restricted range of motion.

13.3 Imaging Findings

13.3.1 Radiograph

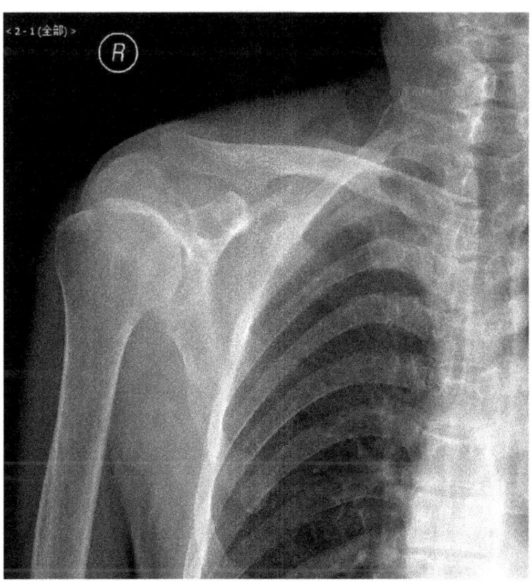

Fig. 13.1 Frontal view of the right shoulder

X. Cheng et al., *Imaging of Bone Tumors in Shoulder and Elbow*,
https://doi.org/10.1007/978-981-33-6150-8_13

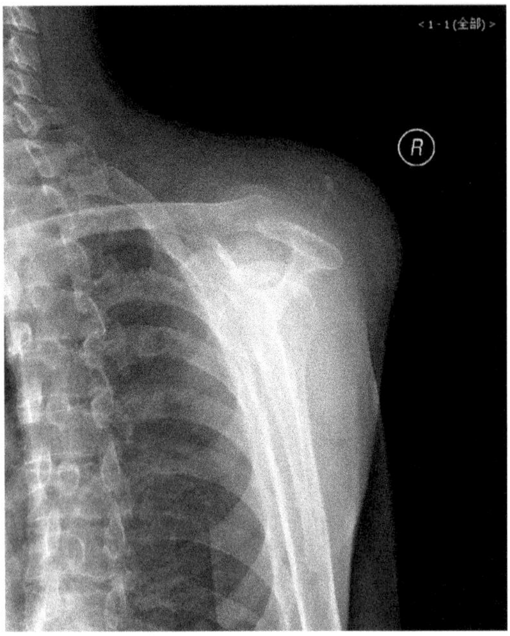

Fig. 13.2 Lateral view of the right shoulder

Radiographs of the right shoulder demonstrate bony destruction around the right scapula with adjacent high-density soft tissue mass and internal calcification.

13.3.2 CT Imaging

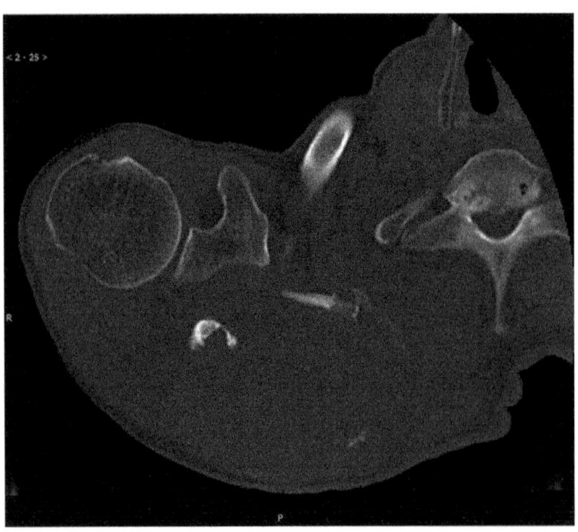

Fig. 13.3 Axial CT image of the right shoulder in bone window

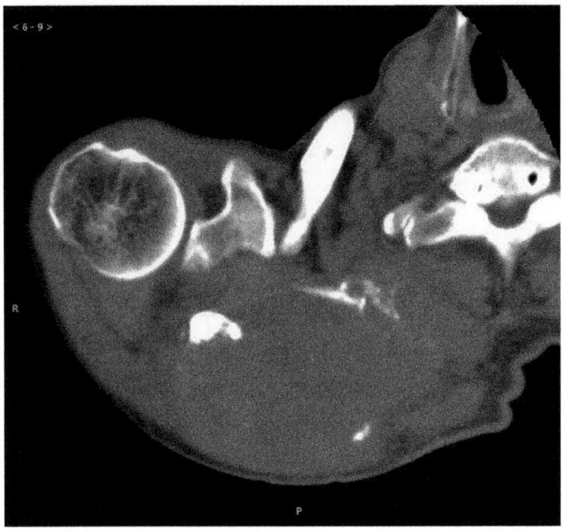

Fig. 13.4 Axial CT image of the right shoulder in soft tissue window

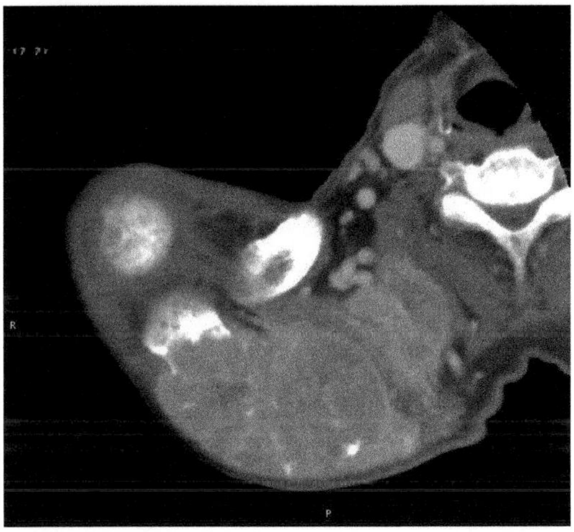

Fig. 13.5 Axial post-contrast CT image of the right shoulder in soft tissue window

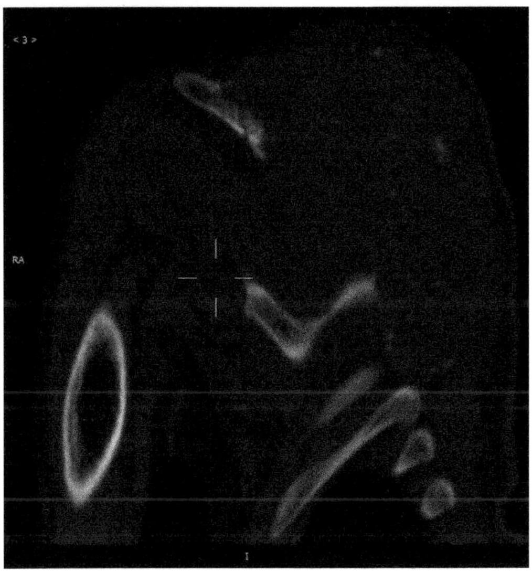

Fig. 13.6 Coronal CT image of the right shoulder in bone window

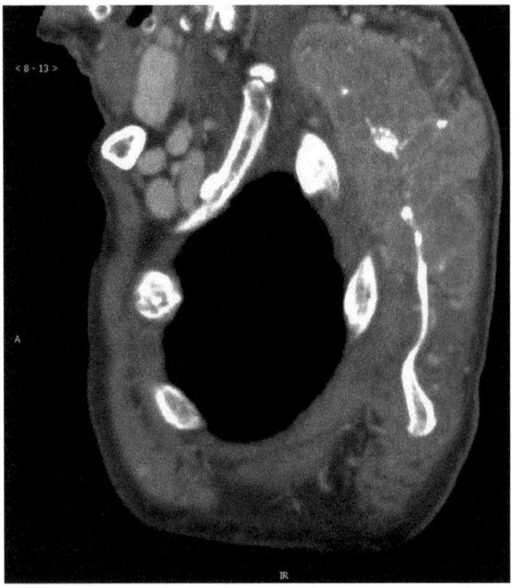

Fig. 13.7 Sagittal post-contrast CT image of the right shoulder in soft tissue window

CT images of the right shoulder demonstrate extensive lytic osseous destruction of the right scapula with associated large soft tissue mass and internal calcification. There is avid heterogeneous enhancement.

13.4 Description and Discussion from Residents

The patient is an older male. Radiographs demonstrate extensive osseous destruction around the right scapula above and below the scapula spine with high-density adjacent soft tissue mass and internal punctuate high densities noted. On CT scan, there is small lobular calcification in the soft tissue mass with avid solid enhancement mixed with patchy area of low densities, raising concern for metastatic lesion. With this enhancement pattern, this is more likely of mesenchymal chondrosarcoma or dedifferentiated chondrosarcoma than central chondrosarcoma. In mesenchymal chondrosarcoma, there is usually an internal significant amount of calcifications not like the small lobular appearances in this case. In dedifferentiated chondrosarcoma, usually, there are regions demonstrating features of typical low-grade chondrosarcoma. Additionally, undifferentiated high-grade pleomorphic sarcoma usually does not show the above imaging features. Given the patient's age, imaging features, the top consideration is metastatic lesion with primary from liver or renal source.

13.5 Analysis and Comments from Professor Xiaoguang Cheng

The patient is an older male. There is no clear abnormality on the front view radiograph of the shoulder. On the lateral view, there is expansile bony destruction of the scapula body with large soft tissue mass. On the CT scan, there are internal punctuate calcifications, raising concern for chondrosarcoma. However, avid enhancement noted of the soft tissue mass is not consistent with typical chondrosarcoma. Thus, the metastatic lesion is at the top of the differential diagnosis.

13.6 Diagnosis

Bony metastatic lesion (Renal clear cell carcinoma).

Suggested Reading

Murphy J, Patel A, James SL, et al. "Flow-void" sign in osseous metastatic renal cell carcinoma. Clin Radiol. 2019 Feb;74(2):111–5.

Roberts CC, Daffner RH, Weissman BN, et al. ACR appropriateness criteria on metastatic bone disease. J Am Coll Radiol. 2010 Jun;7(6):400–9.

Diffuse Large B-Cell Lymphoma: Case 14

14

14.1 Medical History

The patient is a 76-year-old male. He presented with pain around the right shoulder with a restricted range of motion for 2 days.

14.2 Physical Examination

The right shoulder is fixed with a brace. There is swelling and painful restricted range of motion of the right shoulder.

14.3 Imaging Findings

14.3.1 Radiograph

X. Cheng et al., *Imaging of Bone Tumors in Shoulder and Elbow*,
https://doi.org/10.1007/978-981-33-6150-8_14

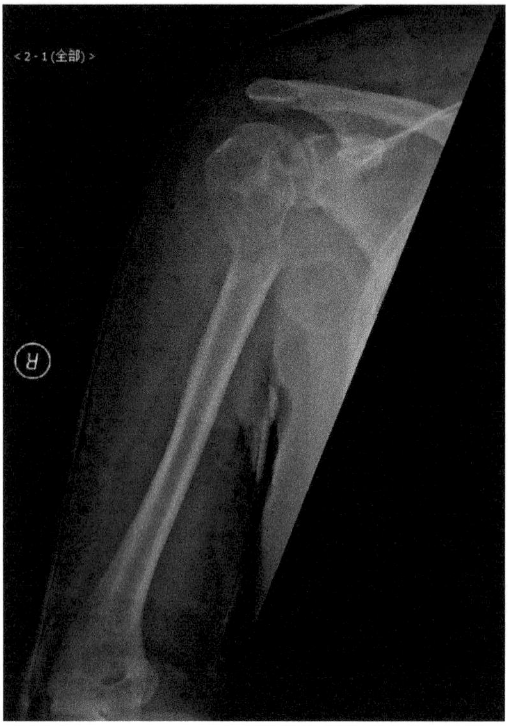

Fig. 14.1 Frontal view of the right shoulder

The radiograph of the right shoulder demonstrates mixed bony destruction around the right proximal humerus with expansile appearance and associated pathologic fracture about the surgical neck.

14.3.2 CT Imaging

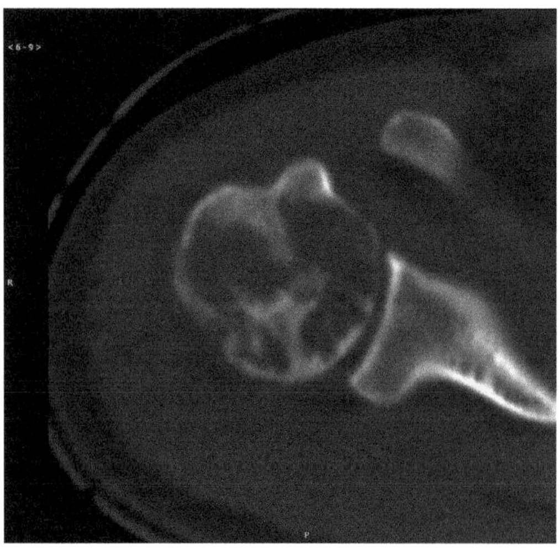

Fig. 14.2 Axial CT image of the right shoulder in bone window

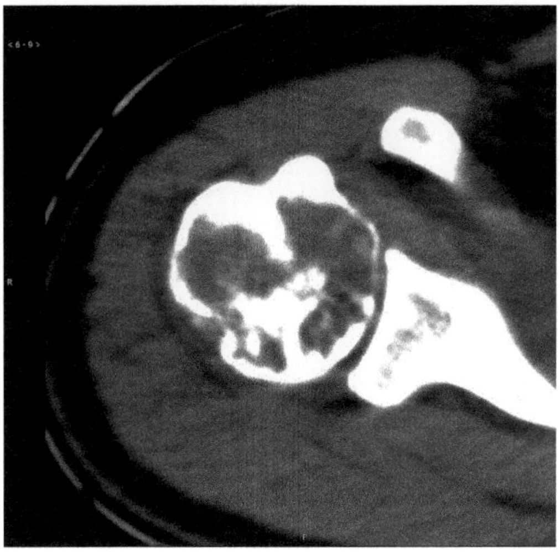

Fig. 14.3 Axial CT image of the right shoulder in soft tissue window

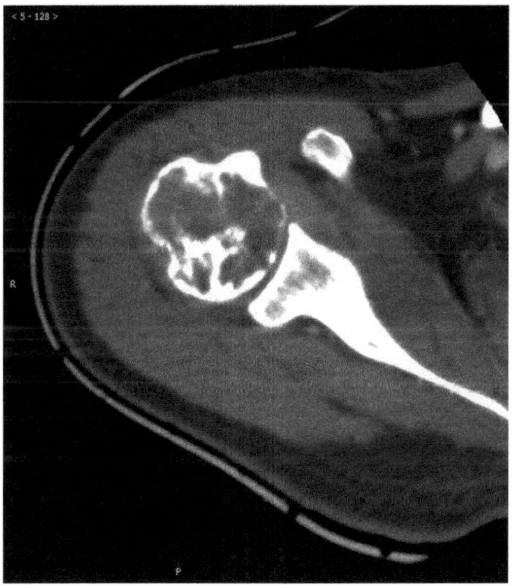

Fig. 14.4 Axial post-contrast CT image of the right shoulder in soft tissue window

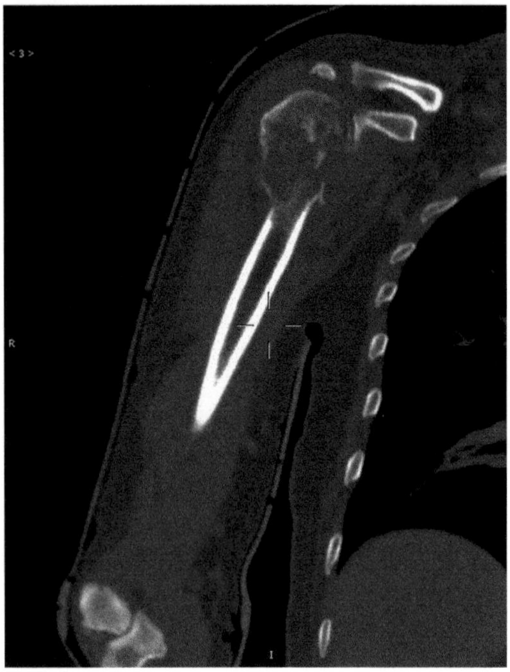

Fig. 14.5 Coronal CT image of the right shoulder in bone window

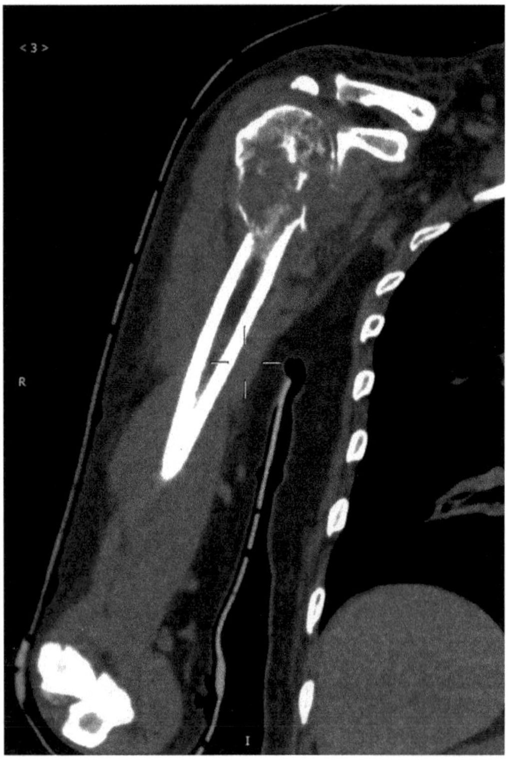

Fig. 14.6 Coronal CT image of the right shoulder in soft tissue window

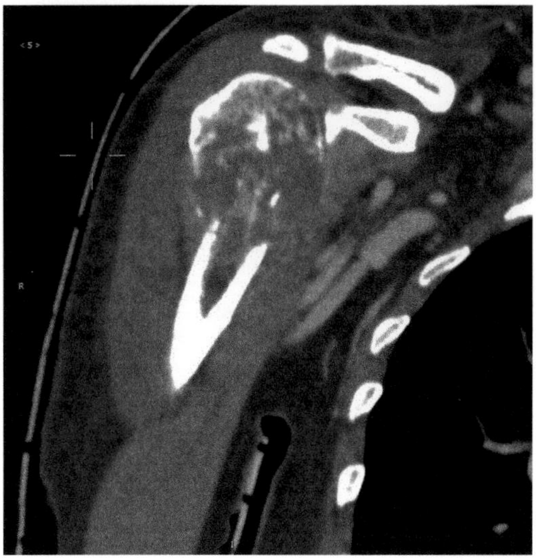

Fig. 14.7 Coronal post-contrast CT image of the right shoulder in soft tissue window

CT images of the right shoulder demonstrate mixed bony destruction involving the proximal right humerus extending to the humeral head with pathological fracture. There is cortical disruption with soft tissue mass extruded. Peripheral enhancement is noted.

14.3.3 MR Imaging

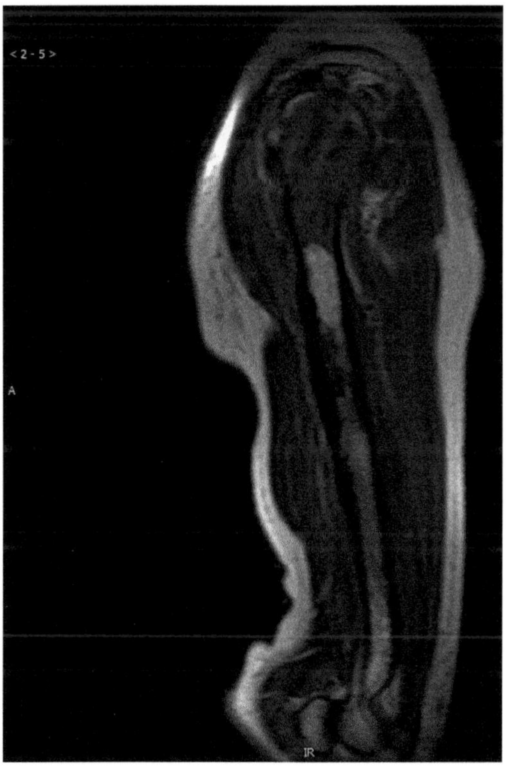

Fig. 14.8 Sagittal T1-weighted MR image of the right shoulder

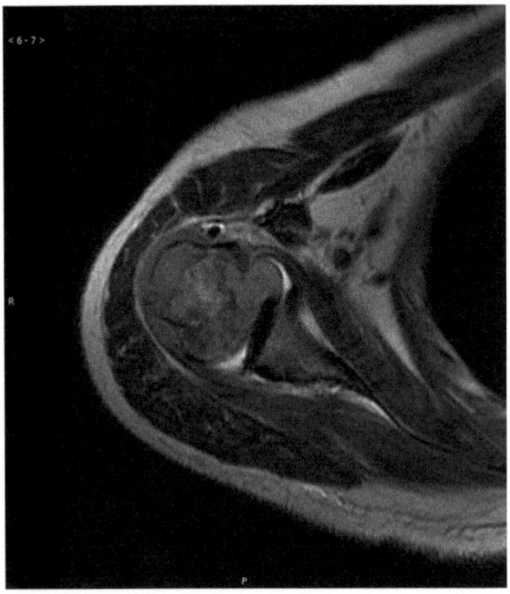

Fig. 14.9 Axial T2-weighted MR image of the right shoulder

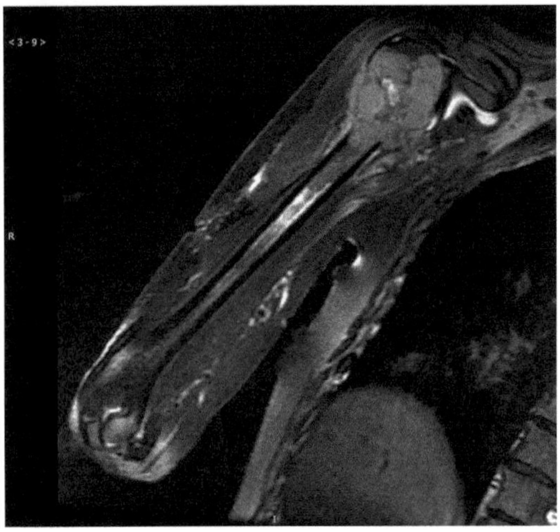

Fig. 14.10 Coronal fat-suppressed T2-weighted MR image of the right shoulder

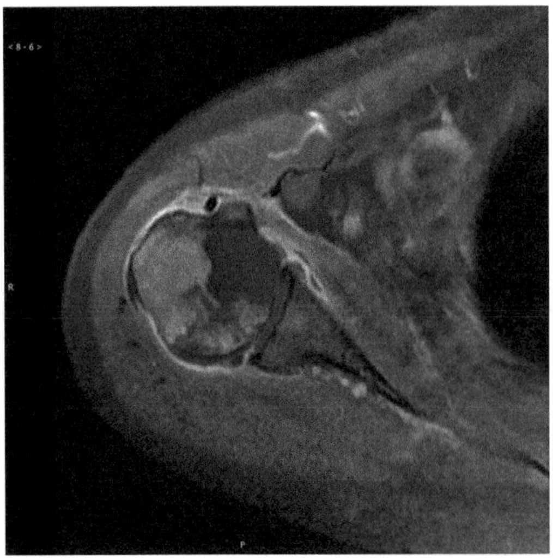

Fig. 14.11 Axial post-contrast fat-suppressed T1-weighted MR image of the right shoulder

MR images of the right shoulder demonstrate the lesion at the proximal right humerus including the humeral head with heterogeneous low T1 signal and iso-intense T2 signal. There is another segment of abnormal low T1 and slightly high T2 signal distally of the right humeral shaft. Internal fluid-like necrosis or cyst is noted. There is heterogeneous enhancement.

14.4 Description and Discussion from Residents

The patient is an older male. Radiograph demonstrates mixed bony destruction with more dominant lytic process with heterogeneous densities and bony septation. There is thinning of the cortex with irregular margin and pathologic fracture. On the CT images, the lesion is slightly expansile with cortical disruption and soft tissue mass. Given the patient's age, metastatic lesion is in the differential diagnosis. However, there is a very mild enhancement in the soft mass, not typical of metastatic lesion. With mild enhancement, chondrosarcoma is included in the differential diagnosis. However, extruded soft tissue mass with no significant osseous destruction is not typical of chondrosarcoma. And, the intra-lesional high densities may not be calcifications. Given the patient's age, lymphoma should be included in the differential diagnosis. MRI images demonstrate intramedullary abnormal signal involving the right humeral shaft, right scapula, and rib with diffuse enhancement. This pattern is suggestive of metastatic disease, lymphoma, and multiple myeloma. Without identification of lobular high T2 signal of chondroid matrix on MR images, chondrosarcoma can be excluded. Lymphoma has complex imaging features. The current case demonstrates density/signal relatively homogeneous soft tissue mass beyond the cortex, suggesting lymphoma.

14.5 Analysis and Comments from Professor Xiaoguang Cheng

The patient is an older male. On imaging, there is right proximal humeral bone destruction with soft tissue mass and no involvement of the joint. MR images demonstrate abnormal signal of the intramedullary cavity of the humeral shaft, scapula, and rib. With multiple sites of involvements, metastatic lesion is at the top of differential diagnosis. However, given the patient's age, there should not be a high T2 signal on fat-suppressed sequence at mid humeral shaft, red marrow conversion would not start in the diaphysis, usually in the metaphysis. Thus, most likely this is a case of lymphoma.

14.6 Diagnosis

Diffuse large B cell lymphoma.

Suggested Reading

Hwang S. Imaging of lymphoma of the musculoskeletal system. Magn Reson Imaging Clin N Am. 2010 Feb;18(1):75–93.

Krishnan A, Shirkhoda A, Tehranzadeh J, et al. Primary bone lymphoma: radiographic-MR imaging correlation. Radiographics. 2003 Nov–Dec;23(6):1371–83.

Murphey MD, Kransdorf MJ. Primary musculoskeletal lymphoma. Radiol Clin N Am. 2016 Jul;54(4):785–95.

Weber MA, Papakonstantinou O, Nikodinovska VV, et al. Ewing's sarcoma and primary osseous lymphoma: spectrum of imaging appearances. Semin Musculoskelet Radiol. 2019 Feb;23(1):36–57.

15 Tuberculosis: Case 15

15.1 Medical History

A 6-year-old boy presented with pain while raising his left arm without a definite inciting event and restricted range of motion.

15.2 Physical Examination

Mild point tenderness around the lateral left upper arm. Restricted abduction and extension of the left shoulder and pain with passive movement. There was also restricted motion of the left elbow and wrist.

15.3 Imaging Findings

15.3.1 Radiograph

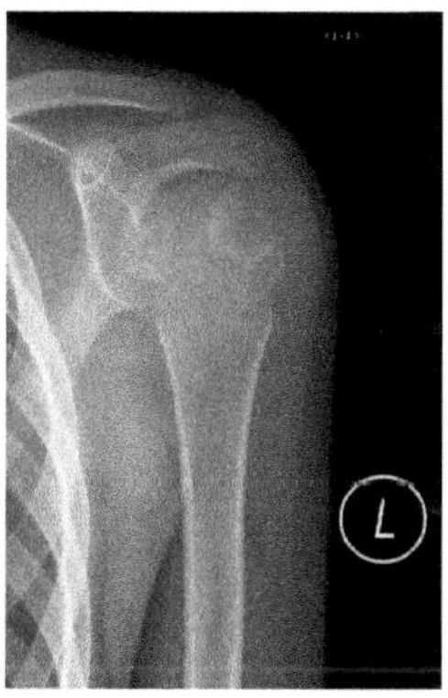

Fig. 15.1 Frontal view of the left shoulder

X. Cheng et al., *Imaging of Bone Tumors in Shoulder and Elbow*,
https://doi.org/10.1007/978-981-33-6150-8_15

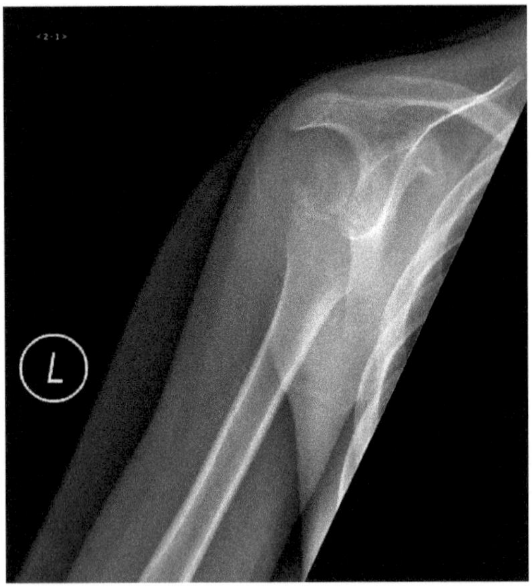

Fig. 15.2 Lateral view of the left shoulder

Radiographs demonstrate semicircular bone destruction around the proximal left humeral epiphysis laterally with peripheral sclerosis. There is soft tissue swelling around the joint.

15.3.2 CT Imaging

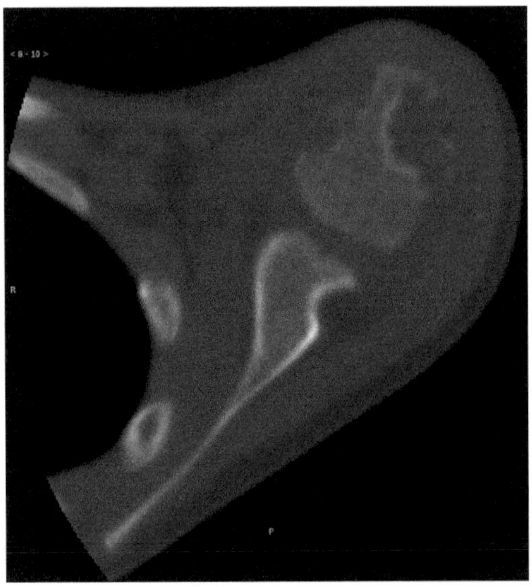

Fig. 15.3 Axial CT image of the left shoulder in bone window

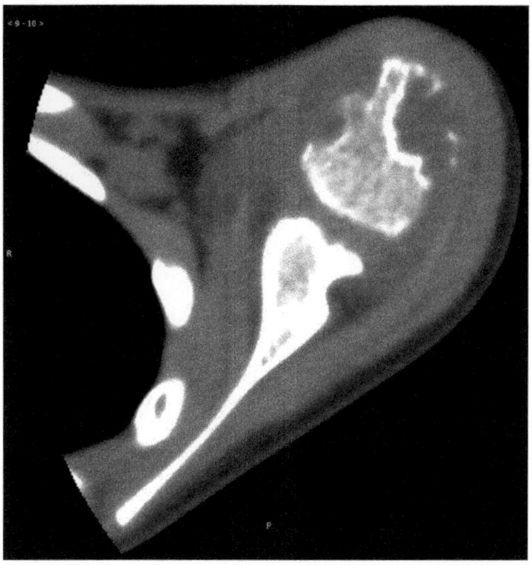

Fig. 15.4 Axial CT image of the left shoulder in soft tissue window

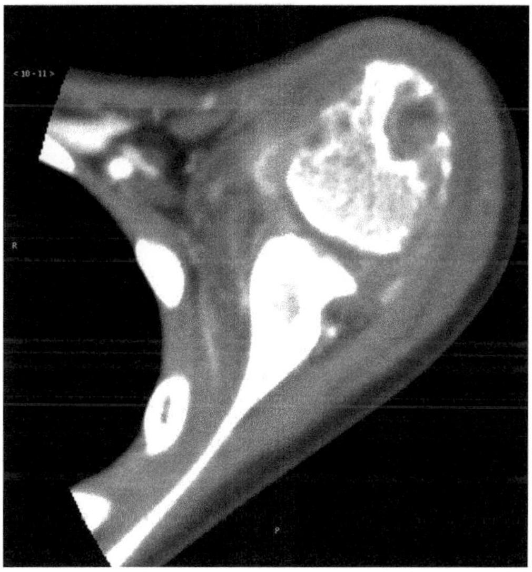

Fig. 15.5 Axial post-contrast CT image of the left shoulder in soft tissue window

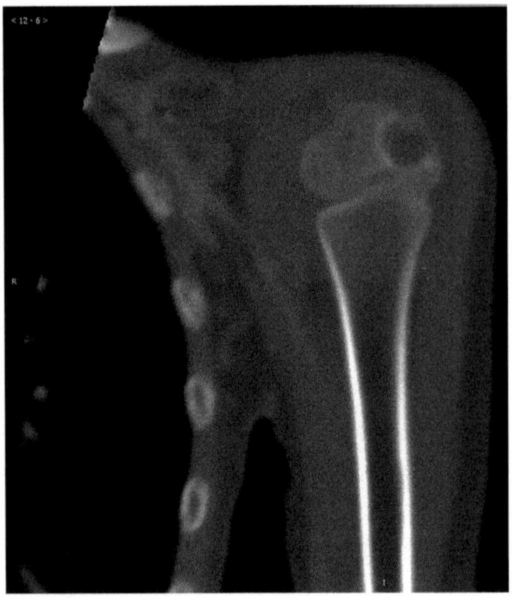

Fig. 15.6 Coronal CT image of the left shoulder in bone window

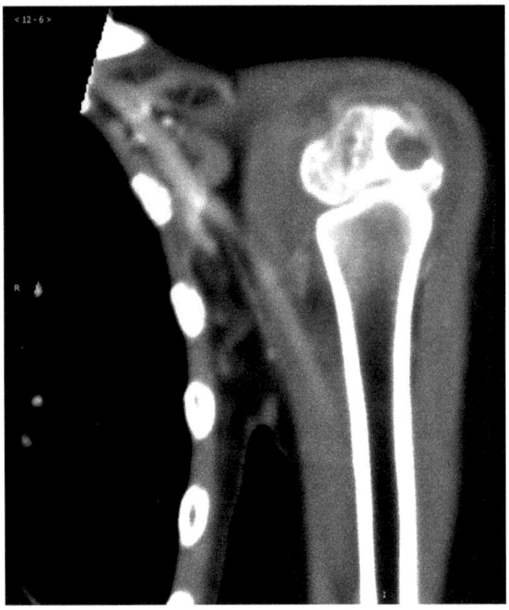

Fig. 15.7 Coronal post-contrast CT image of the left shoulder in soft tissue window

CT scan demonstrates multifocal cortical destruction around the proximal left humeral epiphysis with peripheral sclerosis. And, some erosive changes at the glenoid are noted. Heterogenous enhancement is noted with focal circular morphology. There is joint effusion with preserved joint space.

15.4 Description and Discussion from Residents

Radiographs demonstrate asymmetric bone destruction of the lateral proximal left humeral epiphysis with clear margin and peripheral sclerosis. There is thinning of the cortex but continuous with adjacent soft tissue swelling. On CT scan, there is internal soft tissue low density within the lesion, which does not protrude outside of the cortical margin with peripheral sclerosis of "lace-like" appearances and no periosteal reaction. Heterogeneous enhancement is noted with the distension of the joint capsule. Given the location of the lesion and the patient's age, chondroblastoma is at the top of the consideration.

15.5 Analysis and Comments from Professor Xiaoguang Cheng

Radiographs demonstrate bone destruction around the left humeral head epiphysis. This is a common location for chondroblastoma in children. However, multiple foci of osseous destructions are noted on CT scan with cortical irregularity along the glenoid, not consistent with chondroblastoma. Tuberculosis needs to be considered, correlation with clinical history and laboratory tests is recommended.

15.6 Diagnosis

Tuberculosis.

Suggested Reading

De Backer AI, Mortelé KJ, Vanhoenacker FM, et al. Imaging of extraspinal musculoskeletal tuberculosis. Eur J Radiol. 2006 Jan;57(1):119–30.

Prasad A, Manchanda S, Sachdev N, et al. Imaging features of pediatric musculoskeletal tuberculosis. Pediatr Radiol. 2012 Oct;42(10):1235–49.

Langerhans Cell Histiocytosis: Case 16

16

16.1 Medical History

The patient is a 13-year-old boy. He presented with left shoulder pain for about a month.

16.2 Physical Examination

Point tenderness around the left shoulder with palpable deep mass. The mass appears to have a clear margin, rubbery, and mobile.

16.3 Imaging Findings

16.3.1 Radiograph

X. Cheng et al., *Imaging of Bone Tumors in Shoulder and Elbow*,
https://doi.org/10.1007/978-981-33-6150-8_16

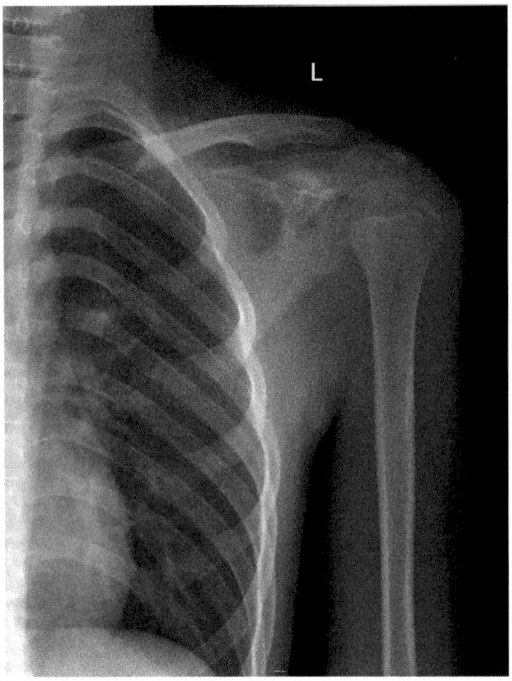

Fig. 16.1 Frontal view of the left scapula

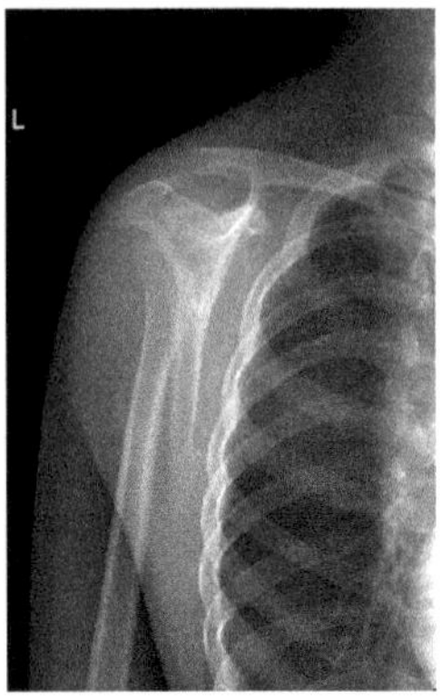

Fig. 16.2 Lateral view of the left scapula

Radiographs of the left scapula demonstrate semicircular lytic osseous destruction with a clear border and no peripheral sclerosis.

16.3.2 CT Imaging

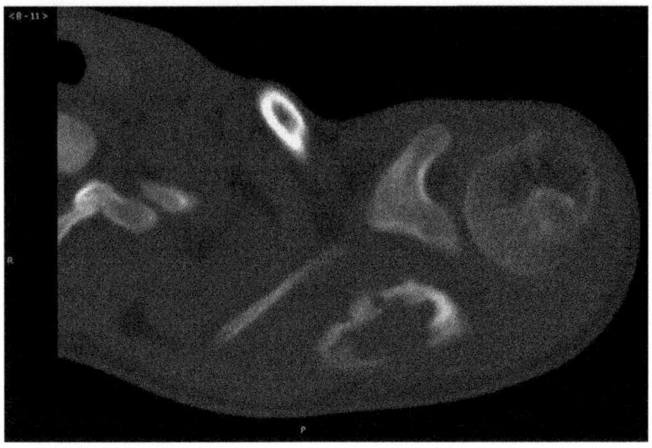

Fig. 16.3 Axial CT image of the left shoulder in bone window

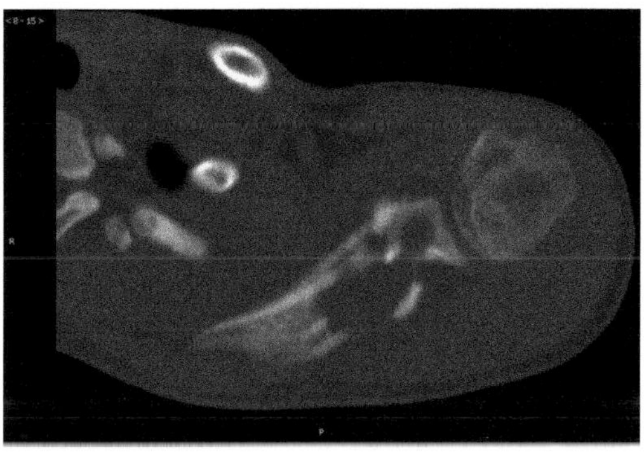

Fig. 16.4 Axial CT image of the left shoulder in bone window

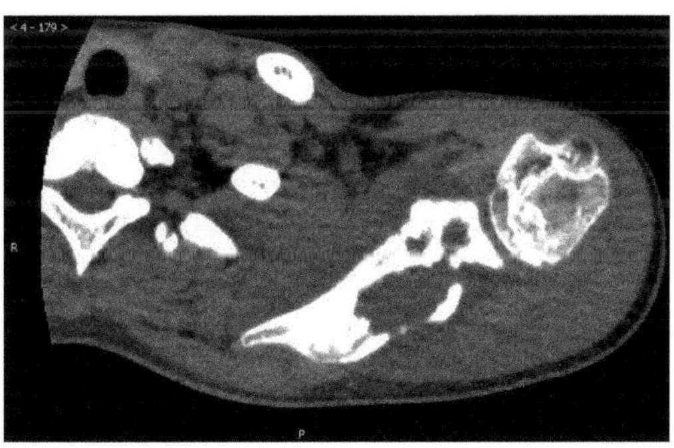

Fig. 16.5 Axial CT image of the left shoulder in soft tissue window

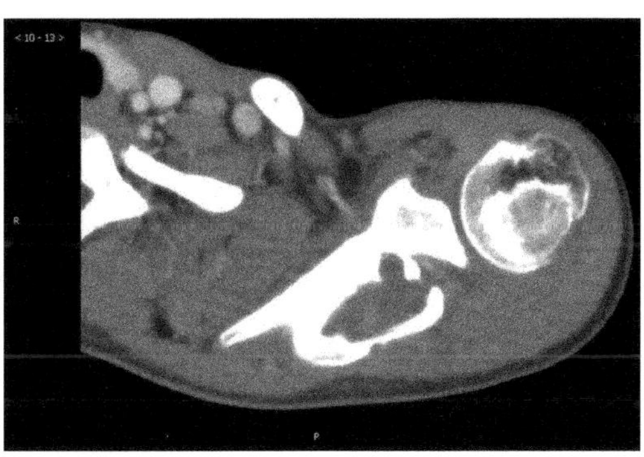

Fig. 16.6 Axial post-contrast CT image of the left shoulder in soft tissue window

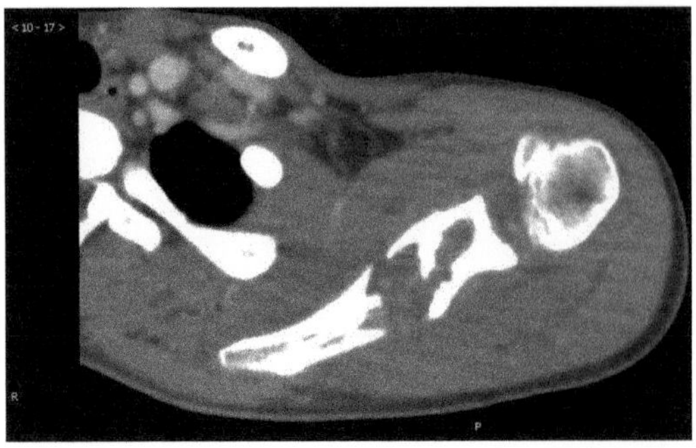

Fig. 16.7 Axial post-contrast CT image of the left shoulder in soft tissue window

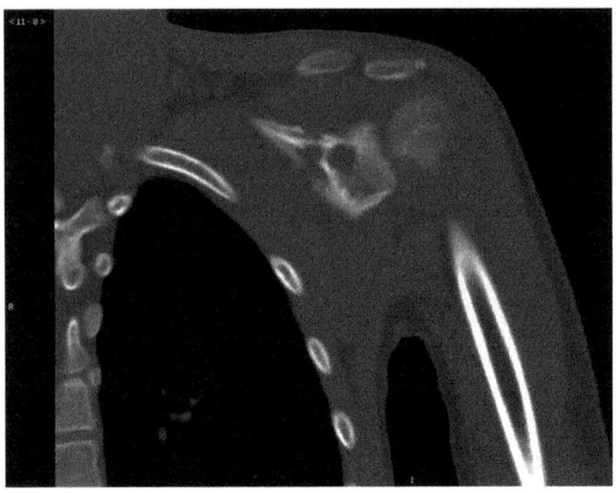

Fig. 16.8 Coronal CT image of the left shoulder in bone window

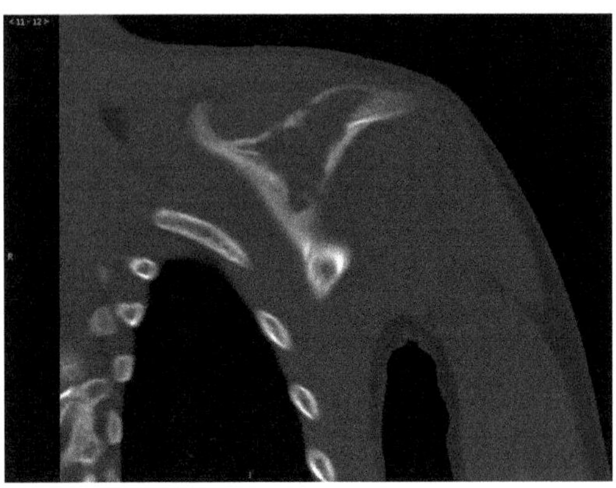

Fig. 16.9 Coronal CT image of the left shoulder in bone window

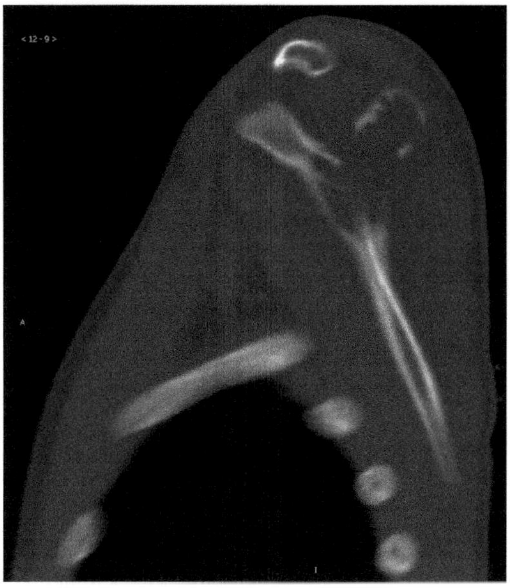

Fig. 16.10 Sagittal CT image of the left shoulder in bone window

CT images of the left shoulder demonstrate lytic osseous destruction around the scapula spine with some peripheral sclerosis. There was continuous laminar periosteal reaction and associated soft tissue mass and heterogeneous mild enhancement.

16.4 Description and Discussion from Residents

The patient is an adolescent. Radiographs demonstrate lytic bone destruction in the left scapula with a clear margin and no peripheral sclerosis with mild prominence of the adjacent soft tissue. The above imaging features are not diagnostic of the aggressiveness of the underlying lesion. On CT images, there is lytic osseous destruction around the left scapula body and spine with some focal peripheral sclerosis and laminar periosteal reaction. The periosteal reaction is not interrupted, likely signaling a reparative process, indicating a chronic course of the lesion. Given the patient's age and imaging features, the top consideration is eosinophilic granuloma. A similar periosteal reaction can be seen in Ewing's sarcoma; however, with that, there is usually a sunburst pattern of the periosteal reaction and large soft tissue mass. In the current case, there is a small soft tissue mass, not typical. Overall, the top consideration is eosinophilic granuloma.

16.5 Analysis and Comments from Professor Xiaoguang Cheng

The patient is an adolescent. There is left scapula lytic osseous destruction without expansile appearances and with peripheral continuous periosteal reaction and some focal disruption. High densities are noted around the disruption, likely representing sequestrums. The soft tissue mass shows mild enhancement. There is mild surrounding soft tissue edema. Given the patient's age, location of the lesion, and imaging features, eosinophilic granuloma is at the top of the differential diagnosis and Ewing's sarcoma needs to be excluded.

16.6 Diagnosis

Langerhans cell histiocytosis (Eosinophilic granuloma).

Suggested Reading

Azouz EM, Saigal G, Rodriguez MM, et al. Langerhans' cell histiocytosis: pathology, imaging and treatment of skeletal involvement. Pediatr Radiol. 2005 Feb;35(2):103–15.

Samet J, Weinstein J, Fayad LM. MRI and clinical features of Langerhans cell histiocytosis (LCH) in the pelvis and extremities: can LCH really look like anything? Skeletal Radiol. 2016 May;45(5):607–13.

Zaveri J, La Q, Yarmish G, et al. More than just Langerhans cell histiocytosis: a radiologic review of histiocytic disorders. Radiographics. 2014 Nov-Dec;34(7):2008–24.

17 Chondroblastoma: Case 17

17.1 Medical History

The patient is a 17-year-old female. She presented with right upper arm pain for 9 months.

17.2 Physical Examination

Pain around the right upper arm proximally with posterior mass.

17.3 Imaging Findings

17.3.1 Radiograph

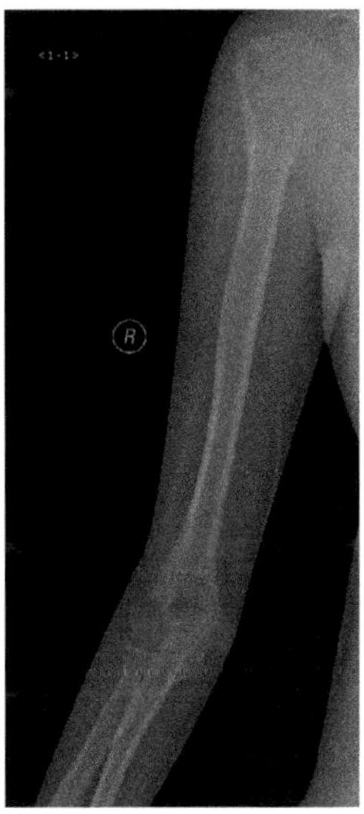

Fig. 17.1 Frontal view of the right shoulder

X. Cheng et al., *Imaging of Bone Tumors in Shoulder and Elbow*,
https://doi.org/10.1007/978-981-33-6150-8_17

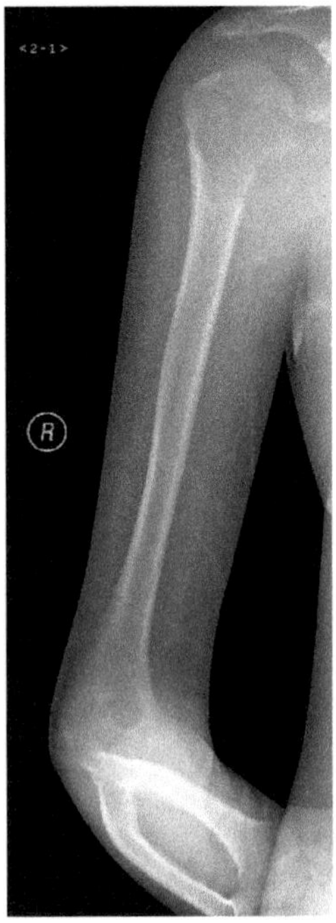

Fig. 17.2 Lateral view of the right shoulder

Radiographs of the right shoulder demonstrate lytic osseous destruction inferior to the humeral head articular surface with cortical thinning and irregular margin.

17.3.2 CT Imaging

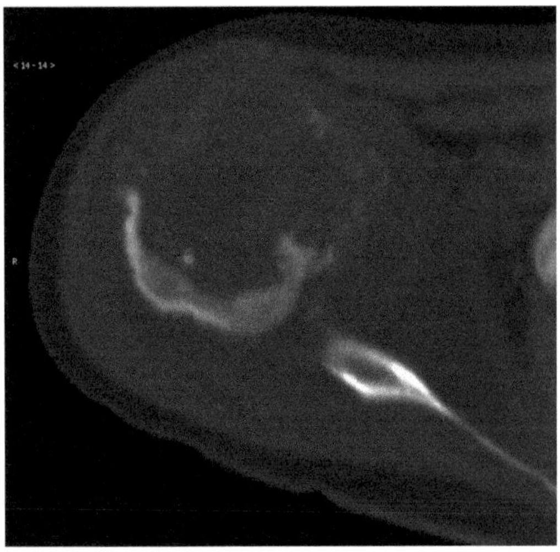

Fig. 17.3 Axial CT image of the right shoulder in bone window

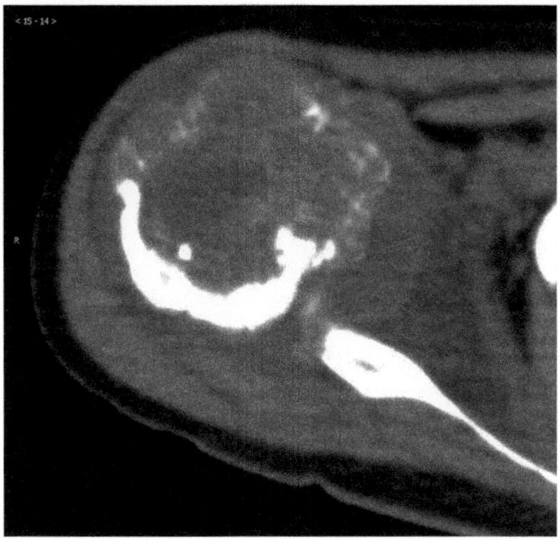

Fig. 17.4 Axial CT image of the right shoulder in soft window

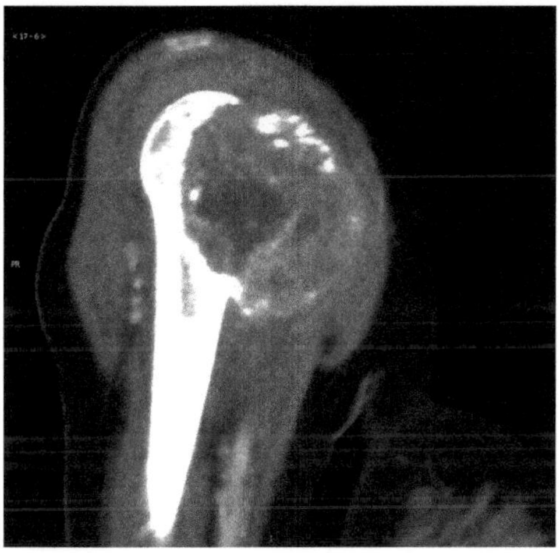

Fig. 17.5 Sagittal post-contrast CT image of the right shoulder in soft tissue window

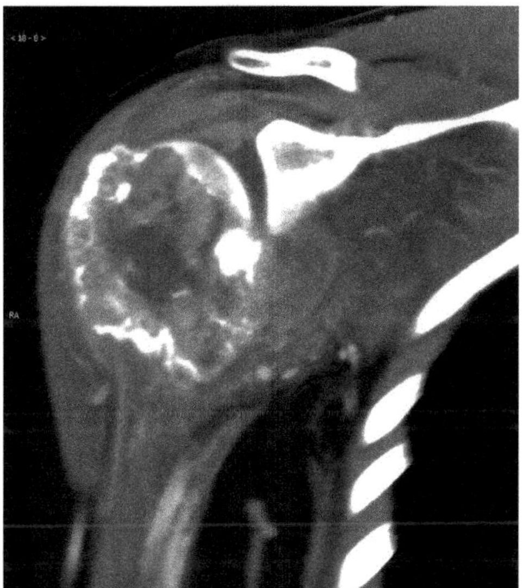

Fig. 17.6 Coronal post-contrast CT image of the right shoulder in soft tissue window

CT images of the right shoulder demonstrate expansile lytic osseous destruction around the right humeral head articular surface with internal calcifications. There is a focal cortical break with extruded soft tissue mass. The lesion demonstrates heterogeneous enhancement with focal avid enhancement.

17.3.3 MR Imaging

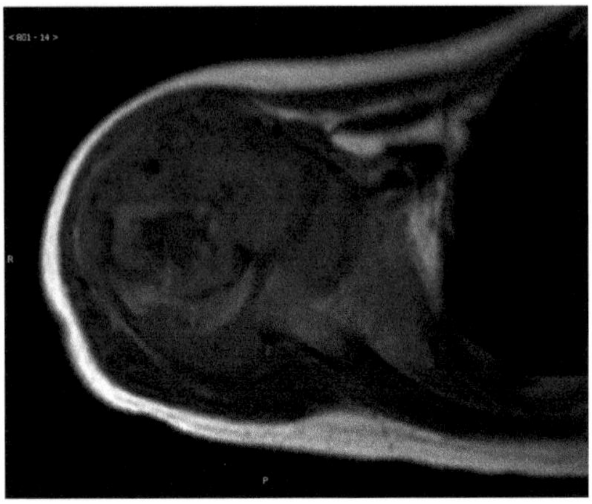

Fig. 17.7 Axial T1-weighted MR image of the right shoulder

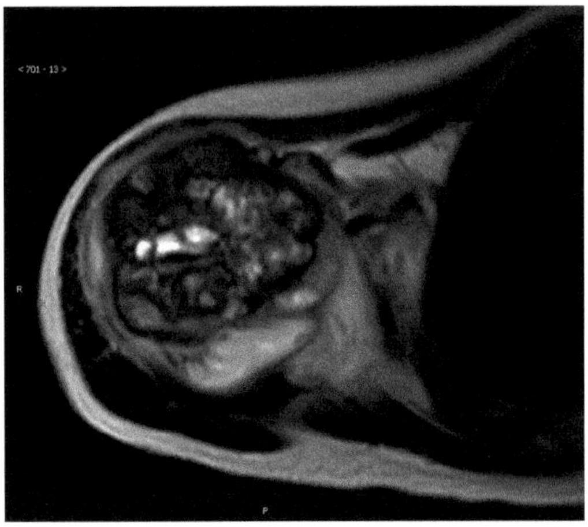

Fig. 17.8 Axial T2-weighted MR image of the right shoulder

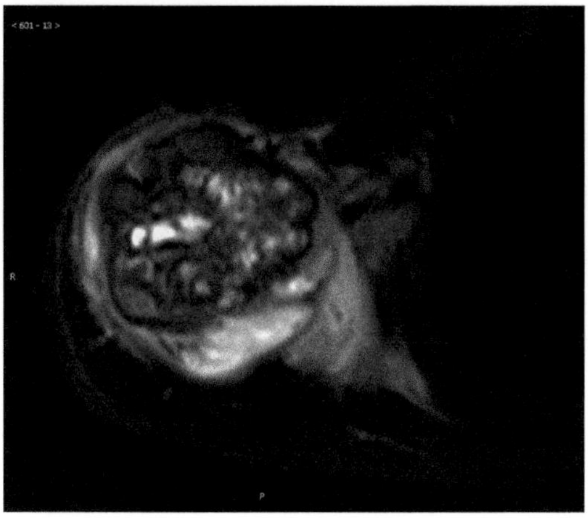

Fig. 17.9 Axial fat-suppressed T2-weighted MR image of the right shoulder

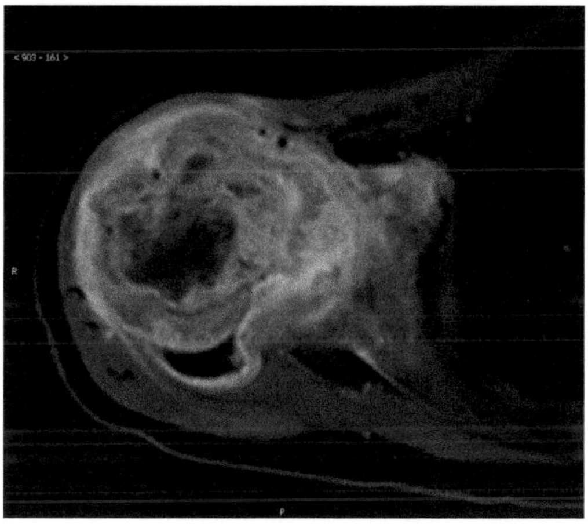

Fig. 17.10 Axial post-contrast fat-suppressed T1-weighted MR image of the right shoulder

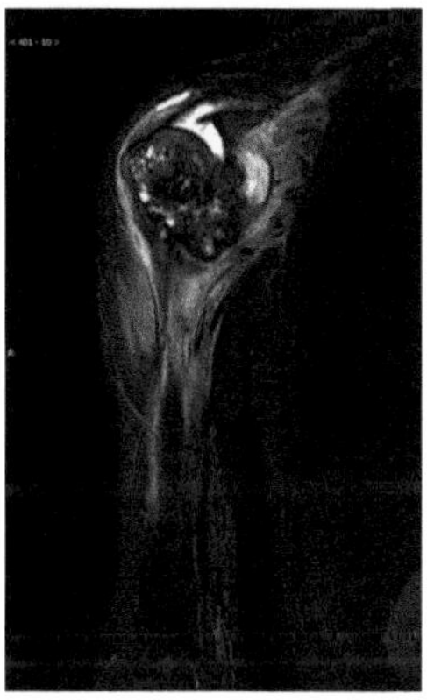

Fig. 17.11 Coronal fat-suppressed T2-weighted MR image of the right shoulder

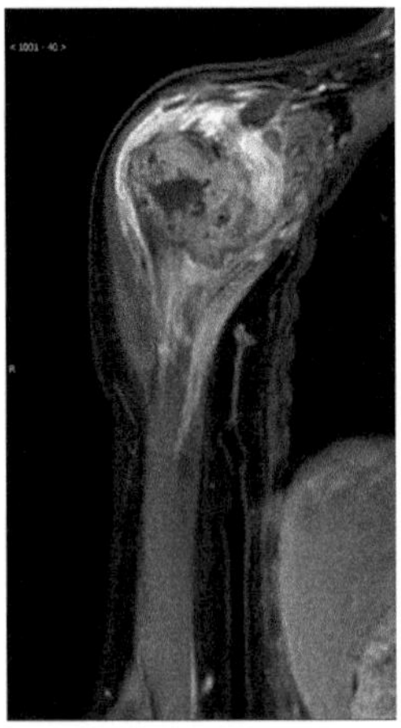

Fig. 17.12 Coronal post-contrast fat-suppressed T1-weighted MR image of the right shoulder

MR images of the right shoulder demonstrate bone destruction of the right humeral head with iso-intense and high T1 signal, heterogeneous T2 signal with internal multiple small cysts, and adjacent extensive soft tissue edema. There is heterogeneous enhancement.

17.4 Description and Discussion from Residents

The imaging features of an asymmetric, lytic lesion in the right proximal humeral head with internal avid enhancement of the solid component are all supportive of the diagnosis of giant cell tumor of bone. However, the patient's age and internal scattered calcifications are not supportive of this diagnosis. With internal calcifications, a chondrogenic tumor has to be included in the differential diagnosis. On the MR images, there is a bony capsule, hemorrhage, and internal cystic changes with small fluid–fluid levels and extensive adjacent soft-tissue edema, and joint effusion. Together with the patient's age, lesion location, chondrogenic tumor is most likely and chondroblastoma with aneurysmal bone cyst (ABC) is at the top of our consideration. Of note, no definite chondroid matrix is noted on the MRI and the enhancement pattern is not typical of chondroblastoma.

17.5 Analysis and Comments from Professor Xiaoguang Cheng

The patient is an adolescent young female with a relatively long clinical history. Images demonstrate lytic osseous destruction of the right humeral head with focal extruded soft tissue mass and soft tissue edema. There is an avid enhancement of the solid component. The above features are indicative of the aggressiveness of the lesion. The presence of internal calcifications supports chondrogenic tumors. Given the patient's age and lesion's location, the top consideration is chondroblastoma. However, the lesion is large with an irregular margin, the possibility of malignancy is raised and chondroblastoma-like osteosarcoma has to be excluded.

17.6 Diagnosis

Chondroblastoma.

Suggested Reading

Harish K, Janaki MG, Alva NK. "Primary" aggressive chondroblastoma of the humerus: a case report. BMC Musculoskelet Disord. 2004 Mar 17;5:9.

Tonogai I, Takahashi M, Manabe H, et al. A massive chondroblastoma in the proximal humerus simulating malignant bone tumors. Case Rep Orthop. 2013;2013:673576.

Weatherall PT, Maale GE, Mendelsohn DB, et al. Chondroblastoma: classic and confusing appearance at MR imaging. Radiology. 1994 Feb;190(2):467–74.

Ewing Sarcoma: Case 18

18

18.1 Medical History

The patient is a 34-year-old male. He presented with a left shoulder mass for 2 months.

18.2 Physical Examination

Palpable mass around the left scapula, hard with irregular margin, non-mobile with point tenderness.

18.3 Imaging Findings

18.3.1 Radiograph

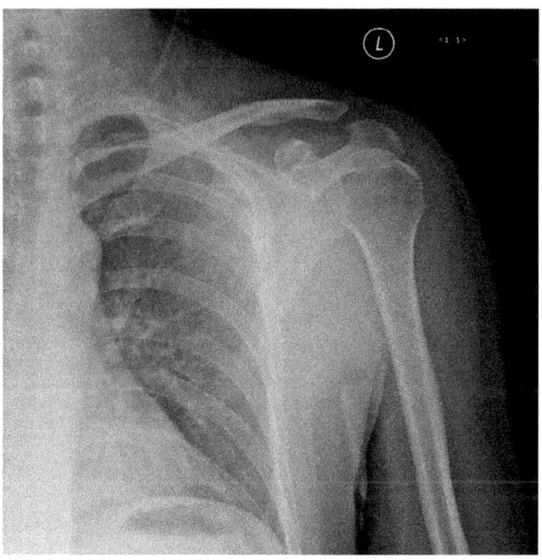

Fig. 18.1 Frontal view of the left shoulder

X. Cheng et al., *Imaging of Bone Tumors in Shoulder and Elbow*,
https://doi.org/10.1007/978-981-33-6150-8_18

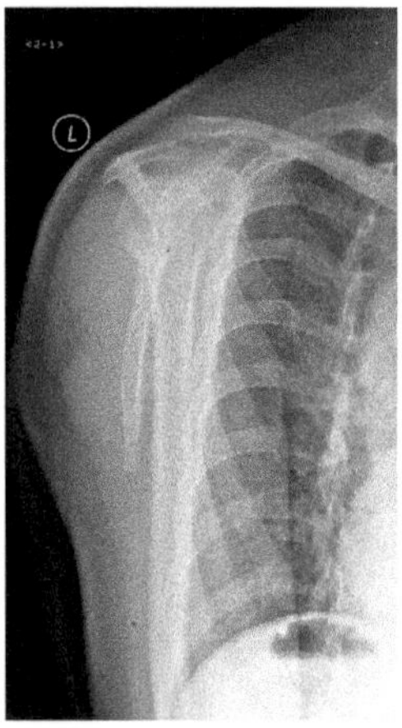

Fig. 18.2 Lateral view of the left scapula

Radiographs of the left shoulder demonstrate irregular shaped soft tissue mass around the left shoulder.

18.3.2 CT Imaging

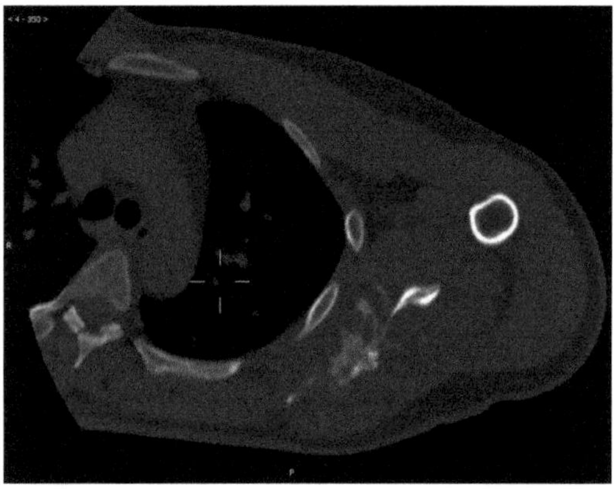

Fig. 18.3 Axial CT image of the left shoulder in bone window

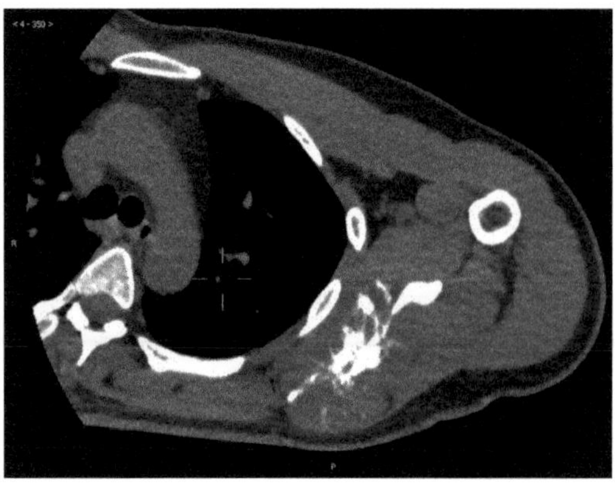

Fig. 18.4 Axial CT image of the left shoulder in soft tissue window

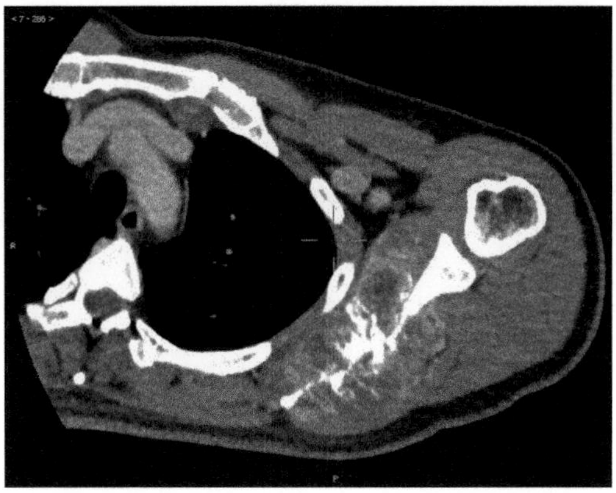

Fig. 18.5 Axial post-contrast CT image of the left shoulder in soft tissue window

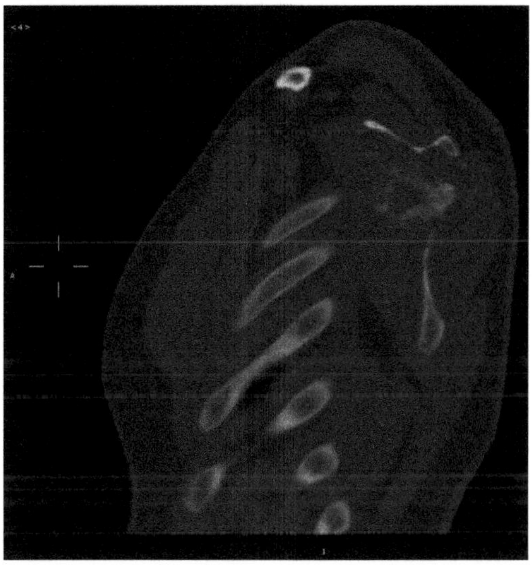

Fig. 18.6 Sagittal CT image of the left shoulder in bone window

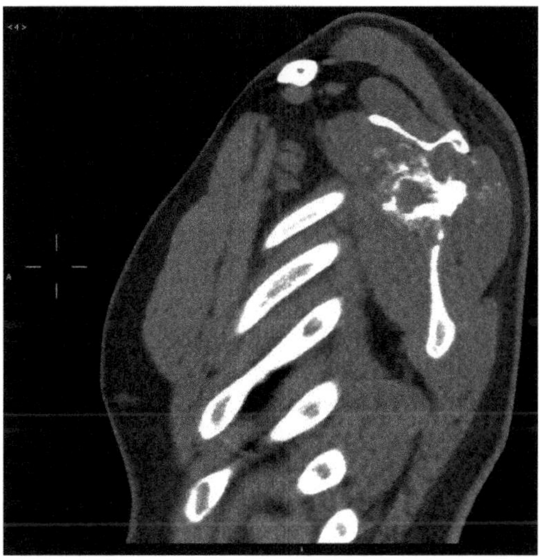

Fig. 18.7 Sagittal CT image of the left shoulder in soft tissue window

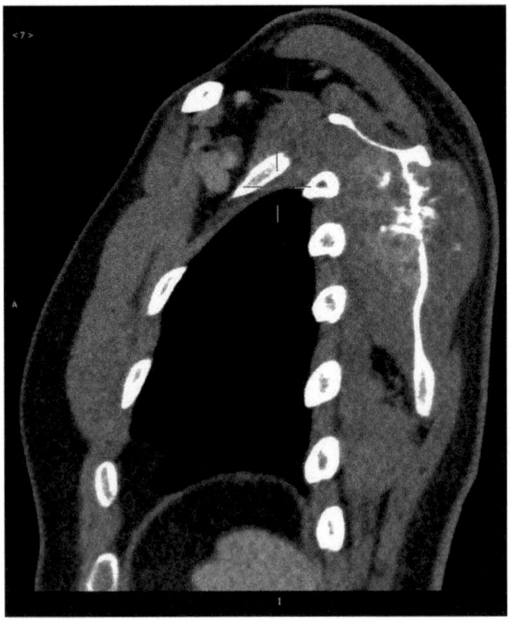

Fig. 18.8 Sagittal post-contrast CT image of the left shoulder in soft tissue window

CT images of the left shoulder demonstrate bone destruction around the body of the left scapula with a sun-burst pattern of periosteal reaction. There is a large associated soft tissue mass, with avid, heterogeneous enhancement.

18.3.3 MR Imaging

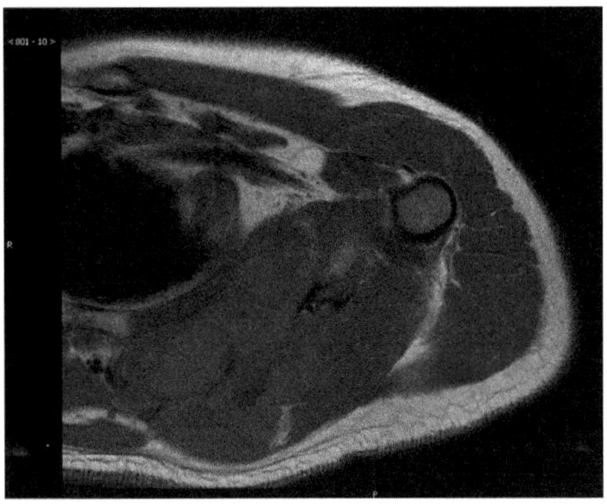

Fig. 18.9 Axial T1-weighted MR image of the left shoulder

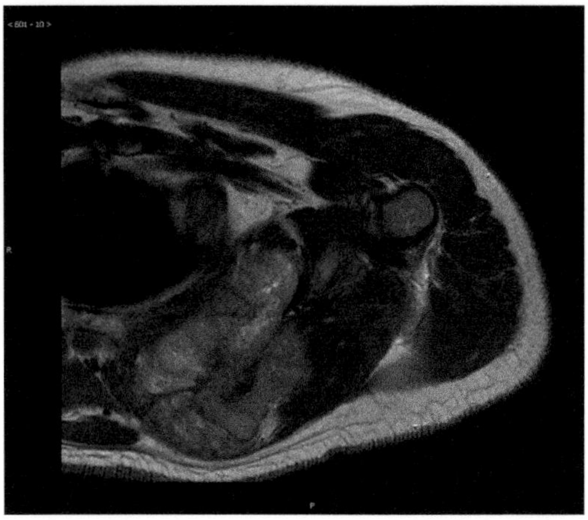

Fig. 18.10 Axial T2-weighted MR image of the left shoulder

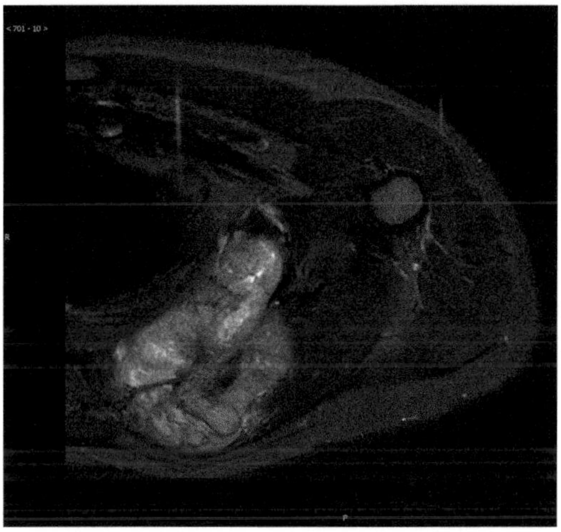

Fig. 18.11 Axial fat-suppressed T2-weighted MR image of the left shoulder

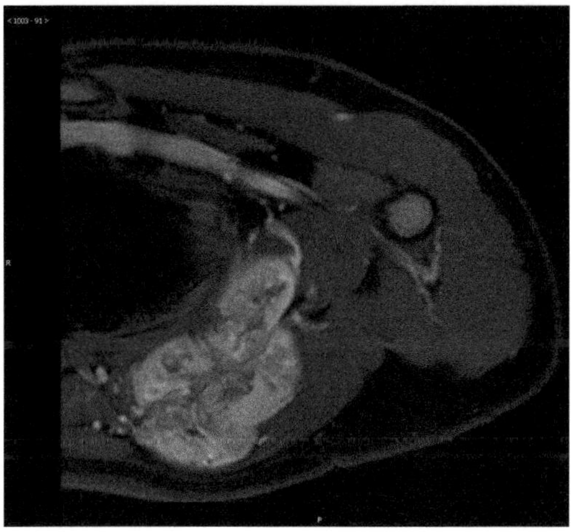

Fig. 18.12 Axial post-contrast fat-suppressed T1-weighted MR image of the left shoulder

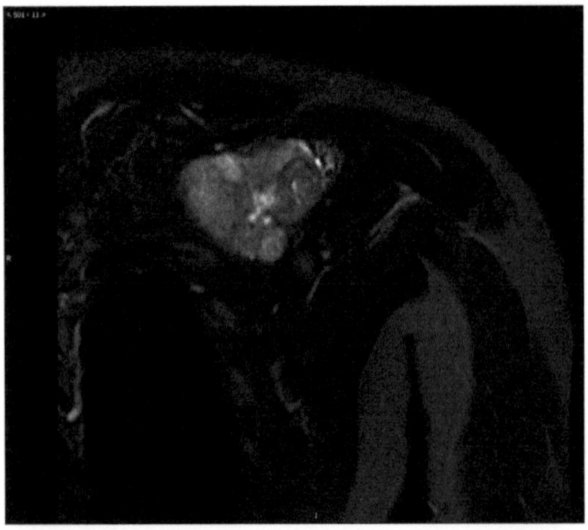

Fig. 18.13 Coronal fat-suppressed T2-weighted MR image of the left shoulder

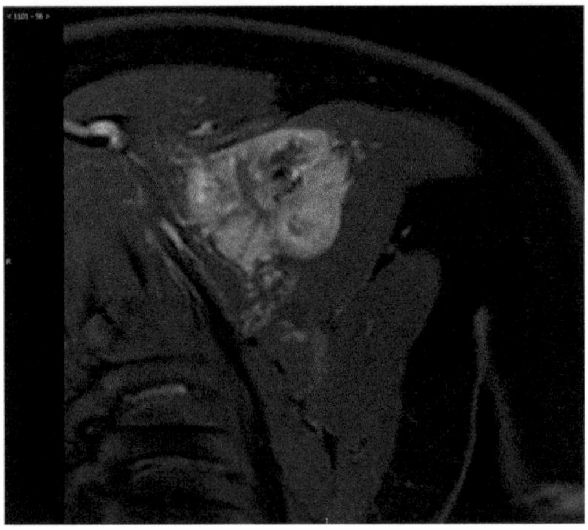

Fig. 18.14 Coronal post-contrast fat-suppressed T1-weighted MR image of the left shoulder

MR images of the left shoulder demonstrate bone destruction around the left scapula body with large soft tissue mass. The soft tissue mass shows T1 iso-intense signal and slightly high T2 signal with internal linear low T1 and low T2 signal areas. There is heterogeneous enhancement of the soft tissue mass.

18.4 Description and Discussion from Residents

The imaging features of bone destruction around the left scapula body with large soft tissue mass; sun-burst pattern of the periosteal reaction; irregular margin and heterogeneous enhancement of the soft tissue mass are indicative of aggressive malignant processes, such as Ewing sarcoma or osteosarcoma. Even though the patient is a young male, not of typical age for Ewing sarcoma or osteosarcoma, the involvement of a flat bone tends to happen in older patients in Ewing sarcoma and osteosarcoma. Since there is no significant osteoblastic process noted in the lesion but large soft tissue mass, the top consideration is Ewing sarcoma.

18.5 Analysis and Comments from Professor Xiaoguang Cheng

The patient is a young male with short clinical history. Imaging shows left scapula bone destruction with large soft tissue mass and needle-like periosteal reaction, all indicating a malignant process. MR images do not provide more diagnostic information. There is long T1 and long T2 signal change along the left proximal humerus which likely represents red marrow conversion after chemotherapy. The patient is older for typical Ewing sarcoma, but with the involvement of a flat bone, the top consideration is still Ewing sarcoma, statistically speaking. Osteosarcoma is in the differential diagnosis.

18.6 Diagnosis

Ewing sarcoma.

Suggested Reading

Murphey MD, Senchak LT, Mambalam PK, et al. From the radiologic pathology archives: ewing sarcoma family of tumors: radiologic-pathologic correlation. Radiographics. 2013 May;33(3):803–31.

Shahid M, Varshney M, Maheshwari V, et al. Ewing's sarcoma of scapula: a rare entity. BMJ Case Rep. 2011 Mar 10; https://doi.org/10.1136/bcr.02.2011.3810.

19 SAPHO Syndrome: Case 19

19.1 Medical History

The patient is a 64-year-old female. She presented with pain around the sternoclavicular joint with swelling for a year.

19.2 Physical Examination

She has palmoplantar pustulosis.

19.3 Imaging Findings

19.3.1 Radiograph

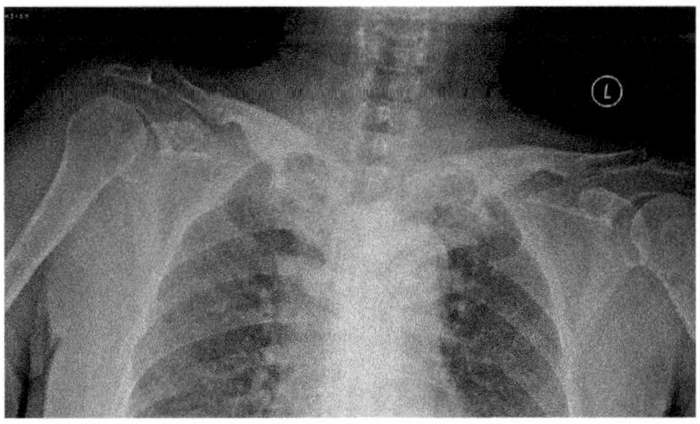

Fig. 19.1 Frontal view of the sternoclavicular joint

Radiograph demonstrates bilateral symmetrical diffuse osseous abnormalities involving the medial portions of the bilateral clavicles and the manubrium. Bone expansions with sclerosis are noted. There are multiple areas of low densities within the sclerosis.

X. Cheng et al., *Imaging of Bone Tumors in Shoulder and Elbow*,
https://doi.org/10.1007/978-981-33-6150-8_19

19.3.2 CT Imaging

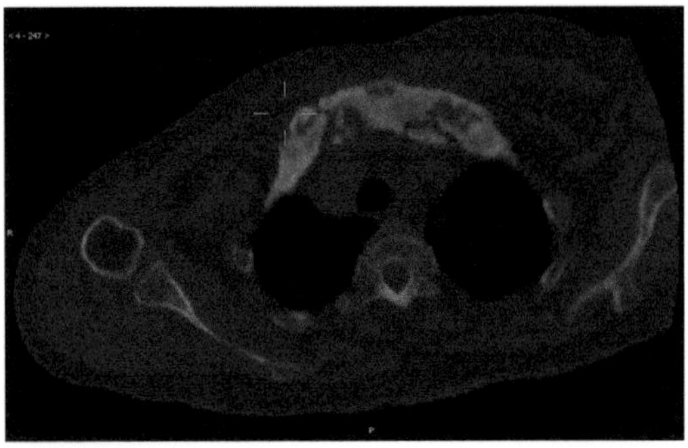

Fig. 19.2 Axial CT image of the sternoclavicular joint in bone window

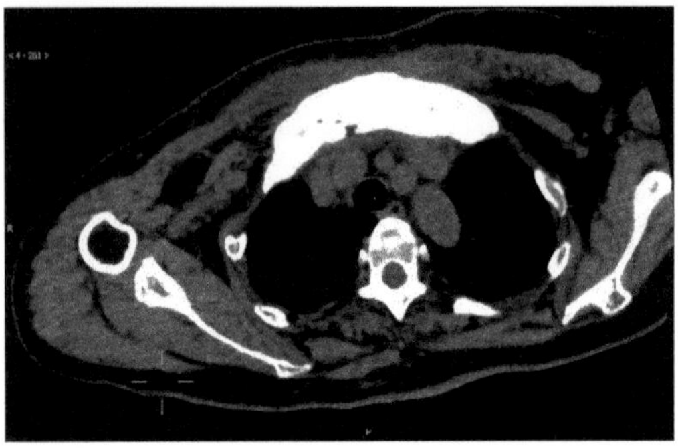

Fig. 19.3 Axial CT image of the sternoclavicular joint in soft tissue window

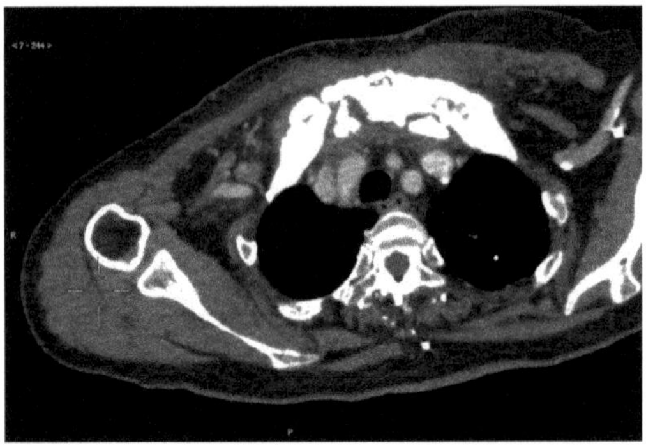

Fig. 19.4 Axial post-contrast CT image of the sternoclavicular joint in soft tissue window

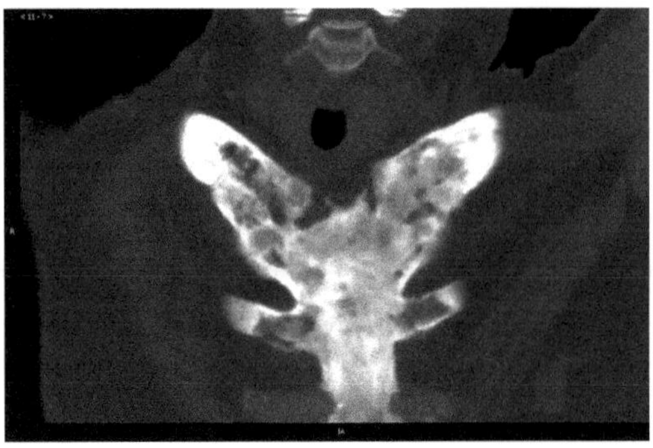

Fig. 19.5 Coronal CT image of the sternoclavicular joint in bone window

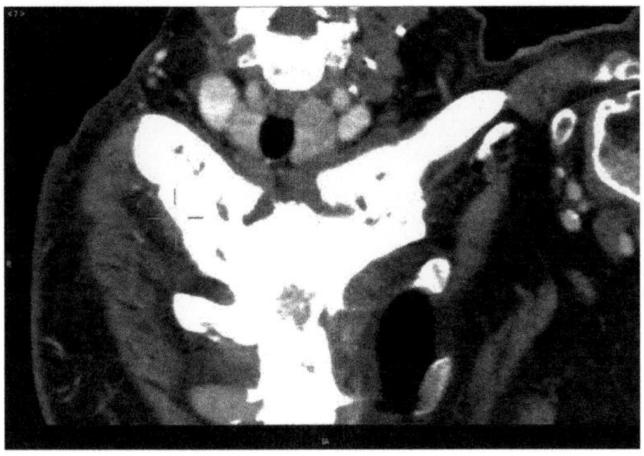

Fig. 19.6 Coronal post-contrast CT image of the sterno-clavicular joint in soft tissue window

CT images of the sternoclavicular joint demonstrate similar findings as noted on the radiograph with adjacent soft tissue swelling. There are enhancements in the areas of low densities within the sclerosis.

19.4 Description and Discussion from Residents

The patient is an older female. Radiograph demonstrates symmetrical, diffuse abnormality of the osseous structures, mainly involves the proximal and mid clavicles, sternum with expansion, and low densities areas within the sclerosis. On CT images, there is adjacent soft tissue swelling with mild enhancements in the low-density areas within the sclerosis. The differential diagnosis includes: chronic recurrent multifocal osteomyelitis (CRMO)/infectious process (osteomyelitis) or SAPHO syndrome (synovitis–acne–pustulosis–hyperostosis–osteomyelitis syndrome). SAPHO syndrome is a clinical diagnosis based on clinical history and physical examination.

19.5 Analysis and Comments from Professor Xiaoguang Cheng

The patient is an older female with prolonged clinical history. Radiograph shows bilateral symmetrical, diffuse bone abnormality, involving the mid and proximal clavicles, manubrium with sclerosis, and peripheral soft tissue swelling. Overall, the differential diagnosis includes: SAPHO syndrome and arthritis. Further evaluation with clinical history, physical examination, and laboratory testing would be helpful.

19.6 Diagnosis

SAPHO syndrome.

Suggested Reading

Cotten A, Flipo RM, Mentre A, et al. SAPHO syndrome. Radiographics. 1995 Sep;15(5):1147–54.

Greenwood S, Leone A, Cassar-Pullicino VN. SAPHO and recurrent multifocal osteomyelitis. Radiol Clin North Am. 2017 Sep;55(5):1035–53.

Okuno H, Watanuki M, Kuwahara Y, et al. Clinical features and radiological findings of 67 patients with SAPHO syndrome. Mod Rheumatol. 2018 Jul;28(4):703–8.

20 Fibrous Dysplasia: Case 20

20.1 Medical History

An 18-year-old female with left upper extremity pain after a fall 5 months ago with restricted motion.

20.2 Physical Examination

Not significant.

20.3 Imaging Findings

20.3.1 Radiograph

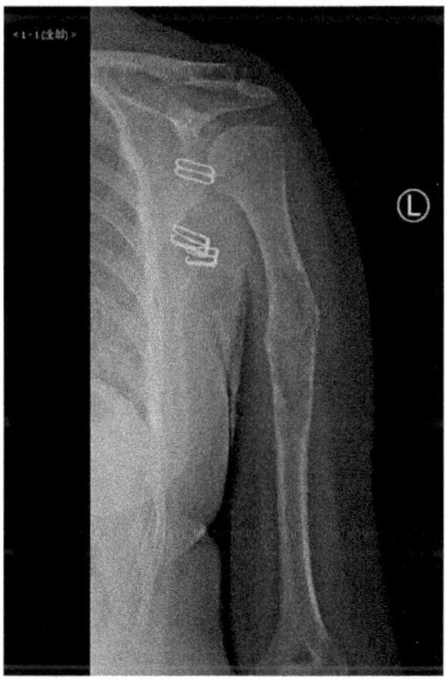

Fig. 20.1 Frontal view of the left humerus

X. Cheng et al., *Imaging of Bone Tumors in Shoulder and Elbow*,
https://doi.org/10.1007/978-981-33-6150-8_20

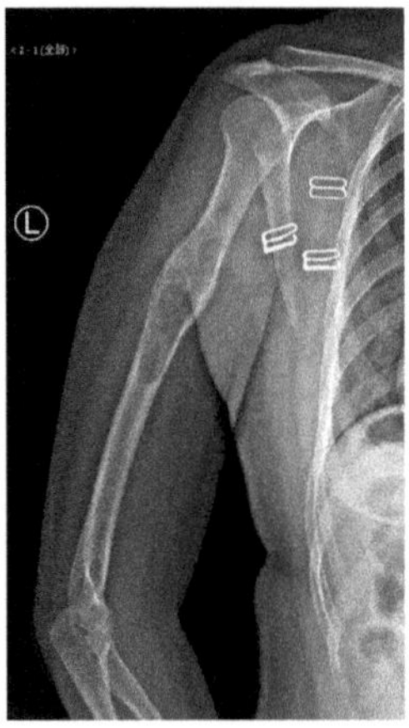

Fig. 20.2 Lateral view of the left humerus

Radiographs demonstrate focal expansile lytic lesion at the midshaft of the left humerus with the long axis of the lesion parallel to the bone shaft. Osteoid is noted within the lesion and there is focal irregularity of the cortex.

20.3.2 CT Imaging

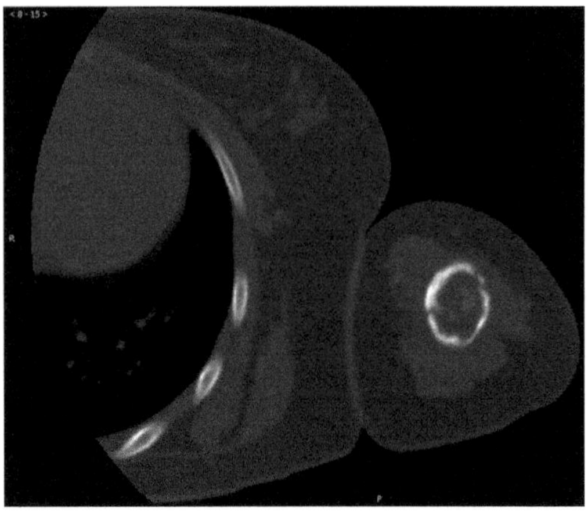

Fig. 20.3 Axial CT image of the left humerus in bone window

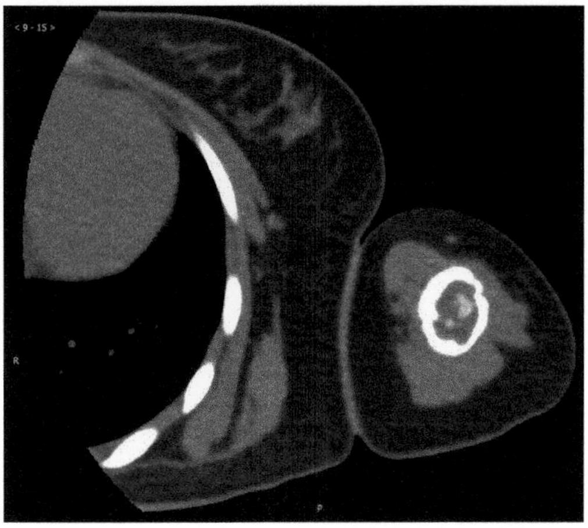

Fig. 20.4 Axial CT image of the left humerus in soft tissue window

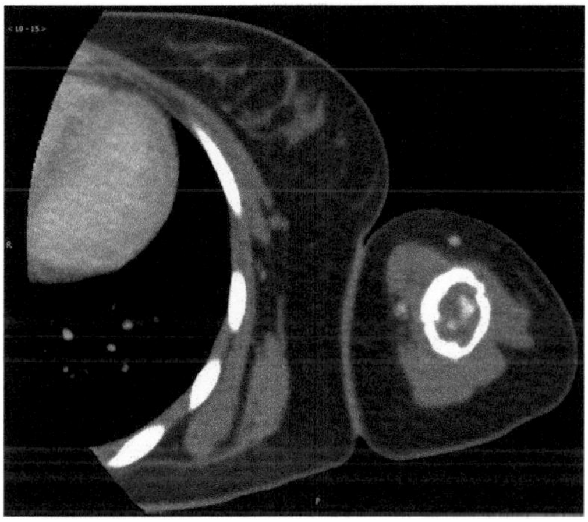

Fig. 20.5 Axial post-contrast CT image of the left humerus in soft tissue window

CT scan demonstrates expansile lytic lesion at the left humeral midshaft with thinning of the cortex and cortical break. Focal high densities are noted in the medullary cavity and there is no enhancement.

20.3.3 MR Imaging

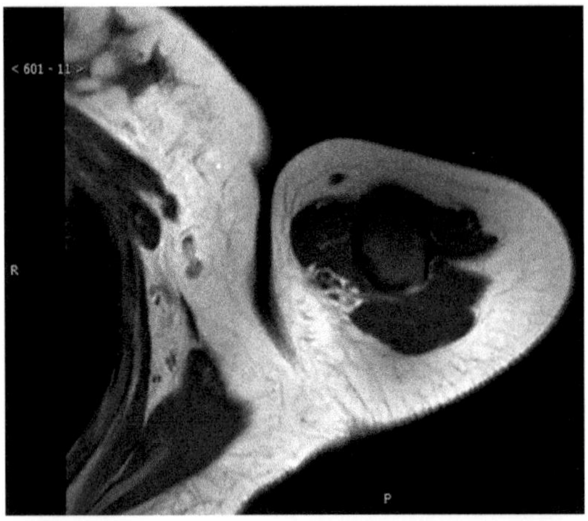

Fig. 20.6 Axial T1-weighted MR image of the left humerus

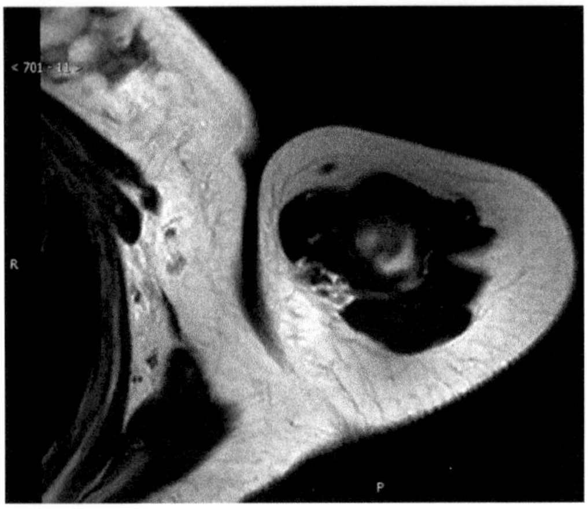

Fig. 20.7 Axial T2-weighted MR image of the left humerus

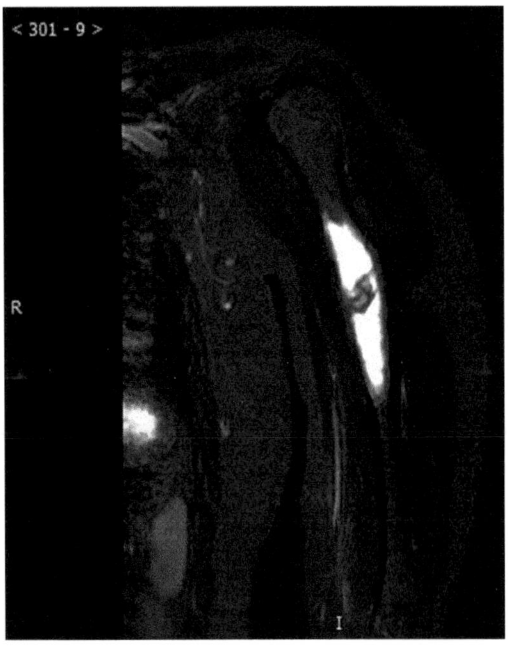

Fig. 20.8 Coronal fat-suppressed T2-weighted MR image of the left humerus

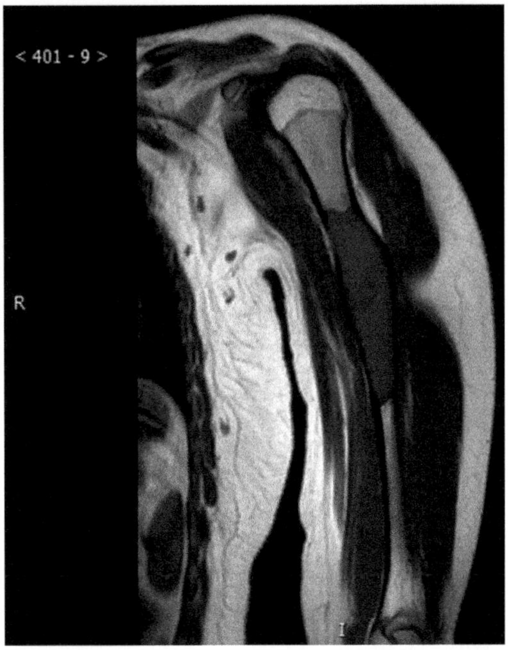

Fig. 20.9 Coronal T1-weighted MR image of the left humerus

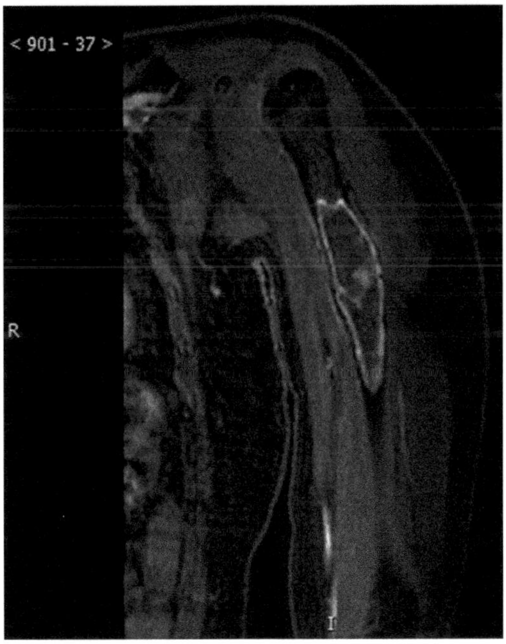

Fig. 20.10 Coronal post-contrast fat-suppressed T1-weighted MR image of the left humerus

MRI scan demonstrates focal abnormal signal within the medullary cavity of the midshaft of the left humerus. There is a low T1 signal and high T2 signal with and without fat suppression and internal patchy linear low signal with peripheral enhancement.

20.4 Description and Discussion from Residents

Radiographs demonstrate a lytic lesion at the midshaft of the left humerus parallel to the long axis of the shaft with mild expansion and clear margin. There is thinning of the cortex and osteoid noted in the lesion. This could be a chondrogenic lesion, intra-osseous cyst, or cystic fibrous dysplasia. Pathologic fracture from the latter two entities could cause hemorrhage, degeneration leading to inhomogeneous density within the lesion. The cortex is mostly intact on CT scan with patchy bone densities in the lesion, rare in intra-osseous cyst. The lesion demonstrates low T1 signal, high T2 signal with and without fat suppression with internal linear patchy low signal and peripheral enhancement on MRI. Overall, the above findings favor fibrous dysplasia with pathologic fracture.

20.5 Analysis and Comments from Professor Xiaoguang Cheng

The patient is a young female. Imaging demonstrates expansile lytic lesion at the midshaft of the left humerus with pathologic fracture, thinning of the cortex, and clear margin. The lesion appears nonaggressive, with differential diagnosis includes intra-osseous cyst, fibrous dysplasia, and chondrogenic lesion. Patchy high densities noted within the lesion on CT scan, likely relate to injury. This could also be calcifications in chondrogenic lesions; however, the morphology does not support it. Solid component is noted within the lesion, uncommon in intra-osseous cyst. The lesion is well-circumscribed on MR images with the majority demonstrating high T2 signal on fat-suppressed sequence. Based on the pattern of enhancement, chondrogenic lesions can be excluded. Given the patient's age, the top consideration is intra-osseous cyst and cystic fibrous dysplasia is in the differential diagnosis.

20.6 Diagnosis

Fibrous dysplasia.

Suggested Reading

Jee WH, Choi KH, Choe BY, et al. Fibrous dysplasia: MR imaging characteristics with radiopathologic correlation. AJR Am J Roentgenol. 1996 Dec;167(6):1523–7.

Kransdorf MJ, Moser RP Jr, Gilkey FW. Fibrous dysplasia. Radiographics. 1990 May;10(3):519–37.

Telangiectatic Osteosarcoma: Case 21

21

21.1 Medical History

The patient is an 8-year-old boy. He presented with right upper arm pain and swelling for over a month.

21.2 Physical Examination

Mild swelling around the right proximal humerus with significant point tenderness and some restricted range of motion around the right shoulder.

21.3 Imaging Findings

21.3.1 Radiograph

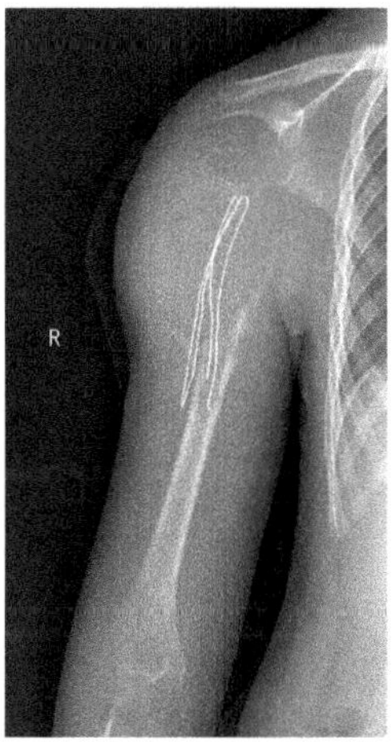

Fig. 21.1 Frontal view of the right shoulder

X. Cheng et al., *Imaging of Bone Tumors in Shoulder and Elbow*,
https://doi.org/10.1007/978-981-33-6150-8_21

Radiograph of the right shoulder demonstrates lytic osseous destruction of the right proximal humerus (sparing the epiphysis) with irregular margin, periosteal reaction, and soft tissue mass.

21.3.2 CT Imaging

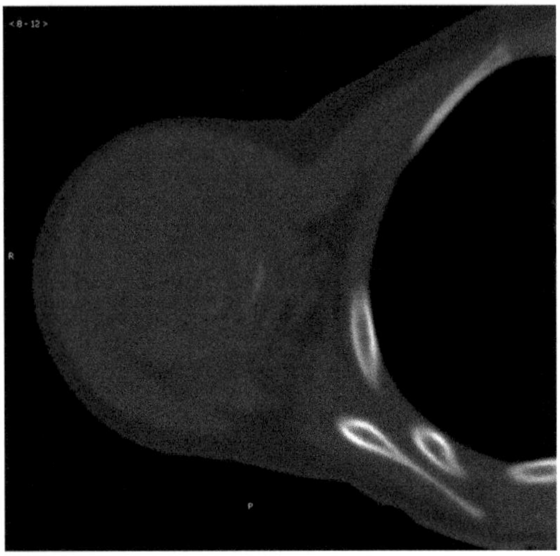

Fig. 21.2 Axial CT image of the right shoulder in bone window

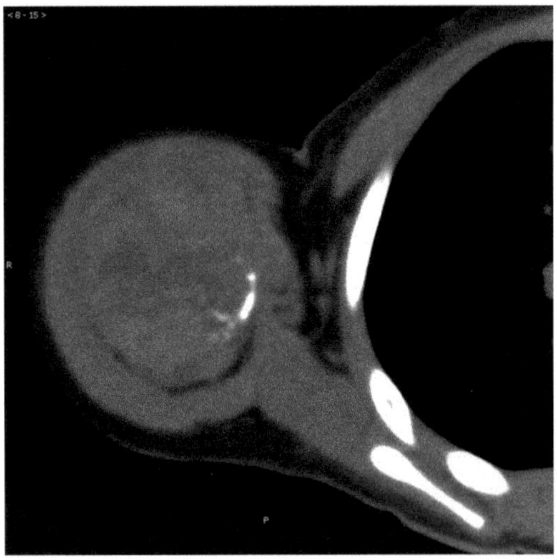

Fig. 21.3 Axial CT image of the right shoulder in soft tissue window

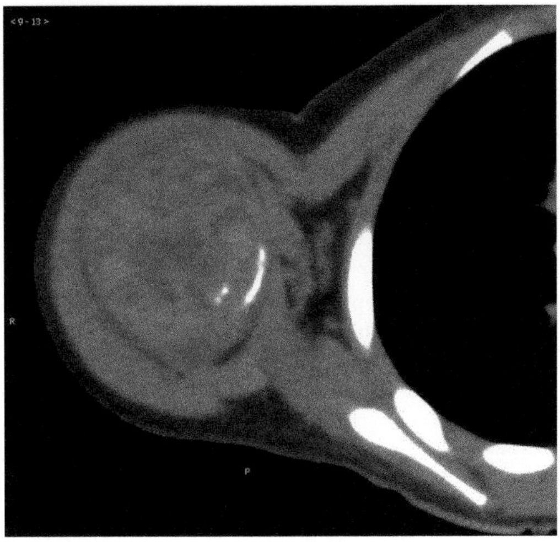

Fig. 21.4 Axial CT image of the right shoulder in soft tissue window

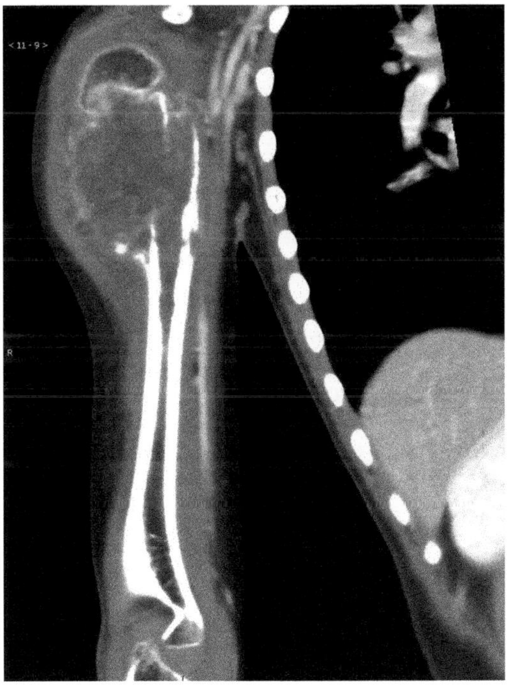

Fig. 21.5 Coronal post-contrast CT image of the right shoulder in soft tissue window

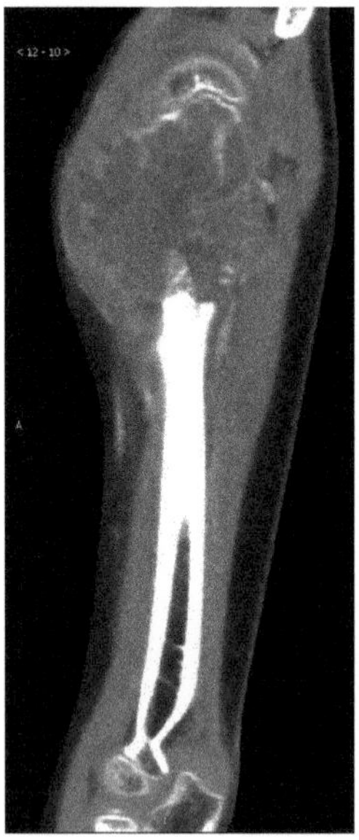

Fig. 21.6 Sagittal post-contrast CT image of the right shoulder in soft tissue window

CT images of the right shoulder demonstrate lytic osseous destruction around the proximal humerus with irregular margin and interrupted periosteal reaction and soft tissue mass. There is heterogeneous density within the mass and heterogeneous enhancement.

21.3.3 MR Imaging

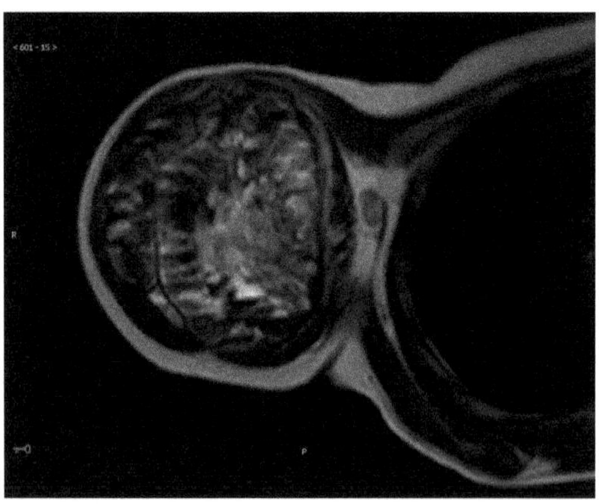

Fig. 21.7 Axial T2-weighted MR image of the right shoulder

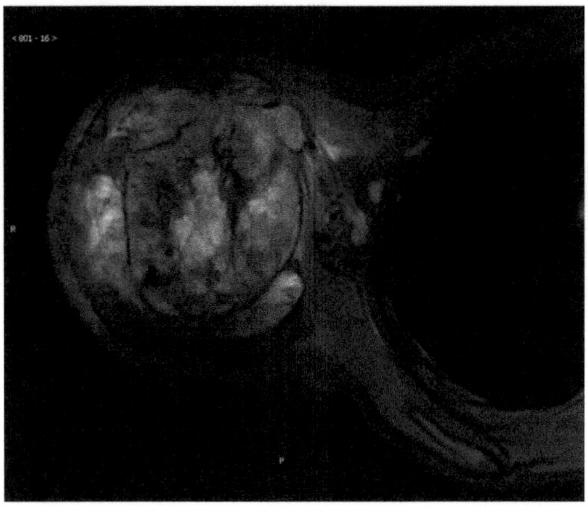

Fig. 21.8 Axial fat-suppressed T2-weighted MR image of the right shoulder

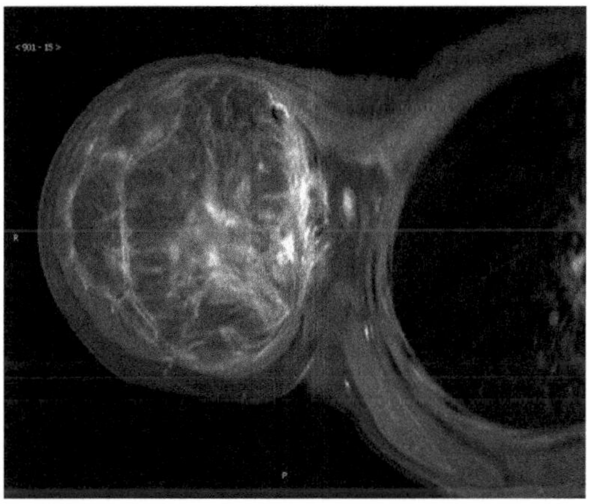

Fig. 21.9 Axial post-contrast fat-suppressed T1-weighted MR image of the right shoulder

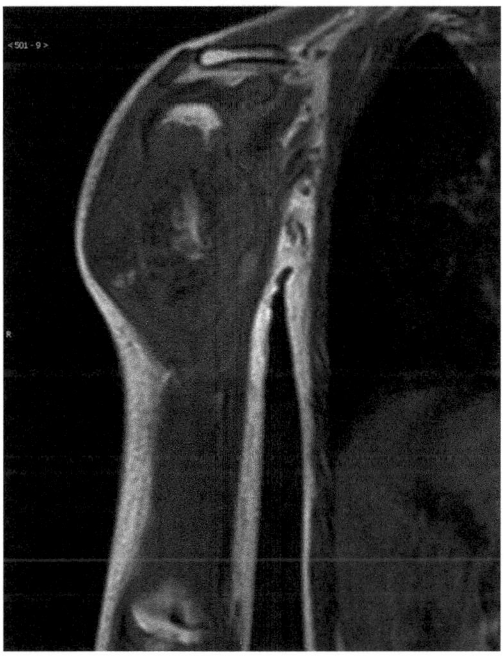

Fig. 21.10 Coronal T1-weighted MR image of the right shoulder

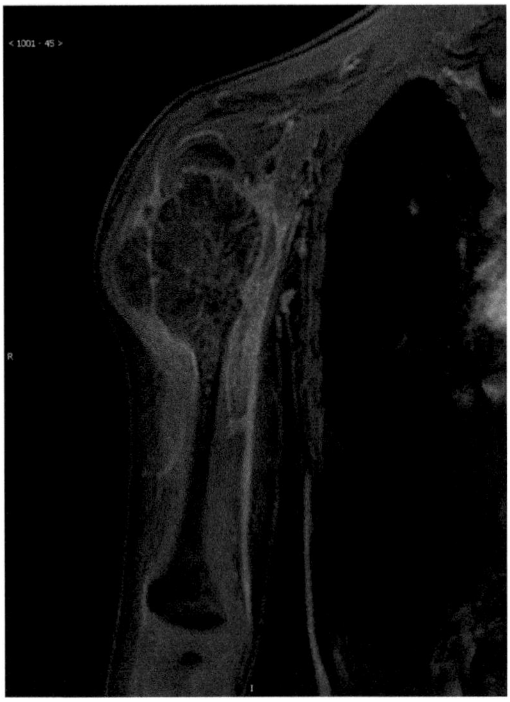

Fig. 21.11 Coronal post-contrast fat-suppressed T1-weighted MR image of the right shoulder

MR images of the right shoulder demonstrate extensive osseous destruction around the proximal humerus with heterogeneous T1 and T2 signals. Fluid–fluid levels are noted.

21.4 Description and Discussion from Residents

The patient is a child. The radiograph demonstrates osseous destruction around the proximal right humerus with irregular margin and sparing of the epiphysis. Periosteal reaction and soft tissue mass are noted. On the CT images, there are right proximal humeral lytic osseous destruction and interruption of the cortex. There is periosteal reaction but discontinuous with large associated soft tissue mass. The mass demonstrates inhomogeneous densities with heterogeneous enhancement and internal patchy necrosis. Given the lack of osseous production within the lesion and the patient's age and short clinical course, osteolytic osteosarcoma is the consideration with Ewing sarcoma in the differential diagnosis. MR images demonstrate the destruction of the right proximal humerus with heterogeneous T1 and T2 signals and multiple fluid–fluid levels. Additionally, there are patchy high T1 and T2 signals which remain high signal after fat suppression. Overall, the lesion is most consistent with aggressive lesion, favoring osteosarcoma, likely telangiectatic osteosarcoma.

21.5 Analysis and Comments from Professor Xiaoguang Cheng

The patient is a boy with a rapid clinical course. Lytic osseous destruction around the metaphysis of the right proximal humerus with periosteal reaction and soft tissue mass are most suggestive of osteosarcoma. However, there is a large soft tissue mass with heterogeneous enhancement and no osteoid production, not consistent with conventional osteosarcoma, and it could be telangiectatic osteosarcoma. Ewing sarcoma and aneurysmal bone cyst have to be excluded. The soft tissue mass seen in Ewing sarcoma is usually more solid. Aneurysmal bone cyst is a benign entity, with nonaggressive features.

21.6 Diagnosis

Telangiectatic osteosarcoma.

Suggested Reading

Angelini A, Mavrogenis AF, Trovarelli G, et al. Telangiectatic osteosarcoma: a review of 87 cases. J Cancer Res Clin Oncol. 2016 Oct;142(10):2197–207.

Murphey MD, Jaovisidha SW, Temple HT, et al. Telangiectatic osteosarcoma: radiologic-pathologic comparison. Radiology. 2003 Nov;229(2):545–53.

Synovial Sarcoma: Case 22

22

22.1 Medical History

The patient is a 19-year-old male. He presented with right shoulder mass for 8 months with subsequent open biopsy and chemotherapy.

22.2 Physical Examination

Skin protuberance around the right shoulder in the back with palpable mass, point tenderness, nonmobile, and without clear margin.

22.3 Imaging Findings

22.3.1 Radiograph

X. Cheng et al., *Imaging of Bone Tumors in Shoulder and Elbow*,
https://doi.org/10.1007/978-981-33-6150-8_22

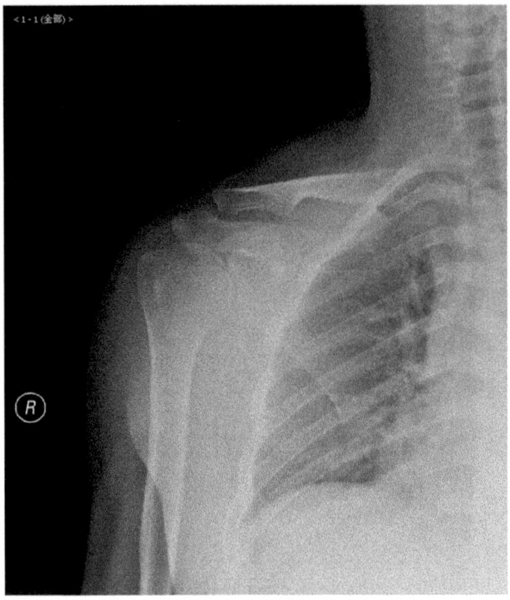

Fig. 22.1 Frontal view of the right scapula

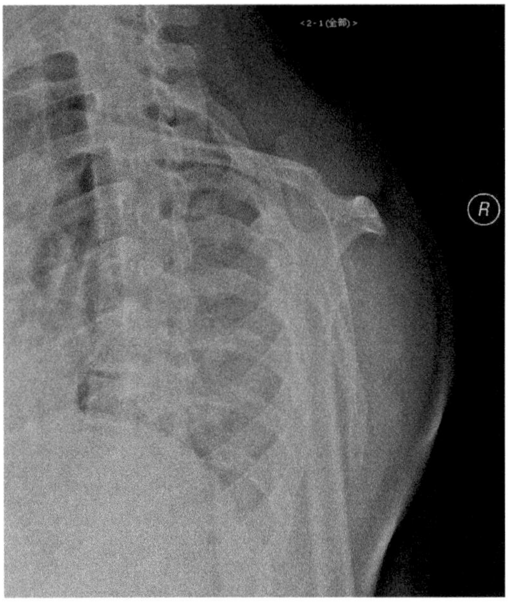

Fig. 22.2 Lateral view of the right scapula

Radiographs demonstrate soft tissue mass around the right scapula without osseous abnormalities.

22.3.2 CT Imaging

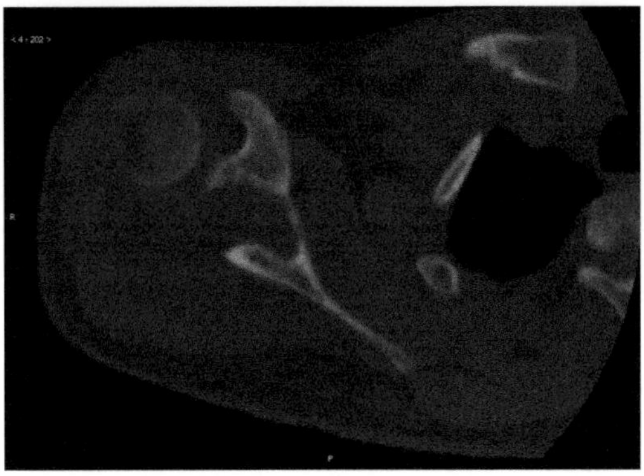

Fig. 22.3 Axial CT image of the right shoulder in bone window

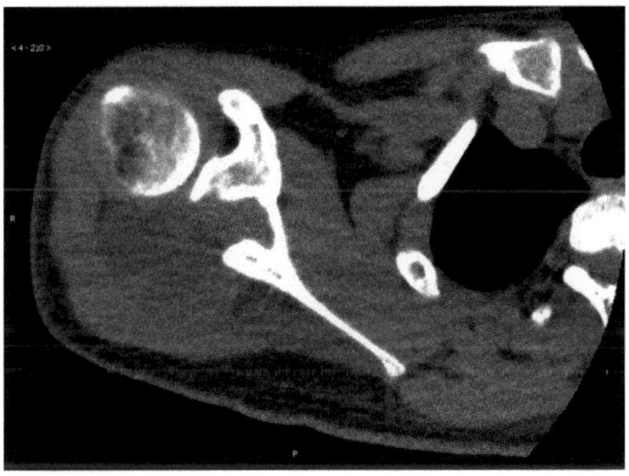

Fig. 22.4 Axial CT image of the right shoulder in soft tissue window

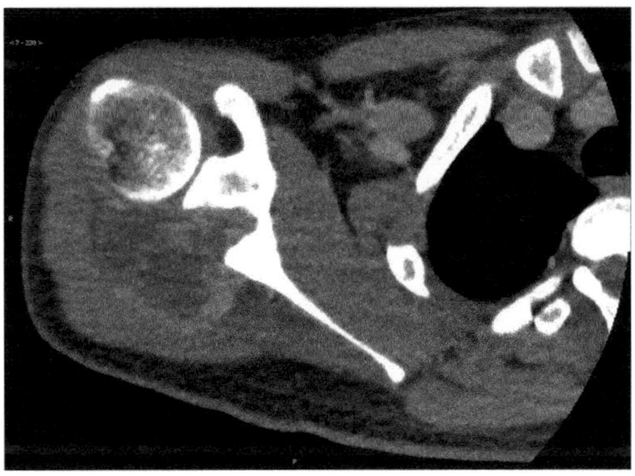

Fig. 22.5 Axial post-contrast CT image of the right shoulder in soft tissue window

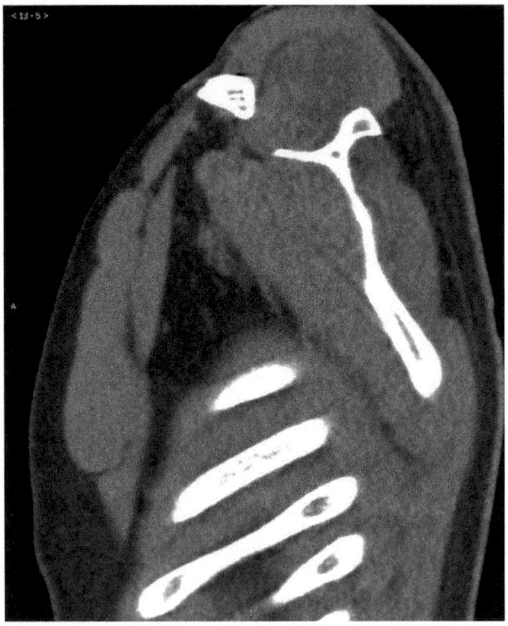

Fig. 22.6 Sagittal CT image of the right shoulder in soft tissue window

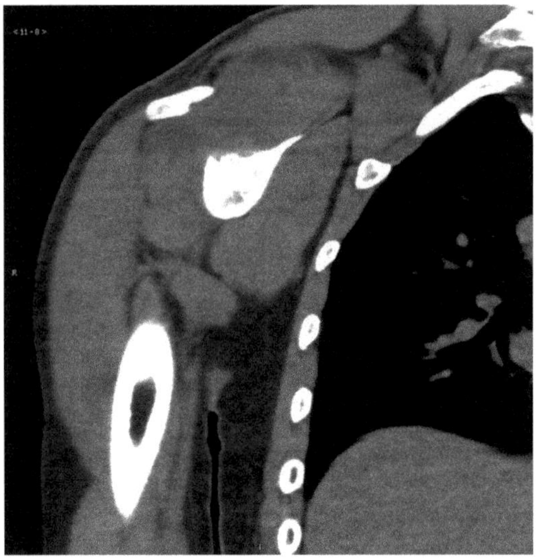

Fig. 22.7 Coronal CT image of the right shoulder in soft tissue window

CT images of the right shoulder demonstrated soft tissue mass around the right scapula involving the supraspinatus, infraspinatus, and subscapularis muscles. The lesion demonstrated an irregular margin with inhomogeneous densities. There was heterogeneous enhancement with internal liquefying necrosis after contrast administration.

22.3.3 MR Imaging

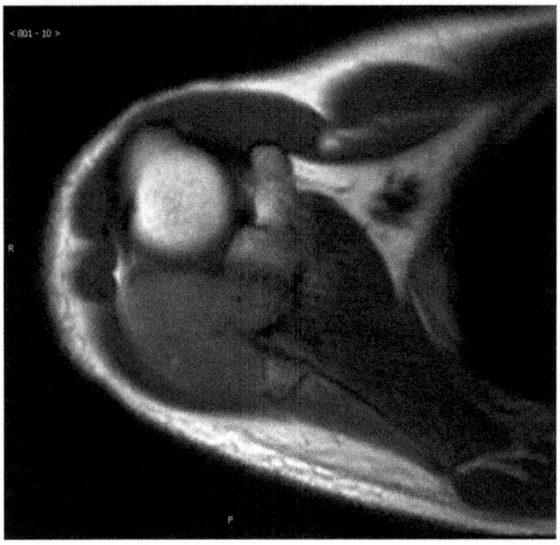

Fig. 22.8 Axial T1-weighted MR image of the right shoulder

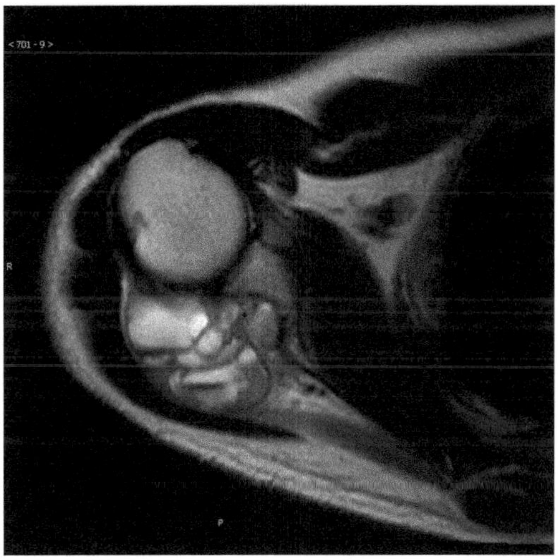

Fig. 22.9 Axial T2-weighted MR image of the right shoulder

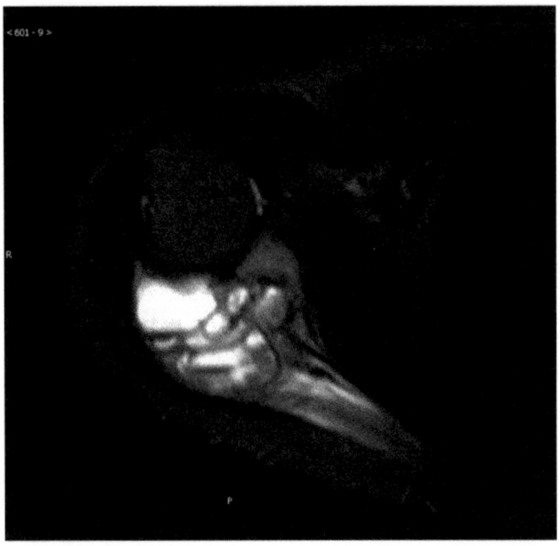

Fig. 22.10 Axial fat-suppressed T2-weighted MR image of the right shoulder

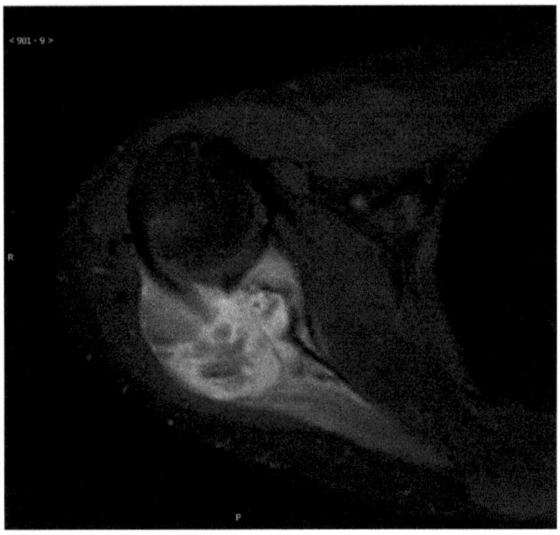

Fig. 22.11 Axial post-contrast fat-suppressed T1-weighted MR image of the right shoulder

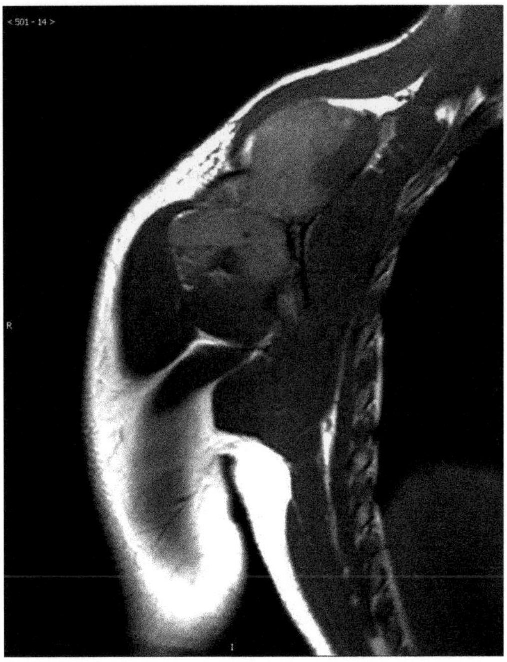

Fig. 22.12 Coronal T1-weighted MR image of the right shoulder

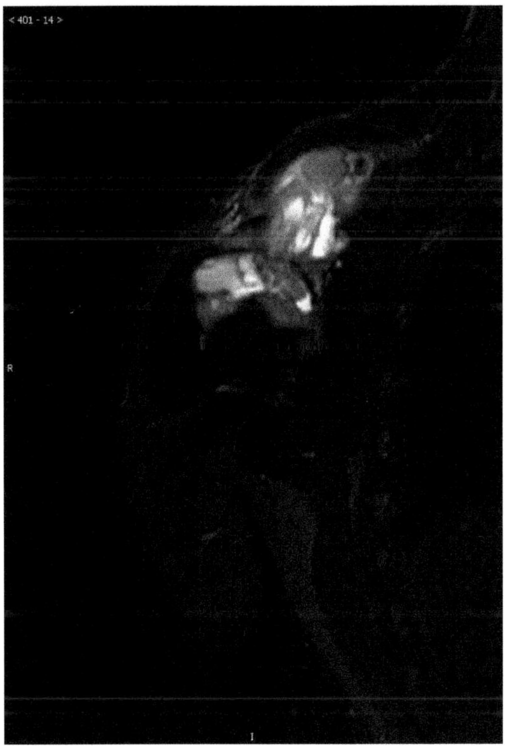

Fig. 22.13 Coronal fat-suppressed T2-weighted MR image of the right shoulder

MR images of the right shoulder demonstrate heterogeneous signal within the lesion, of predominant high T1 signal and heterogeneous high T2 signal and internal multiple fluid–fluid levels. An abnormal marrow signal is noted in the right scapula.

22.4 Description and Discussion from Residents

The patient is a young male. The radiographs demonstrate soft tissue mass around the supraspinatus and infraspinatus regions with thinning of the subcutaneous fat from compression. The osseous change of the right scapula appears unremarkable. This is most consistent with a soft tissue mass. On the CT images, the soft tissue mass involves the supraspinatus, infraspinatus, and subscapularis muscles with unclear margin and heterogeneous densities and heterogeneous enhancement with necrosis. Focal sclerosis is noted around the scapula body and glenoid. The differential diagnosis includes: (1) malignant bone tumor, patient has history of chemotherapy, Ewing sarcoma is of top consideration, and necrosis could be related to chemotherapy; (2) soft tissue tumor, with involvement of the scapula. Multiple fluid–fluid levels are noted on the MR images with abnormal marrow signal of the scapula. Given the large size of the soft tissue mass, again Ewing sarcoma is at the top of the consideration.

22.5 Analysis and Comments from Professor Xiaoguang Cheng

The patient is a young male with a history of chemotherapy. Radiographs demonstrate soft tissue mass without clear osseous changes. CT images show a large area of necrosis within the mass and possible involvement of the adjacent cortex. It is difficult to decide the origin of the lesion as osseous or from soft tissue. MR images clearly demonstrate the cystic necrosis within the mass and abnormal marrow edema of the glenoid on fat-suppressed fluid sensitive sequences, consistent with malignant lesion, such as Ewing sarcoma. Here, we need to discuss how to evaluate chemotherapy response on imaging. Good responses on imaging are: (1) decreasing in size of the soft tissue mass, liquefying necrosis; (2) increasing sclerosis around bone destruction. Overall, the differential diagnosis: (1) post-chemotherapy of Ewing sarcoma; (2) soft tissue tumor cannot be excluded.

22.6 Diagnosis

Synovial sarcoma (treatment response of bone and soft tissue tumor can affect the diagnosis).

Suggested Reading

Bakri A, Shinagare AB, Krajewski KM, et al. Synovial sarcoma: imaging features of common and uncommon primary sites, metastatic patterns, and treatment response. AJR Am J Roentgenol. 2012 Aug;199(2):W208–15.

Murphey MD, Gibson MS, Jennings BT, et al. From the archives of the AFIP: imaging of synovial sarcoma with radiologic-pathologic correlation. Radiographics. 2006 Sep-Oct;26(5):1543–65.

Giant Cell Tumor of Bone: Case 23

23

23.1 Medical History

The patient is a 31-year-old male. He presented with a right upper arm restricted range of motion after a twisting injury 3 weeks ago.

23.2 Physical Examination

Swelling with point tenderness of the right upper arm with significantly restricted range of motion.

23.3 Imaging Findings

23.3.1 Radiograph

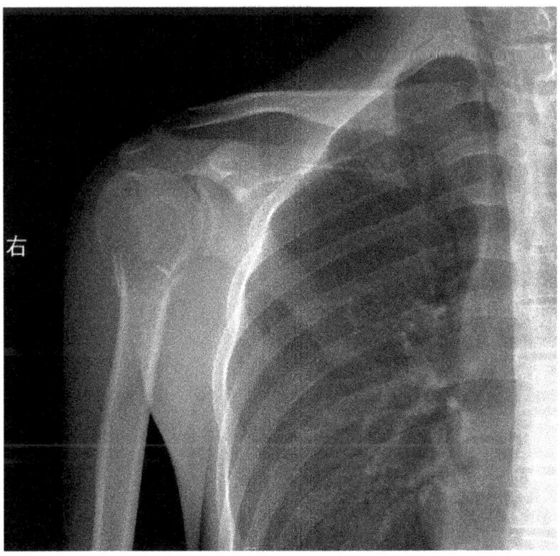

Fig. 23.1 Frontal view of the right shoulder

X. Cheng et al., *Imaging of Bone Tumors in Shoulder and Elbow*,
https://doi.org/10.1007/978-981-33-6150-8_23

Radiograph demonstrates lytic bone destruction around the proximal right humerus with irregular margin and associated pathologic fracture at the surgical neck.

23.3.2 CT Imaging

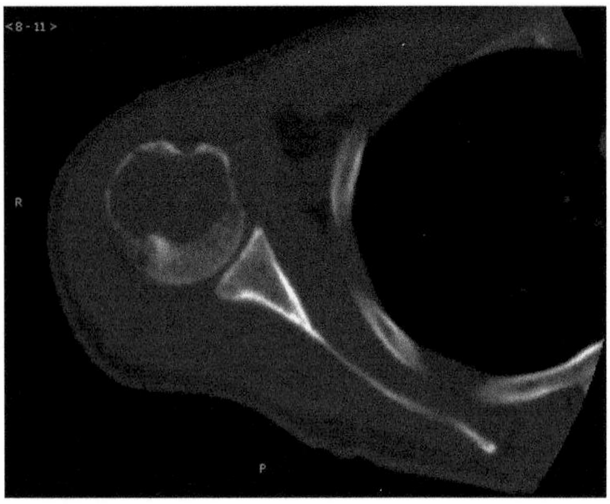

Fig. 23.2 Axial CT image of the right shoulder in bone window

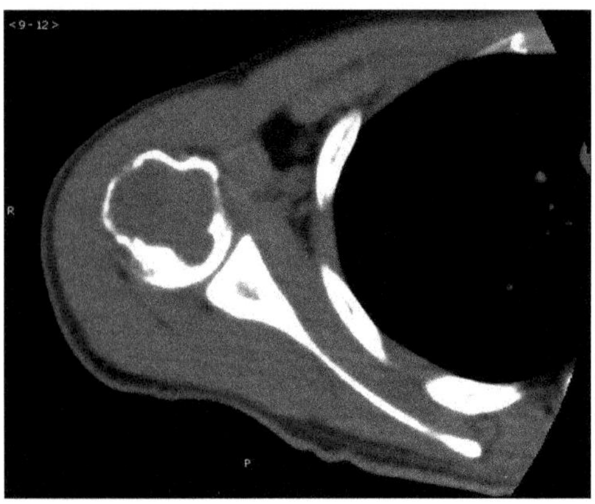

Fig. 23.3 Axial CT image of the right shoulder in soft tissue window

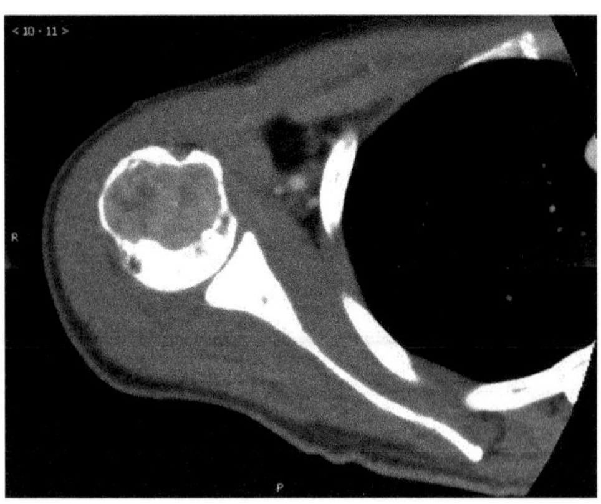

Fig. 23.4 Axial post-contrast CT image of the right shoulder in soft tissue window

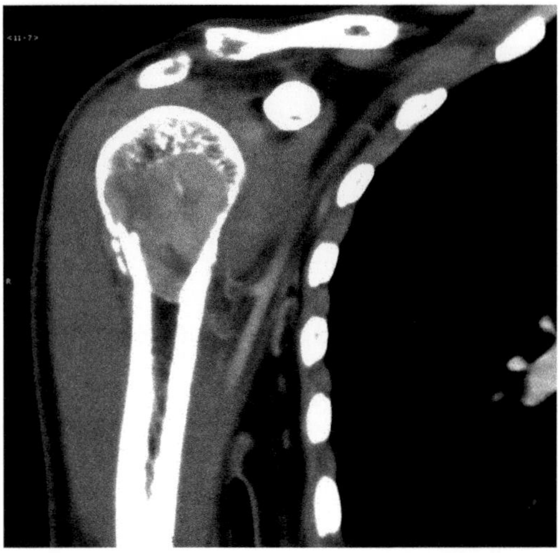

Fig. 23.5 Coronal post-contrast CT image of the right shoulder in soft tissue window

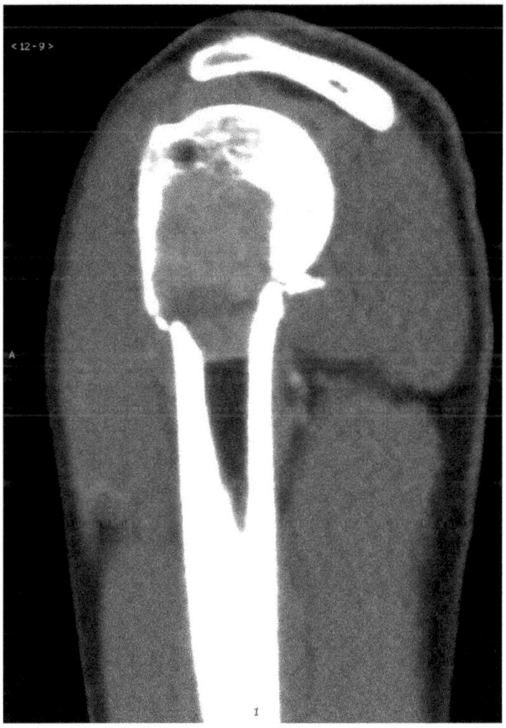

Fig. 23.6 Sagittal post-contrast CT image of the right shoulder in soft tissue window

CT images of the right shoulder demonstrate the lesion at the metaphysis of the right proximal humerus with a clear margin. There are homogeneous internal densities within the lesion, with no periosteal reaction. There is avid heterogeneous enhancement.

23.3.3 MR Imaging

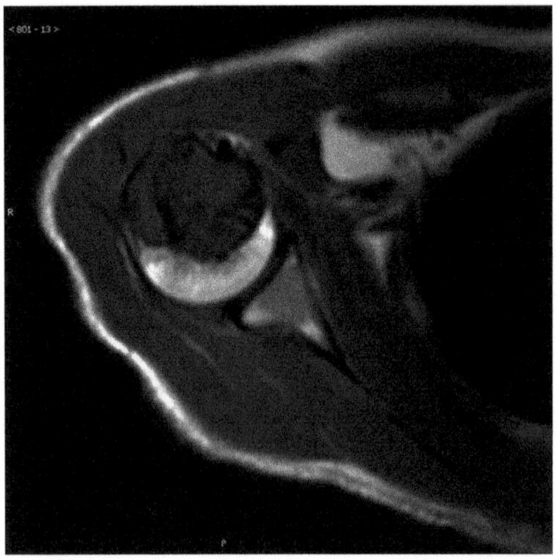

Fig. 23.7 Axial T1-weighted MR image of the right shoulder

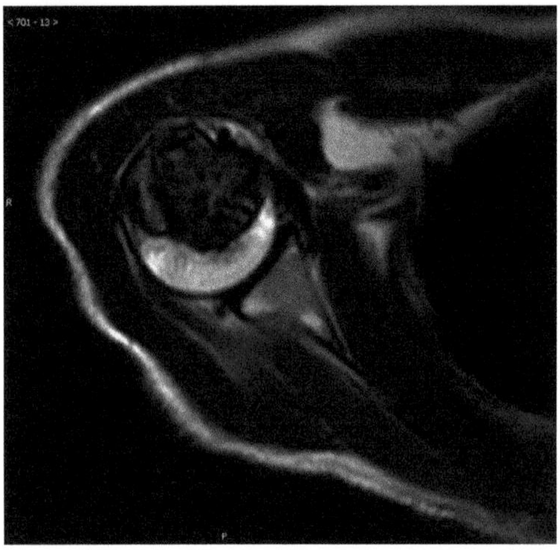

Fig. 23.8 Axial T2-weighted MR image of the right shoulder

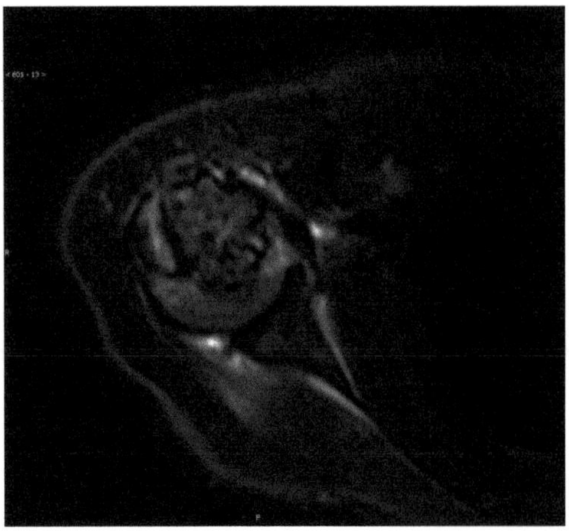

Fig. 23.9 Axial fat-suppressed T2-weighted MR image of the right shoulder

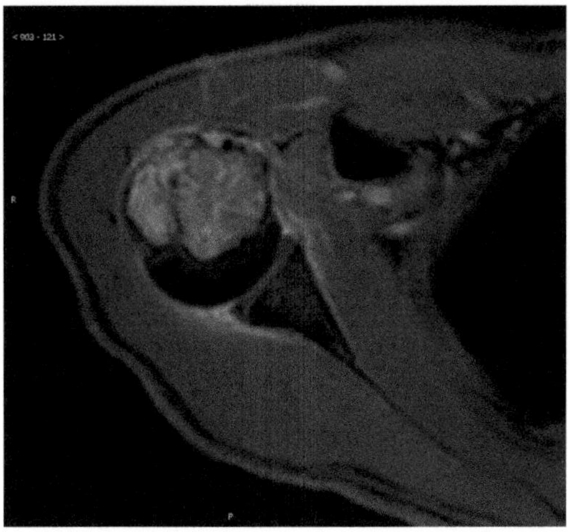

Fig. 23.10 Axial post-contrast fat-suppressed T1-weighted MR image of the right shoulder

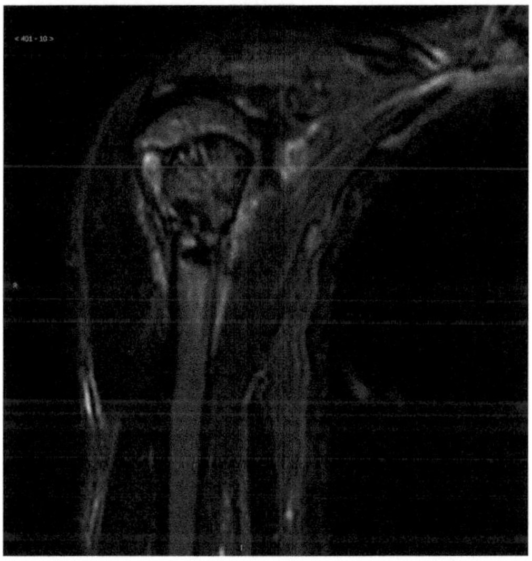

Fig. 23.11 Coronal fat-suppressed T2-weighted MR image of the right shoulder

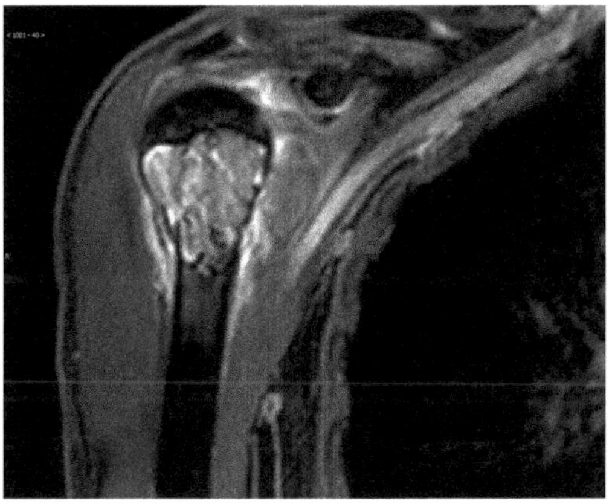

Fig. 23.12 Coronal post-contrast fat-suppressed T1-weighted MR image of the right shoulder

MR images of the right shoulder demonstrate heterogeneous signal within the lesion, of low T1 and relatively low T2 signal with internal band-like patchy low signals and adjacent soft tissue edema. The solid portion of the lesion demonstrates avid enhancement.

23.4 Description and Discussion from Residents

The patient is a young male with a history of trauma. The radiograph demonstrates lytic osseous destruction around the right proximal humerus with unclear margin, associated pathologic fracture, and fallen fragment sign with no surrounding soft tissue abnormality. It is hard to judge the aggressiveness of the process based on radiographic findings alone. CT images show the lesion at proximal metaphysis of the humerus with a clear margin and minimal sclerosis on the border with homogeneous densities. No periosteal reaction is seen and the presence of a fallen fragment sign is noted. After contrast administration, the focal CT value is measured at 120 HU. Given the patient's age, the enhancement pattern, giant cell tumor of bone is at the top of the differential diagnosis. However, giant cell tumor tends to occur around the epiphysis after closing of the physis, not consistent with the current case. Thus, vascular supply rich lesion needs to be excluded, such as plasmacytoma. Relatively low T1 signal and iso-intense to low T2 signal on fat-suppressed T2 sequences are noted on MR images with inflammation of the surrounding soft tissues, again the top differential diagnosis is giant cell tumor of bone, eosinophilic granuloma cannot be totally excluded.

23.5 Analysis and Comments from Professor Xiaoguang Cheng

The patient is a young male with a history of trauma 3 weeks ago. Radiograph demonstrates bone destruction around the metaphysis of the right proximal humerus without clear border but CT images show clear margin. There is periosteal reaction after the pathologic fracture. CT value is measured at more than 100 HU after enhancement. Focal low signal is noted on fat-suppressed T2-weighted MR images, raising concern for hemorrhage. Giant cell tumors should be put at the top of the differential diagnosis. However, with a fuzzy border, the malignant process cannot be excluded; a small blue cell tumor in the medullary cavity should be included in the differential diagnosis. Overall, this is most consistent with an intermediate (locally aggressive) or low-grade malignant tumor.

23.6 Diagnosis

Giant cell tumor of bone.

Suggested Reading

Chakarun CJ, Forrester DM, Gottsegen CJ, et al. Giant cell tumor of bone: review, mimics, and new developments in treatment. Radiographics. 2013 Jan-Feb;33(1):197–211.

Murphey MD, Nomikos GC, Flemming DJ, et al. Imaging of giant cell tumor and giant cell reparative granuloma of bone: radiologic-pathologic correlation. Radiographics. 2001 Sep-Oct;21(5):1283–309.

Chondrosarcoma (Grade II): Case 24

24

24.1 Medical History

The patient is a 19-year-old female. She presented with mass around the proximal left humerus for 4 months.

24.2 Physical Examination

Palpable, egg-sized mass around the medial aspect of the left proximal humerus, hard, non-mobile, and without restricted range of motion of the left shoulder.

24.3 Imaging Findings

24.3.1 Radiograph

X. Cheng et al., *Imaging of Bone Tumors in Shoulder and Elbow*,
https://doi.org/10.1007/978-981-33-6150-8_24

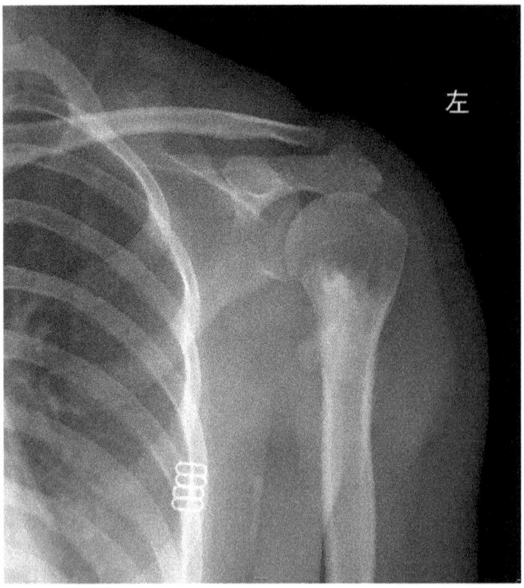

Fig. 24.1 Frontal view of the left shoulder

The radiograph demonstrates a large area of patchy high densities around the medullary cavity of the left proximal humerus. Focal bony protuberance is noted medially of the proximal left humerus. Mild adjacent soft tissue swelling is seen.

24.3.2 CT Imaging

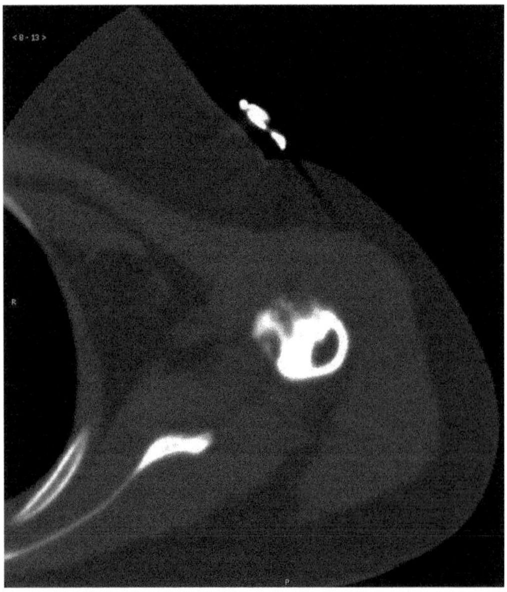

Fig. 24.2 Axial CT image of the left shoulder in bone window

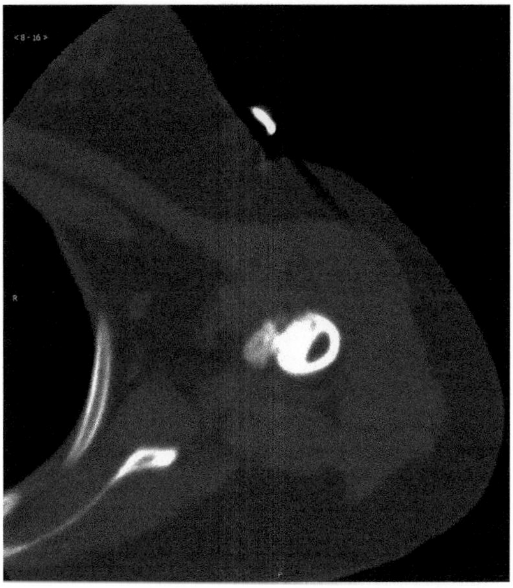

Fig. 24.3 Axial CT image of the left shoulder in bone window

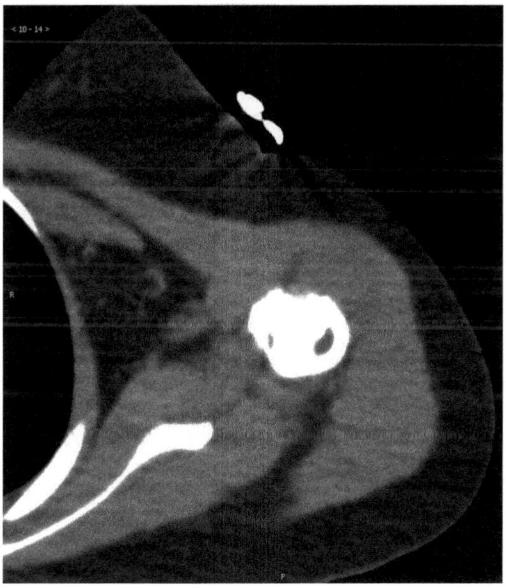

Fig. 24.4 Axial CT image of the left shoulder in soft tissue window

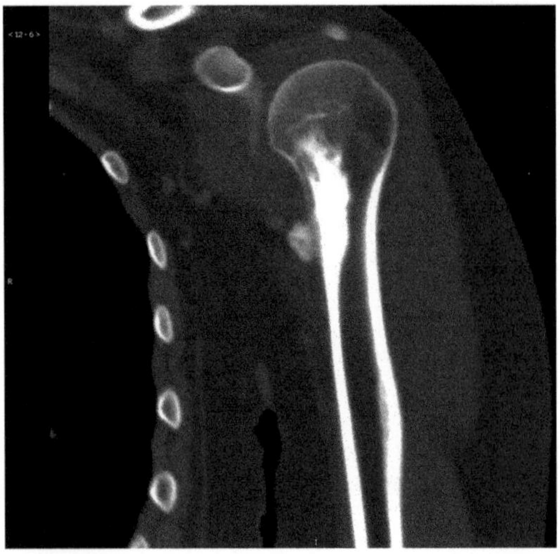

Fig. 24.5 Coronal CT image of the left shoulder in bone window

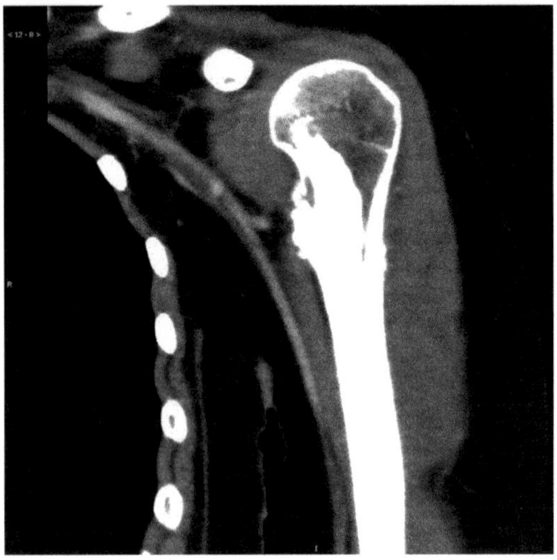

Fig. 24.6 Coronal post-contrast CT image of the left shoulder in soft tissue window

CT images of the left shoulder demonstrate high densities in the left proximal humeral medullary cavity with cortical protuberance of irregular margin and soft tissue mass. Heterogeneous enhancement is noted after contrast administration.

24.3.3 MR Imaging

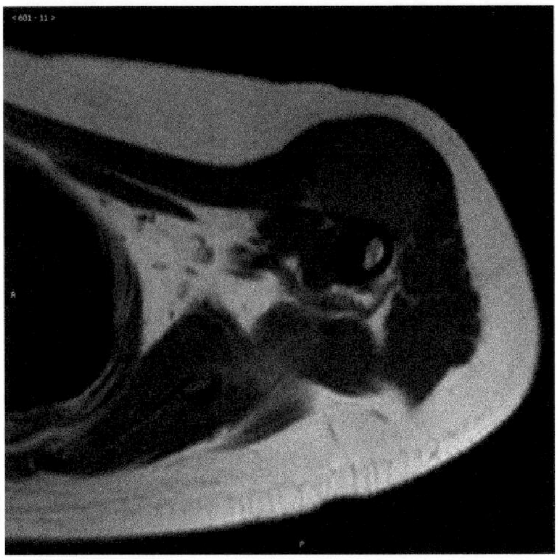

Fig. 24.7 Axial T1-weighted MR image of the left shoulder

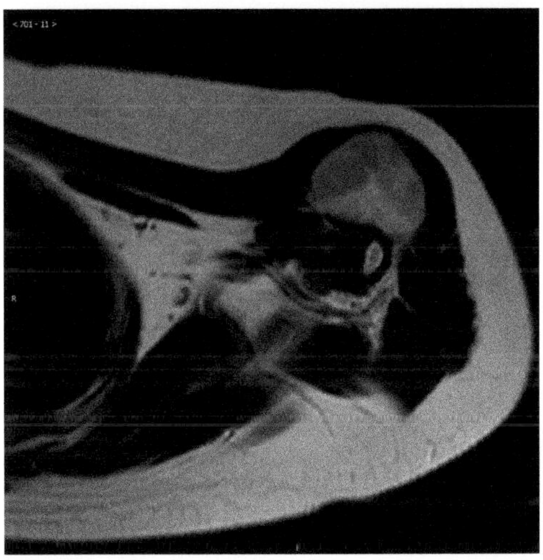

Fig. 24.8 Axial T2-weighted MR image of the left shoulder

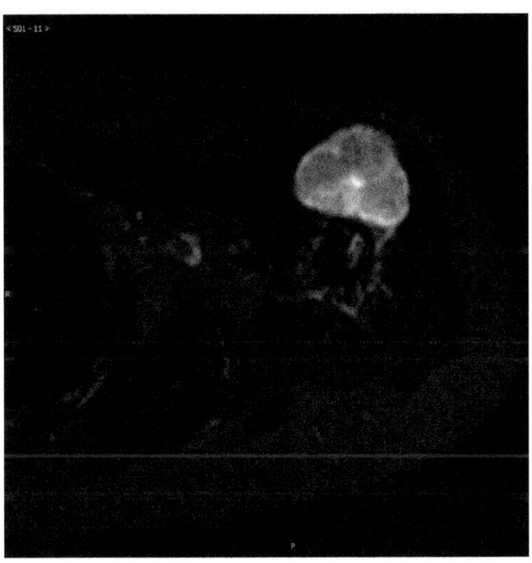

Fig. 24.9 Axial fat-suppressed T2-weighted MR image of the left shoulder

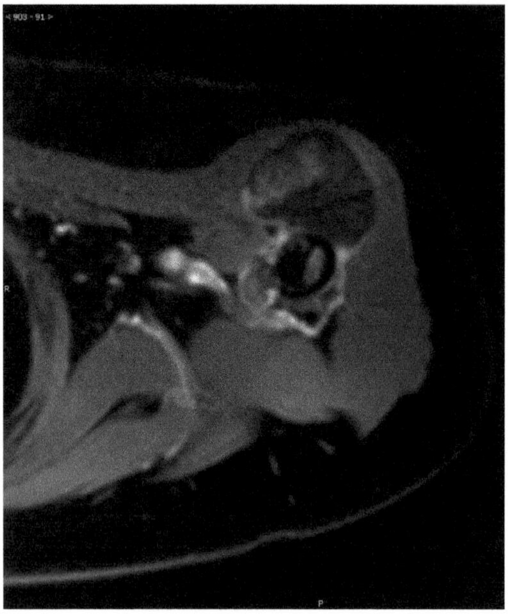

Fig. 24.10 Axial post-contrast fat-suppressed T1-weighted MR image of the left shoulder

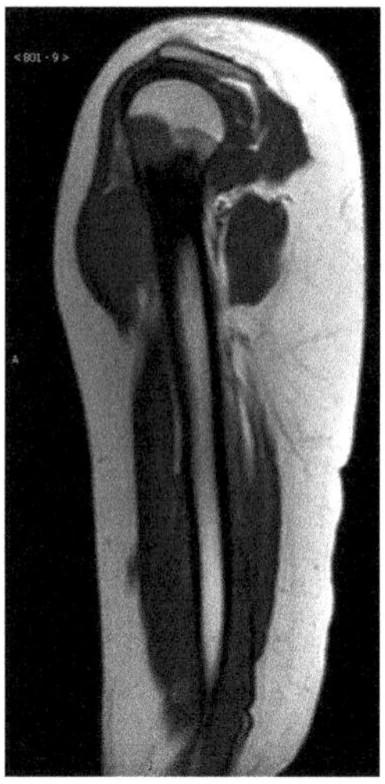

Fig. 24.11 Sagittal T1-weighted MR image of the left shoulder

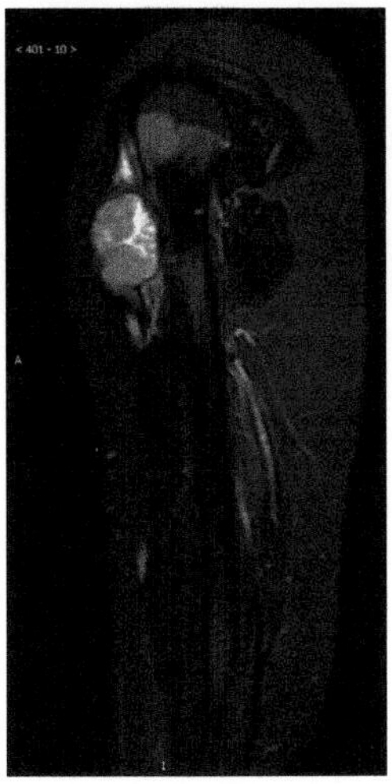

Fig. 24.12 Sagittal fat-suppressed T2-weighted MR image of the left shoulder

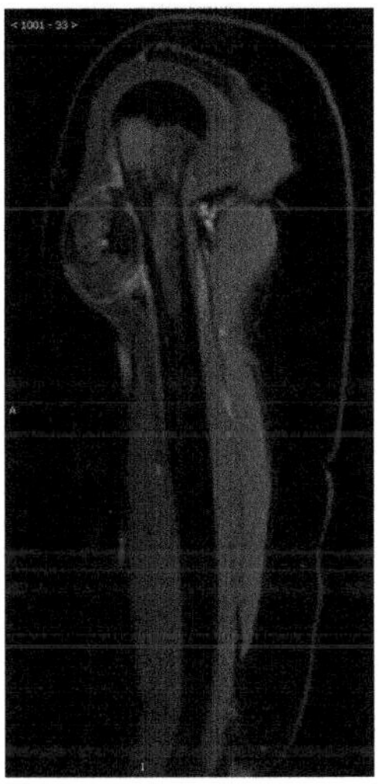

Fig. 24.13 Sagittal post-contrast fat-suppressed T1-weighted MR image of the left shoulder

MR images of the left shoulder demonstrate mild low T1 signal and high T2 signal on fat-suppressed sequences of the lesion at the proximal left humeral meta-diaphysis and the medial osseous protuberance. There is a large soft tissue mass abutting the lateral and anterior cortex of the humerus, adjacent to the area of abnormal marrow changes. Focal enhancements are noted in the proximal medullary cavity, bony protuberance, and soft tissue mass.

24.4 Description and Discussion from Residents

The patient is a young female. Radiograph demonstrates a large area of high densities of the left proximal humeral medullary cavity, very dense, likely represent immature bone. There is medial focal osseous protuberance with mild soft tissue swelling. The top consideration is osteosarcoma. The juxta-cortical protuberance demonstrates irregular margin on CT images with soft tissue mass and heterogeneous enhancement. Given the patient's age, this is likely a parosteal osteosarcoma. MR images demonstrate the larger extent of the lesion with obvious involvement of the medullary cavity and similar enhancement pattern as seen on CT, again support parosteal osteosarcoma.

24.5 Analysis and Comments from Professor Xiaoguang Cheng

The patient is young. Radiograph demonstrates increased densities around the proximal left humeral medullary cavity, bony protuberance, and adjacent soft tissue swelling. The above features are commonly seen in osteosarcoma. And osteoblastoma and osteoid osteoma can have similar features. Increased densities in the medullary cavity, bony protuberance with soft tissue mass are noted on the CT images without identification of a nidus, osteoid osteoma can be excluded. The MR images demonstrate the extent of the soft tissue mass and the intimate relationship with the adjacent cortex, supportive of classic osteosarcoma. The parosteal osteosarcoma suggested by the residents usually would not involve a large area of the medullary cavity, so I would not include it in the differential diagnosis. Overall, this is a malignant process, favoring osteosarcoma.

24.6 Diagnosis

Chondrosarcoma (grade II).

Suggested Reading

Douis H, Saifuddin A. The imaging of cartilaginous bone tumours. II. Chondrosarcoma. Skelet Radiol. 2013 May;42(5):611–26.

Murphey MD, Walker EA, Wilson AJ, et al. From the archives of the AFIP: imaging of primary chondrosarcoma: radiologic-pathologic correlation. Radiographics. 2003 Sep-Oct;23(5):1245–78.

Varma DG, Ayala AG, Carrasco CH, et al. Chondrosarcoma: MR imaging with pathologic correlation. Radiographics. 1992 Jul;12(4):687–704.

25 Giant Cell Tumor of Bone: Case 25

25.1 Medical History

The patient is a 16-year-old female. She presented with right scapula pain with restricted motion of the right shoulder for about 1 year, worsening for one and half months. She had a history of biopsy in the area.

25.2 Physical Examination

Pain around the right shoulder with restricted range of motion.

25.3 Imaging Findings

25.3.1 Radiograph

X. Cheng et al., *Imaging of Bone Tumors in Shoulder and Elbow*,
https://doi.org/10.1007/978-981-33-6150-8_25

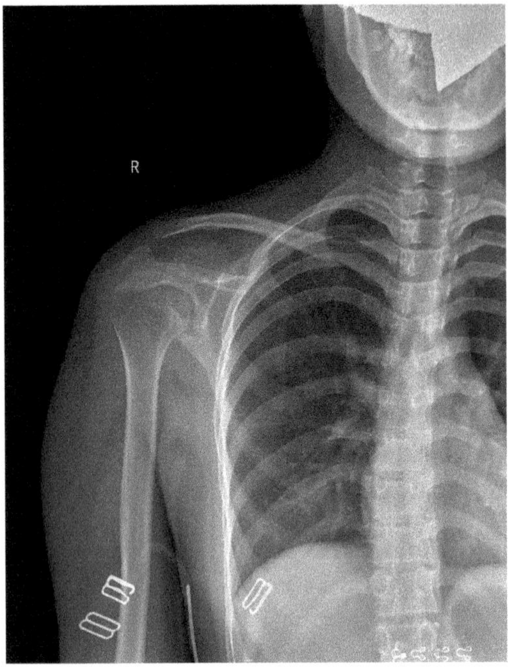

Fig. 25.1 Frontal view of the right scapula

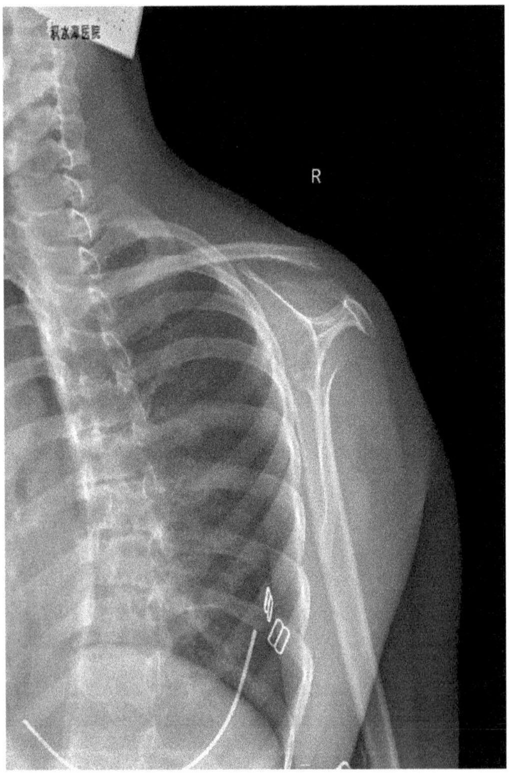

Fig. 25.2 Lateral view of the right scapula

Radiographs demonstrate expansile and lytic osseous destruction around the right glenoid and coracoid process with clear margin and no periosteal reaction or soft tissue mass.

25.3.2 CT Imaging

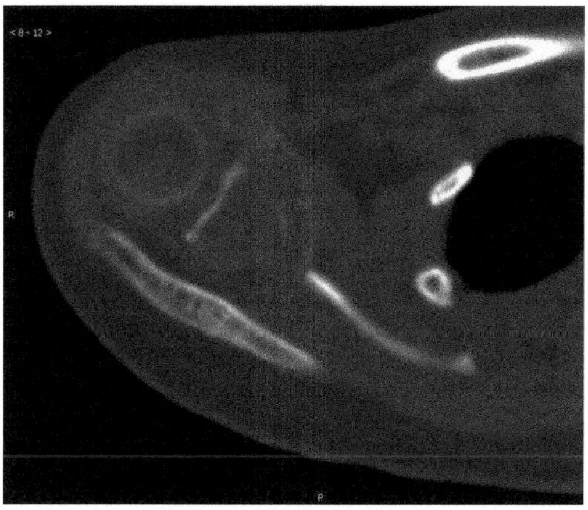

Fig. 25.3 Axial CT image of the right shoulder in bone window

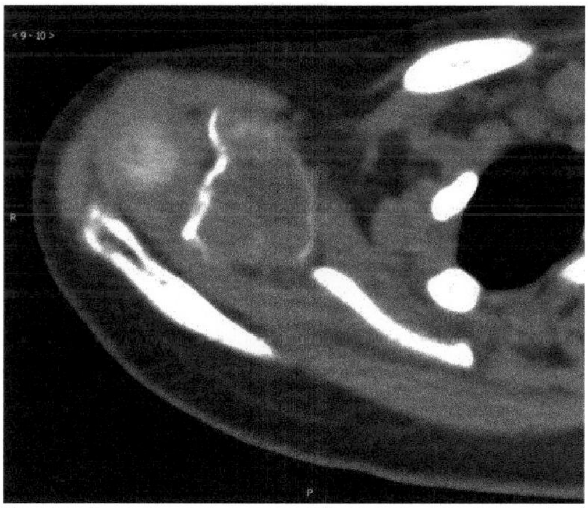

Fig. 25.4 Axial CT image of the right shoulder in soft tissue window

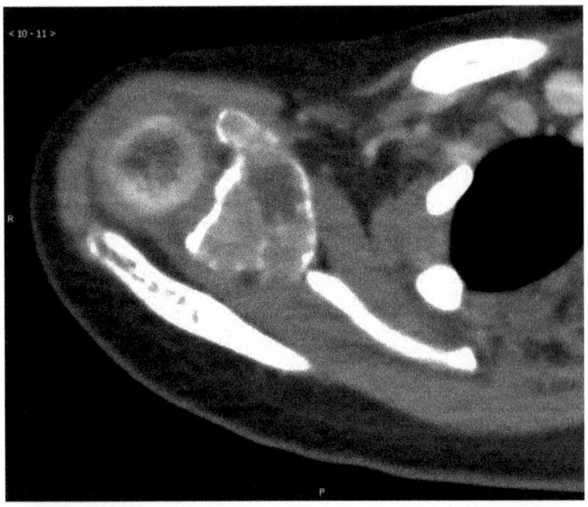

Fig. 25.5 Axial post-contrast CT image of the right shoulder in soft tissue window

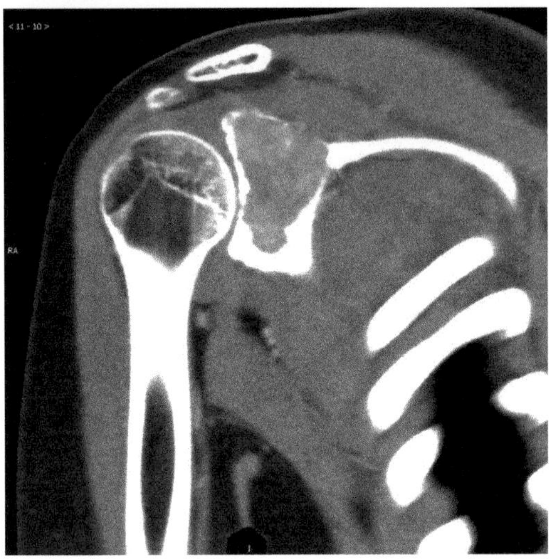

Fig. 25.6 Coronal post-contrast CT image of the right shoulder in soft tissue window

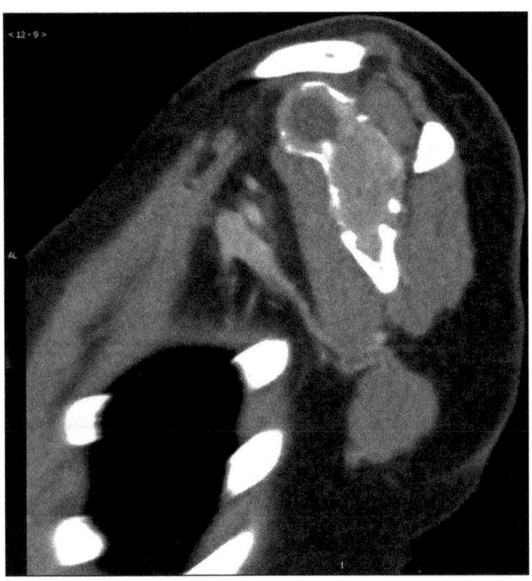

Fig. 25.7 Sagittal post-contrast CT image of the right shoulder in soft tissue window

CT images of the right shoulder demonstrate expansile osseous destruction around the right glenoid and coracoid process with thin outer shell and mild peripheral sclerosis and internal scattered, punctuate, and linear high densities. No periosteal reaction or soft tissue mass is noted. Internal cystic changes and avid enhancement of the solid portion of the lesion are noted after contrast administration.

25.3.3 MR Imaging

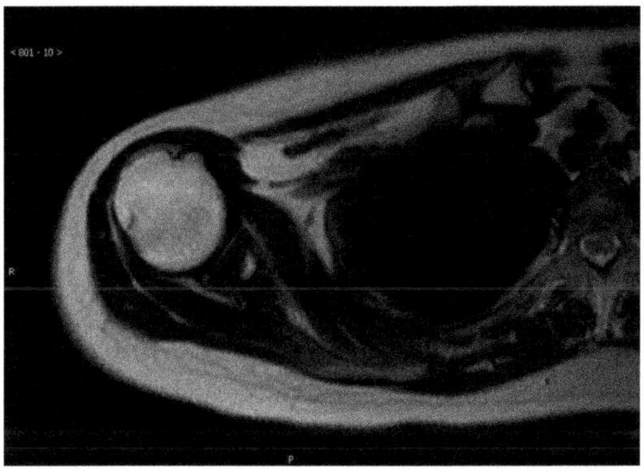

Fig. 25.8 Axial T2-weighted MR image of the right shoulder

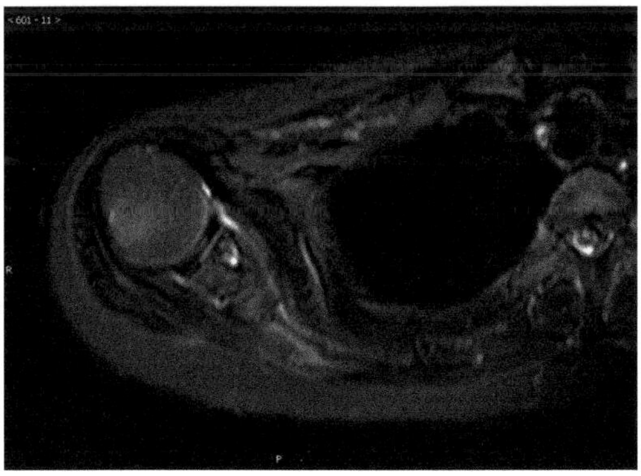

Fig. 25.9 Axial fat-suppressed T2-weighted MR image of the right shoulder

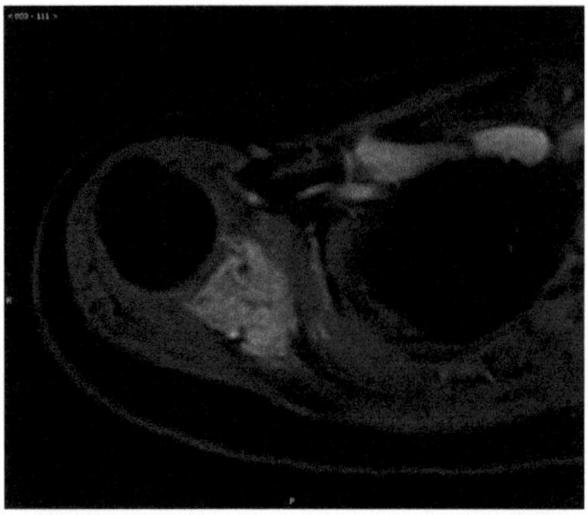

Fig. 25.10 Axial post-contrast fat-suppressed T1-weighted MR image of the right shoulder

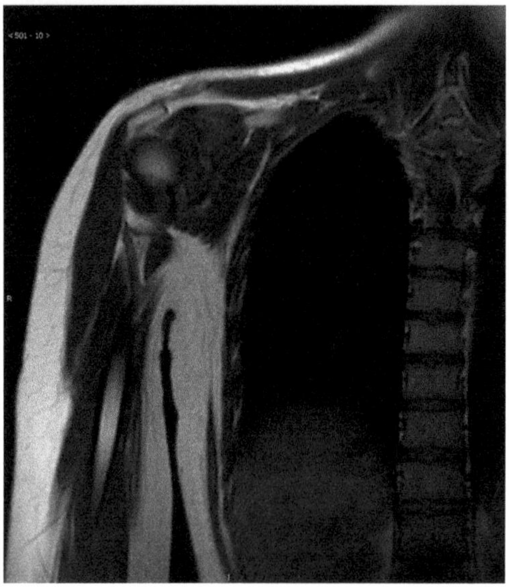

Fig. 25.11 Coronal T1-weighted MR image of the right shoulder

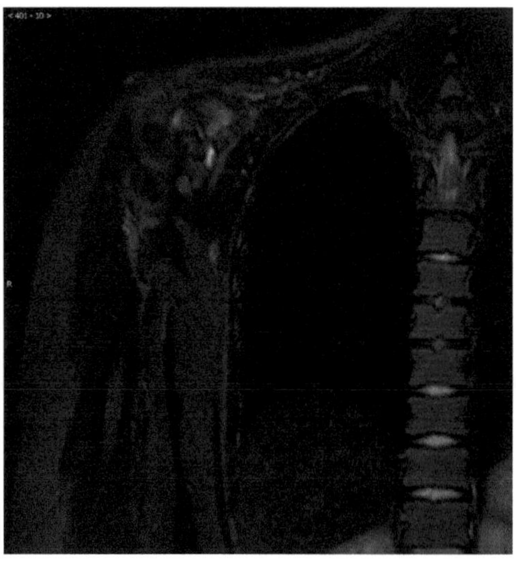

Fig. 25.12 Coronal fat-suppressed T2-weighted MR image of the right shoulder

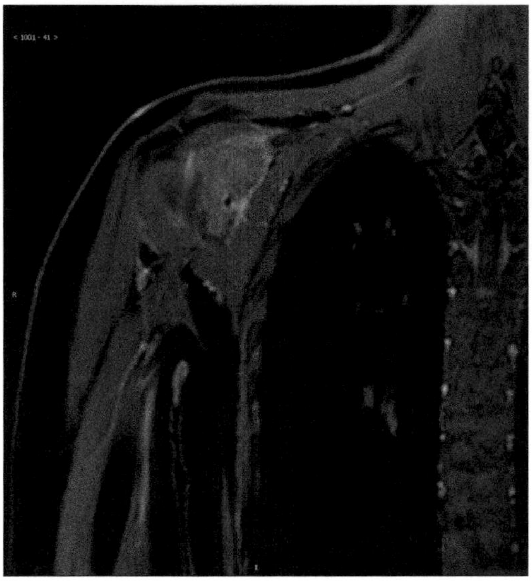

Fig. 25.13 Coronal post-contrast fat-suppressed T1-weighted MR image of the right shoulder

MR images of the right shoulder demonstrate relatively low T1 signal and iso-intense to low T2 signal of the lesion, involving the right glenoid and coracoid process. Internal cystic high signal of the lesion is seen. Enhancement is noted in a large portion of the lesion. No adjacent soft tissue edema is seen.

25.4 Description and Discussion from Residents

The patient is a young female. The radiographs demonstrate expansile and lytic osseous destruction around the right glenoid with irregular margin, thus difficult to exclude malignancy. On the CT images, there is expansile osseous destruction around the glenoid and coracoid process with a clear margin and thin outer shell with mild peripheral sclerosis and no periosteal reaction or soft tissue mass. The solid component of the lesion shows avid enhancement. The expansile morphology of the lesion and enhancement pattern are suggestive of a giant cell tumor of bone; however, the patient's age and location (a flat bone) are not typical. Since the patient is an older adolescent, eosinophilic granuloma needs to be excluded. On the MR images, there is an iso-intense to low T2 signal on the fat-suppressed sequences within the lesion and a relatively low T1 signal with cystic changes. The patient had a history of biopsy 2 months ago, these changes could be related to the prior procedure. There is no adjacent soft tissue edema on MRI, eosinophilic granuloma can be excluded.

25.5 Analysis and Comments from Professor Xiaoguang Cheng

The patient is an adolescent. Radiographs demonstrate expansile changes around the right scapula with a clear margin, favoring a nonaggressive process. The lesion demonstrates a complete border on the CT images with thin outer shell and enhancement of the solid portion. The low-density area on the CT images likely reflects sequela from prior biopsy. No edema is noted around the lesion on MRI, eosinophilic granuloma can be excluded. The expansile morphology and enhancement pattern on CT are all supportive of the diagnosis of giant cell tumor of bone. However, the location is atypical and the patient's age is young. Overall, it is most likely a nonaggressive process.

25.6 Diagnosis

Giant cell tumor of bone.

Suggested Reading

Aoki J, Moser RP Jr, Vinh TN. Giant cell tumor of the scapula. A review of 13 cases. Skelet Radiol. 1989;18(6):427–34.

Chakarun CJ, Forrester DM, Gottsegen CJ, et al. Giant cell tumor of bone: review, mimics, and new developments in treatment. Radiographics. 2013 Jan-Feb;33(1):197–211.

Murphey MD, Nomikos GC, Flemming DJ, et al. Imaging of giant cell tumor and giant cell reparative granuloma of bone: radiologic-pathologic correlation. Radiographics. 2001 Sep-Oct;21(5):1283–309.

Part II

Elbow

26 Ewing Sarcoma: Case 1

26.1 Medical History

The patient is a 31-year-old female. She presented with a mass of the right upper arm for a year with an increase in size. She had a history of biopsy followed by chemotherapy.

26.2 Physical Examination

There is a palpable mass around the midsection of the right upper arm medially, hard, non-mobile without point tenderness. The mass is deep in a location without a clear margin.

26.3 Imaging Findings

26.3.1 Radiograph

X. Cheng et al., *Imaging of Bone Tumors in Shoulder and Elbow*,
https://doi.org/10.1007/978-981-33-6150-8_26

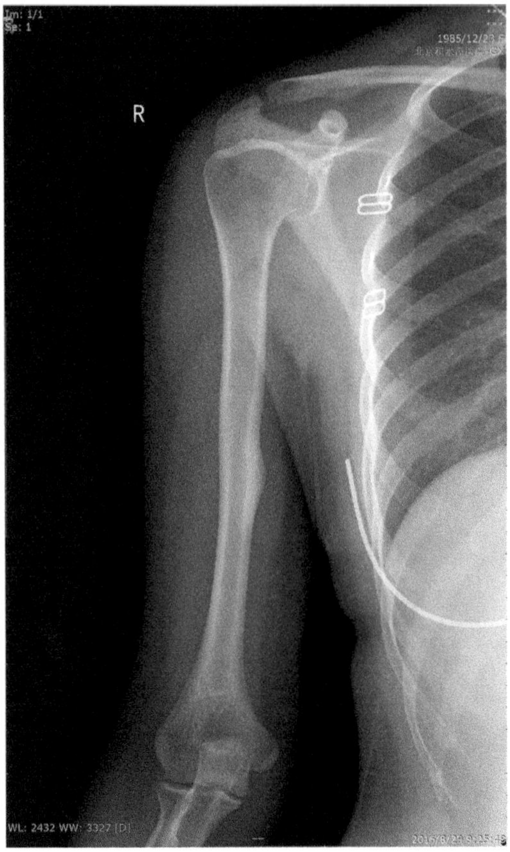

Fig. 26.1 Frontal view of the right upper arm

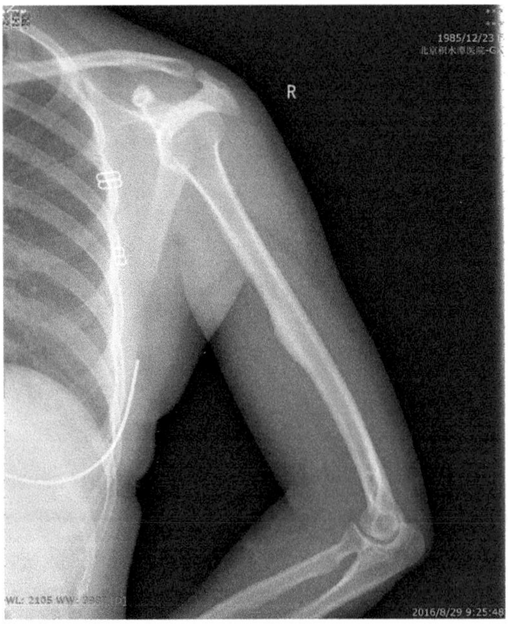

Fig. 26.2 Lateral view of the right upper arm

Radiographs of the right upper arm demonstrate cortical thickening around the mid-right humerus medially with adjacent soft tissue swelling.

26.3.2 CT Imaging

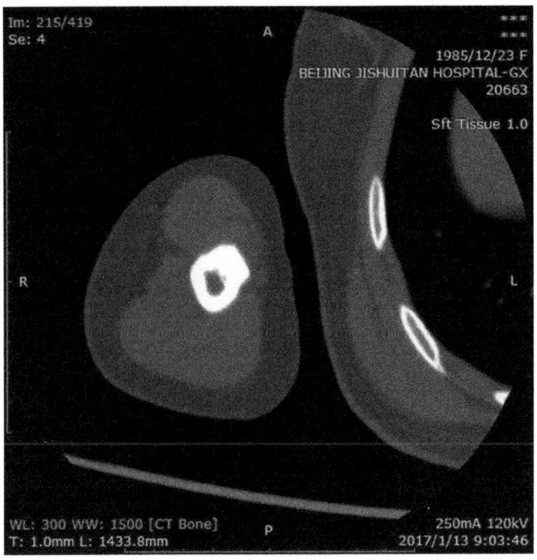

Fig. 26.3 Axial CT image of the right humerus in bone window

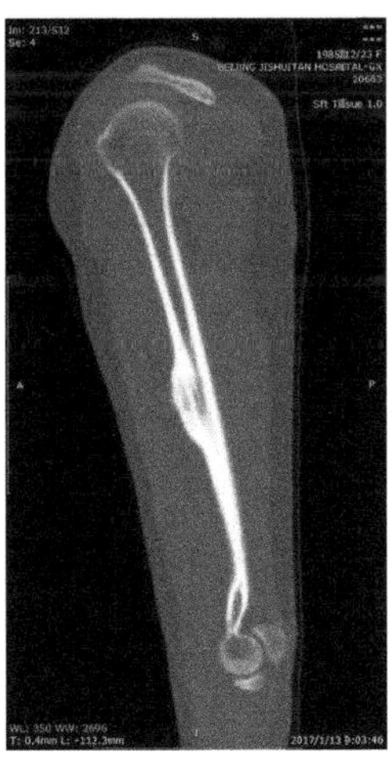

Fig. 26.4 Sagittal CT image of the right humerus in bone window

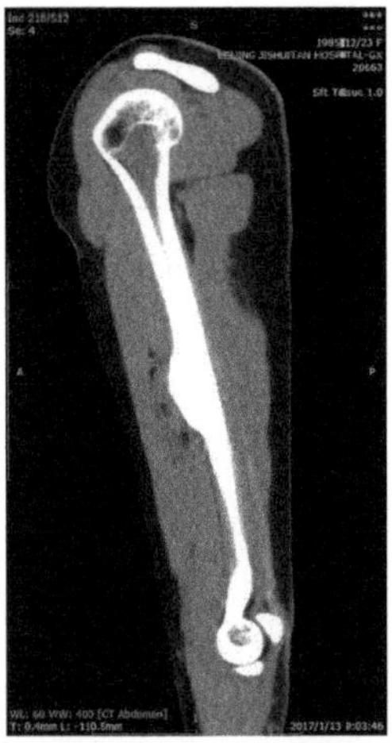

Fig. 26.5 Sagittal CT image of the right humerus in soft tissue window

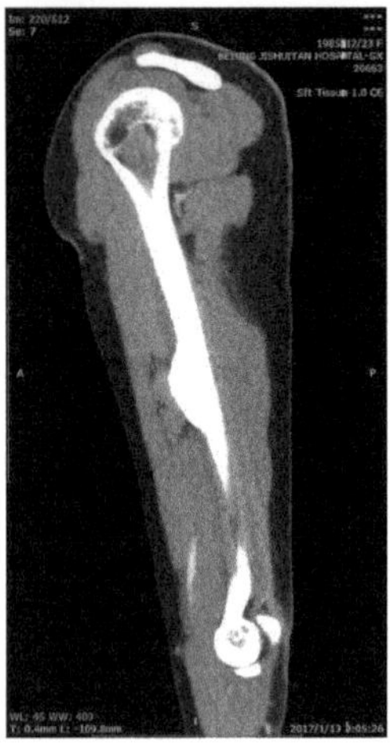

Fig. 26.6 Sagittal post-contrast CT image of the right humerus in soft tissue window

CT images demonstrate focal cortical thickening of the mid-right humerus. There is adjacent soft tissue enhancement after contrast administration.

26.3.3 MR Imaging

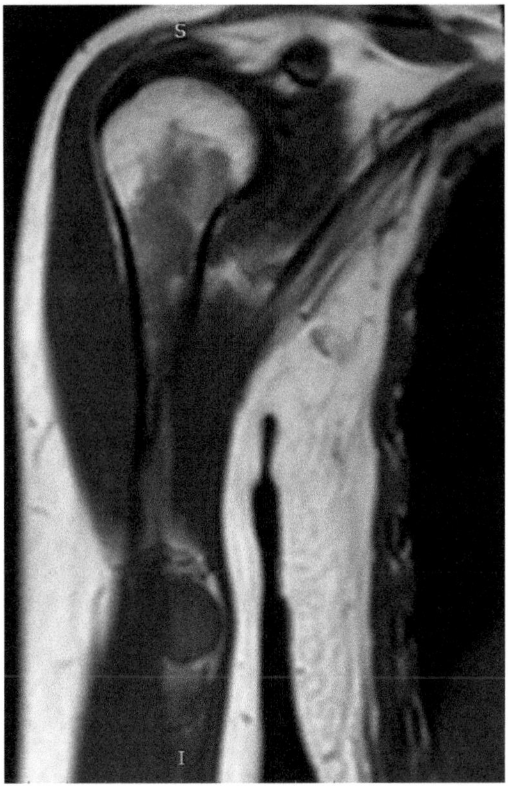

Fig. 26.7 Coronal T1-weighted MR image of the right humerus

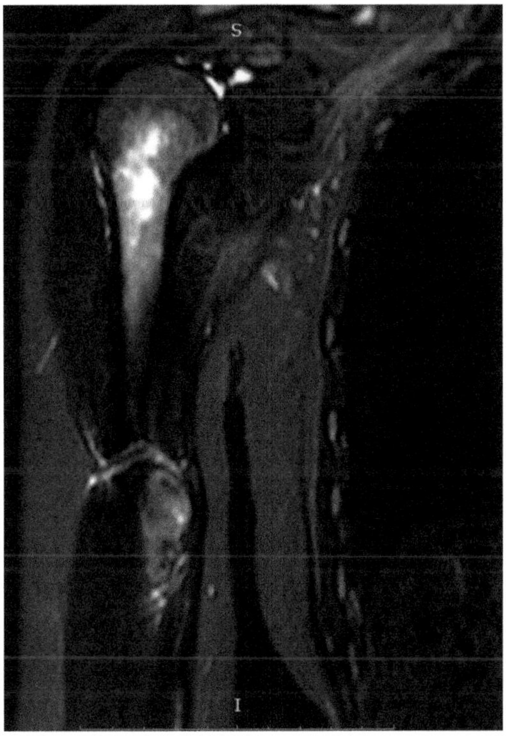

Fig. 26.8 Coronal fat-suppressed T2-weighted MR image of the right humerus

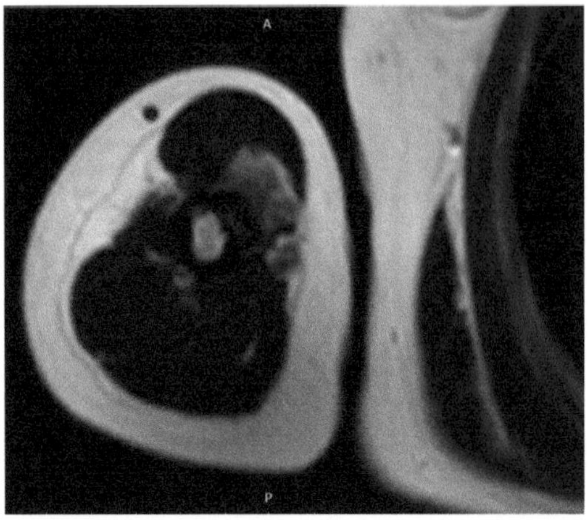

Fig. 26.9 Axial T2-weighted MR image of the right humerus

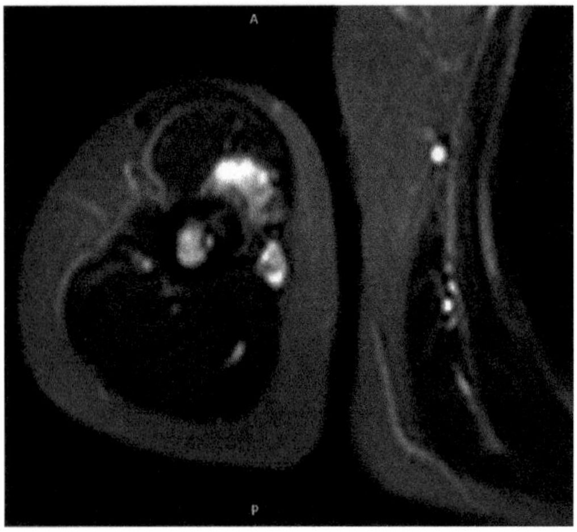

Fig. 26.10 Axial fat-suppressed T2-weighted MR image of the right humerus

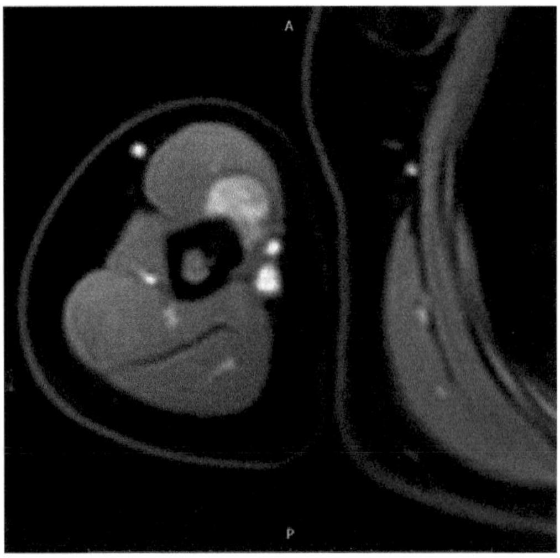

Fig. 26.11 Axial post-contrast fat-suppressed T1-weighted MR image of the right humerus

MR images demonstrate abnormal marrow signal of the right proximal mid humerus. There is adjacent soft tissue mass with enhancement.

26.4 Description and Discussion from Residents

Radiographs of the right humerus show focal mid humeral cortical thickening, without a clear depiction of the architecture of the cortex. There is surrounding soft tissue swelling. On the CT scan, there are osteoblastic changes around the medial aspect of the right proximal and mid humerus with no periosteal reaction. There is adjacent soft tissue mass with avid enhancement. The above findings are most suggestive of an aggressive neoplasm. On the MR scan, there is morphological change of the cortex but no significant cortex signal change, suggestive of parosteal origin of the lesion. However, there is a clear intramedullary abnormal signal of the proximal right humerus.

26.5 Analysis and Comments from Professor Xiaoguang Cheng

The patient has a history of bone biopsy and chemotherapy. There is focal cortical thickening of the right mid humerus with soft tissue mass and an intimate relationship with the underlying bone. On MR images, there is a high T2 signal on fat-suppressed sequences with avid enhancement. In most circumstances, when there is intramedullary abnormality with cortical thickening and soft tissue mass, the possibility of Ewing sarcoma is raised. The patient has a history of chemotherapy, which complicates the imaging findings. For example, periosteal reaction from hemangioma could have similar imaging findings; however, hemangioma is not treated with chemotherapy.

26.6 Diagnosis

Ewing sarcoma.

Suggested Reading

Murphey MD, Senchak LT, Mambalam PK, et al. From the radiologic pathology archives: ewing sarcoma family of tumors: radiologic-pathologic correlation. Radiographics. 2013 May;33(3):803–31.

Wootton-Gorges SL. MR imaging of primary bone tumors and tumor-like conditions in children. Magn Reson Imaging Clin N Am. 2009 Aug;17(3):469–87.

Chondroblastoma: Case 2

27

27.1 Medical History

The patient is a 20-year-old male. He presented with right elbow pain for 11 months and a restricted range of motion for 2 months. He had a history of biopsy.

27.2 Physical Examination

Thcrc is no palpable mass around the right elbow and no point tenderness.

27.3 Imaging Findings

27.3.1 Radiograph

X. Cheng et al., *Imaging of Bone Tumors in Shoulder and Elbow*,
https://doi.org/10.1007/978-981-33-6150-8_27

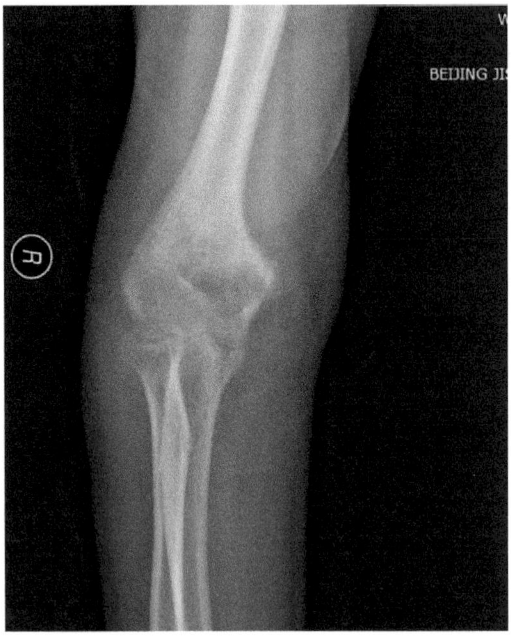

Fig. 27.1 Frontal view of the right elbow

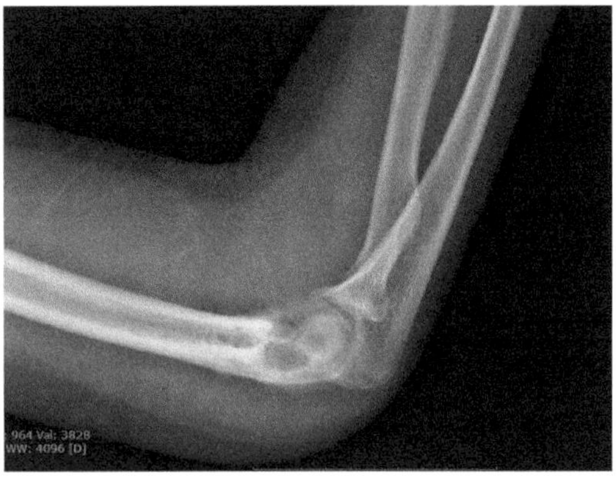

Fig. 27.2 Lateral view of the right elbow

Radiographs of the right elbow demonstrate lytic osseous destruction of the distal humerus with irregular periosteal reaction, and without clear margin. There is decreased osseous density around the right elbow.

27.3.2 CT Imaging

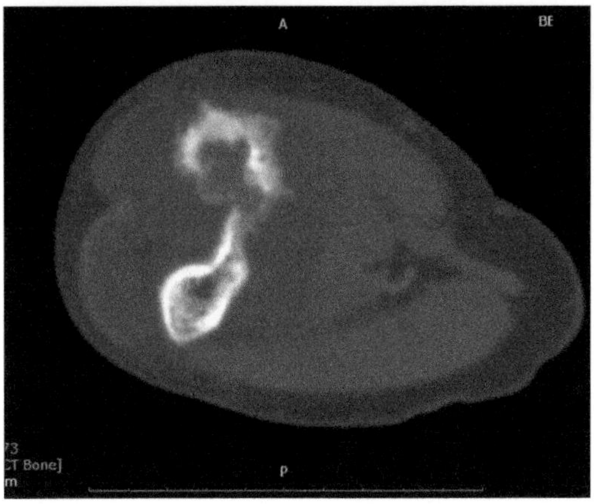

Fig. 27.3 Axial CT image of the right elbow in bone window

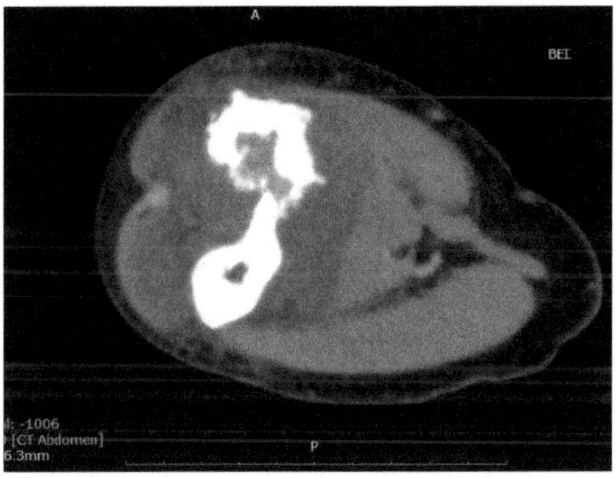

Fig. 27.4 Axial CT image of the right elbow in soft tissue window

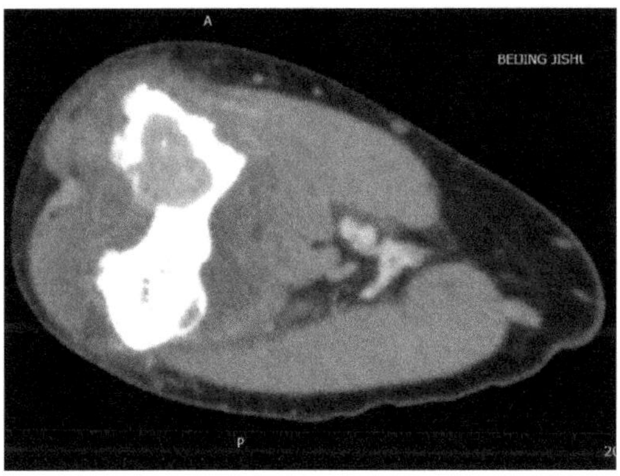

Fig. 27.5 Axial post-contrast CT image of the right elbow in soft tissue window

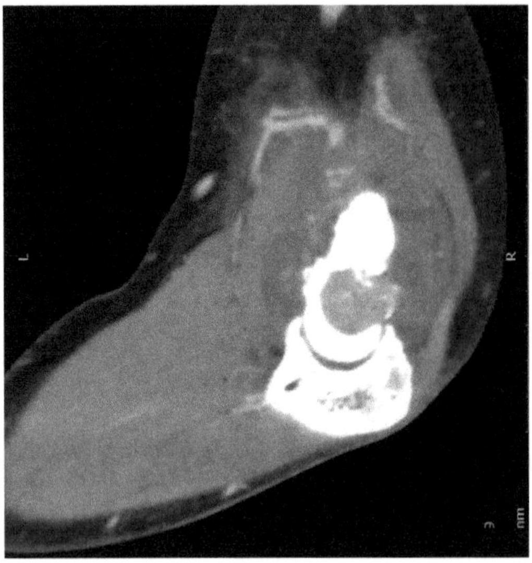

Fig. 27.6 Sagittal post-contrast CT image of the right elbow in soft tissue window

CT images of the right elbow demonstrate osseous destruction of the right distal humerus with internal punctuate calcifications. There is an irregular periosteal reaction. The solid portion of the lesion demonstrates avid enhancement. There is also soft tissue swelling.

27.4 Description and Discussion from Residents

Radiographs of the right elbow show lytic osseous destruction of the distal humerus with irregular periosteal reaction, indistinct margin, and surrounding soft tissue swelling. There are decreased bone densities around the right elbow and secondary osteoarthritis along the articular surface. On the CT images, there is sclerosis around the margin of the lesion with some indistinct margin and internal punctuate calcifications, and irregular periosteal reaction. Avid enhancement is seen. Surrounding soft tissue edema is also noted with internal possible air, very suspicious for infection. Differential diagnosis includes giant cell tumor of bone and chondroblastoma.

27.5 Analysis and Comments from Professor Xiaoguang Cheng

There is asymmetric osseous destruction of the distal right humerus in the ulnar aspect with clear margin, periosteal reaction, and relative preserved joint space of the right elbow. On the CT scan, there are periosteal reaction and internal calcifications. After contrast administration, there is avid enhancement with surrounding soft tissue edema; the differential diagnosis is osteoblastoma or chondroblastoma. Punctate air density likely relates to biopsy.

27.6 Diagnosis

Chondroblastoma.

Suggested Reading

Douis H, Saifuddin A. The imaging of cartilaginous bone tumours. I. Benign lesions. Skeletal Radiol. 2012 Sep;41(10):1195–212.

Yamamura S, Sato K, Sugiura H, et al. Inflammatory reaction in chondroblastoma. Skeletal Radiol. 1996 May;25(4):371–6.

28 Osteoid Osteoma: Case 3

28.1 Medical History

The patient is a 19-year-old male. He presented with right distal upper arm pain (exacerbated in the night) with a restricted range of motion for 1½ years.

28.2 Physical Examination

There is no swelling of the right upper arm with mild asymmetrical atrophy of the muscle and no palpable mass.

28.3 Imaging Findings

28.3.1 Radiograph

X. Cheng et al., *Imaging of Bone Tumors in Shoulder and Elbow*,
https://doi.org/10.1007/978-981-33-6150-8_28

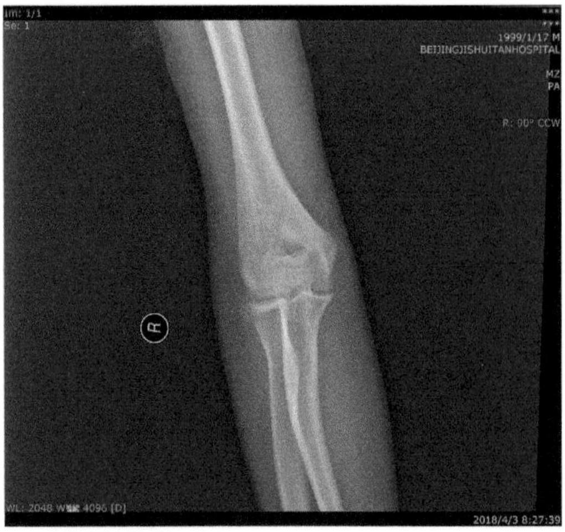

Fig. 28.1 Frontal view of the right elbow

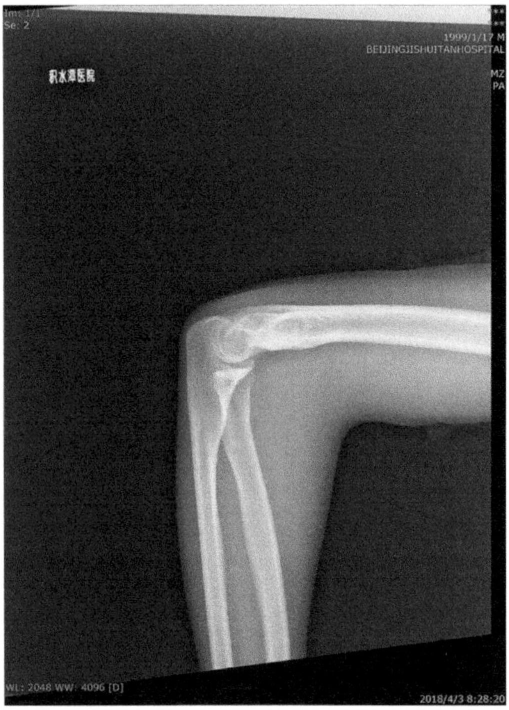

Fig. 28.2 Lateral view of the right elbow

Radiographs of the right elbow demonstrate cortical thickening around the right distal humerus anteriorly and medially with increased densities.

28.3.2 CT Imaging

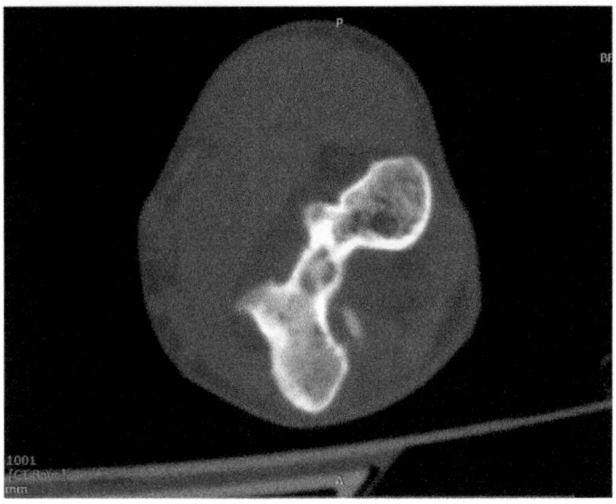

Fig. 28.3 Axial CT image of the right elbow in bone window

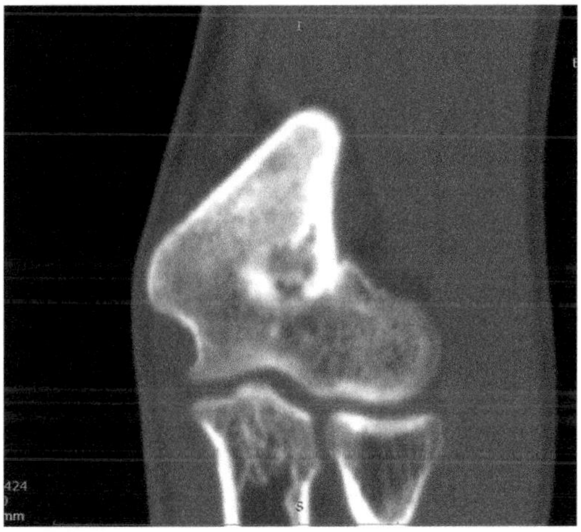

Fig. 28.4 Coronal CT image of the right elbow in bone window

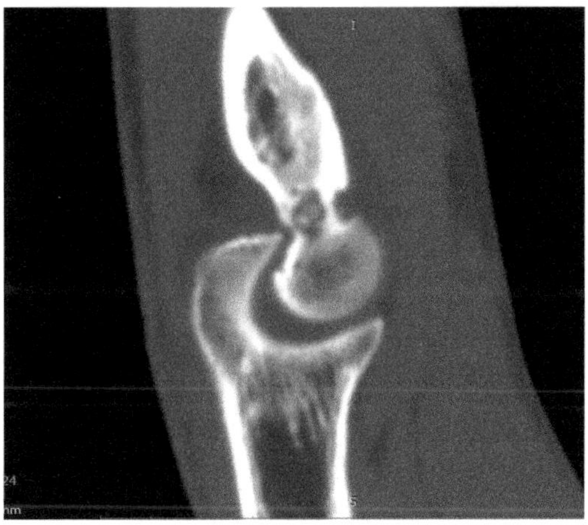

Fig. 28.5 Sagittal CT image of the right elbow in bone window

CT images of the right elbow demonstrate focal lucency in the right distal humerus with internal high densities and peripheral sclerosis.

28.3.3 MR Imaging

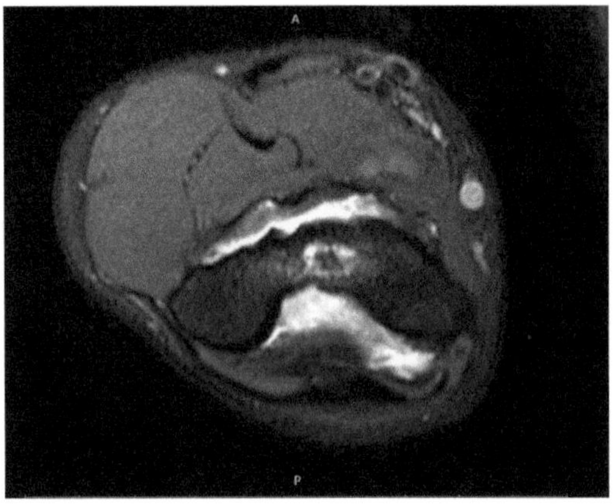

Fig. 28.6 Axial fat-suppressed T2-weighted MR image of the right elbow

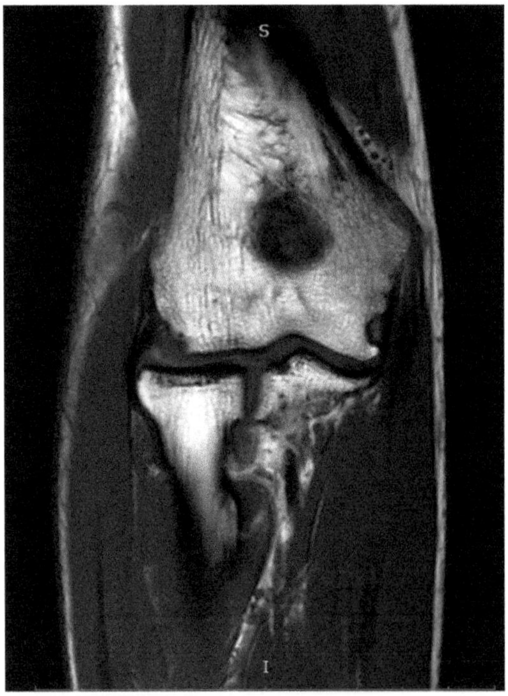

Fig. 28.7 Coronal T1-weighted MR image of the right elbow

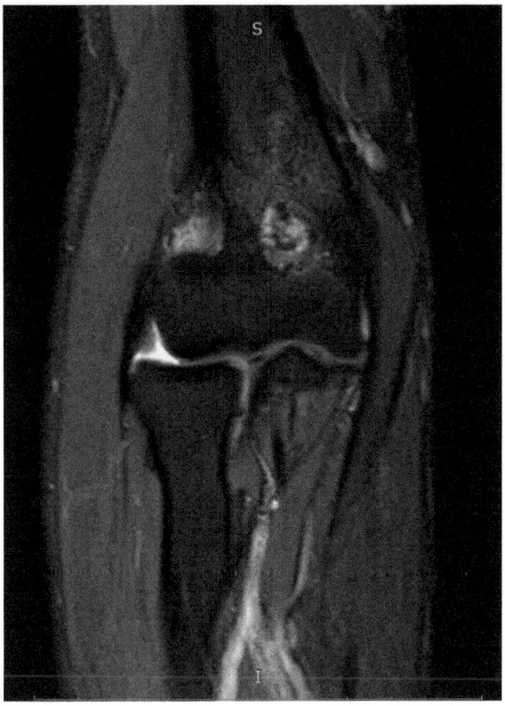

Fig. 28.8 Coronal fat-suppressed T2-weighted MR image of the right elbow

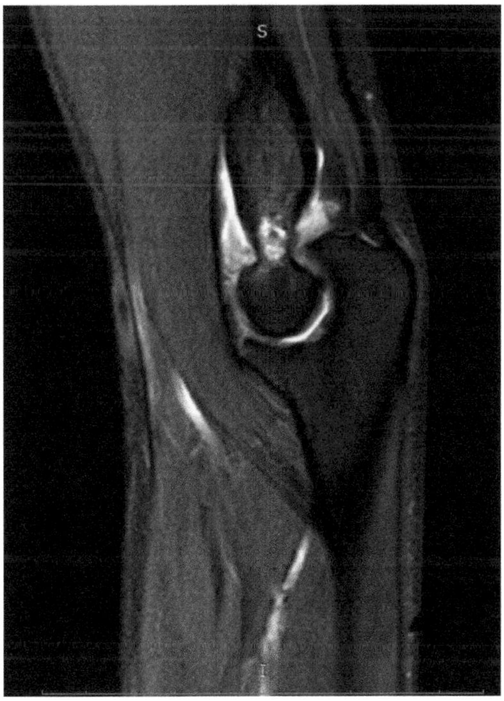

Fig. 28.9 Sagittal fat-suppressed T2-weighted MR image of the right elbow

MR images of the right elbow demonstrate a small lesion with low T1 and high T2 signal at the right distal humerus with internal punctuate low signal. There is extensive surrounding soft tissue edema.

28.4 Description and Discussion from Residents

Radiographs of the right elbow show increased bone density of the distal right humerus anteriorly and medially with cortical thickening and preserved joint space of the elbow. There is no significant soft tissue swelling. On the CT images, there is a low-density lesion in the distal right humerus with internal high densities and peripheral sclerosis. Given the history of night pain, the top consideration is osteoid osteoma. On the MR images, the lesion shows low T1 and high T2 signal with internal low signal and soft tissue edema around the elbow, consistent with the diagnosis of osteoid osteoma.

28.5 Analysis and Comments from Professor Xiaoguang Cheng

There is focal cortical thickening of the distal right humerus with internal lucency. There are high densities inside the lesion (sequestrum? mineralization of the nidus?). Reactive changes are noted around the lesion. This is likely a benign lesion, such as osteoid osteoma with osteoblastoma in the differential diagnosis.

28.6 Diagnosis

Osteoid osteoma.

Suggested Reading

Chai JW, Hong SH, Choi JY, et al. Radiologic diagnosis of osteoid osteoma: from simple to challenging findings. Radiographics. 2010 May;30(3):737–49.

Kransdorf MJ, Stull MA, Gilkey FW, et al. Osteoid osteoma. Radiographics. 1991 Jul;11(4):671–96.

29 Langerhans Cell Histiocytosis (Eosinophilic Granuloma): Case 4

29.1 Medical History

The patient is a 17-year-old female. She presented with right upper arm pain for more than 2 months. She has a history of bone biopsy.

29.2 Physical Examination

There is focal deep point tenderness around the right distal upper arm.

29.3 Imaging Findings

29.3.1 Radiograph

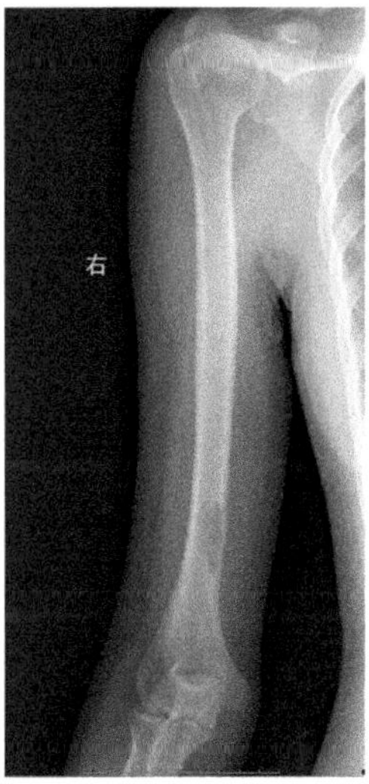

Fig. 29.1 Frontal view of the right upper arm

X. Cheng et al., *Imaging of Bone Tumors in Shoulder and Elbow*,
https://doi.org/10.1007/978-981-33-6150-8_29

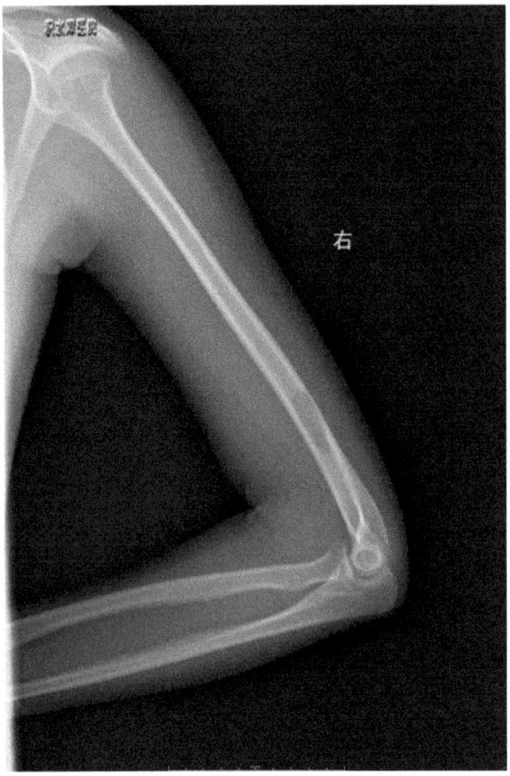

Fig. 29.2 Lateral view of the right upper arm

Radiographs of the right upper arm demonstrate focal osseous destruction at the distal humeral shaft.

29.3.2 CT Imaging

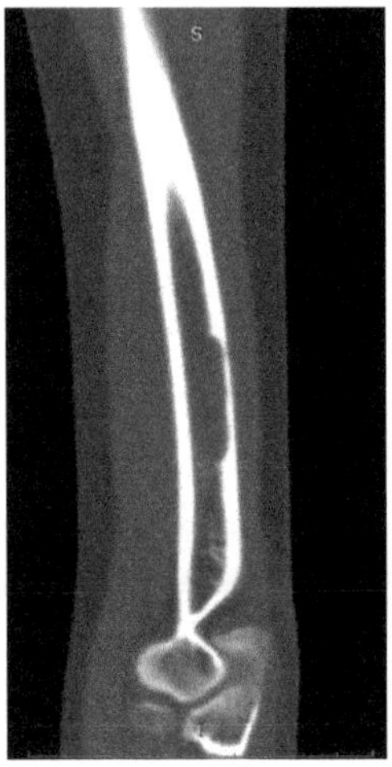

Fig. 29.3 Sagittal CT image of the right humerus in bone window

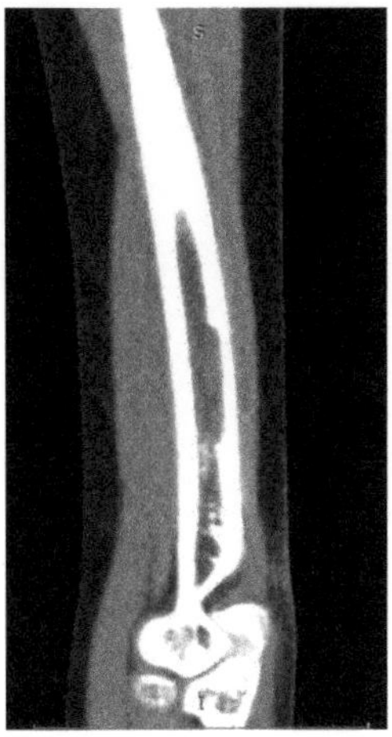

Fig. 29.4 Sagittal CT image of the right humerus in soft tissue window

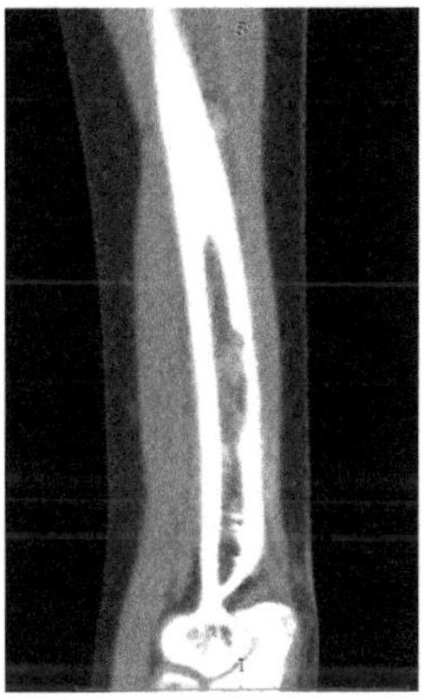

Fig. 29.5 Sagittal post-contrast CT image of the right humerus in soft tissue window

CT images of the right humerus demonstrate focal lytic osseous destruction of the distal humerus with the lesion's long axis parallel to the humerus. The lesion shows a clear margin without associated soft tissue mass. There is irregular enhancement.

29.3.3 MR Imaging

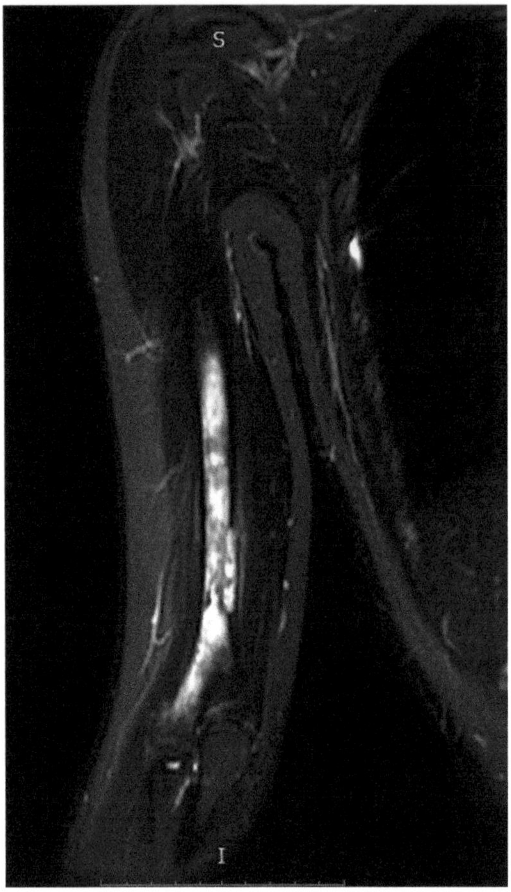

Fig. 29.6 Coronal fat-suppressed T2-weighted MR image of the right humerus

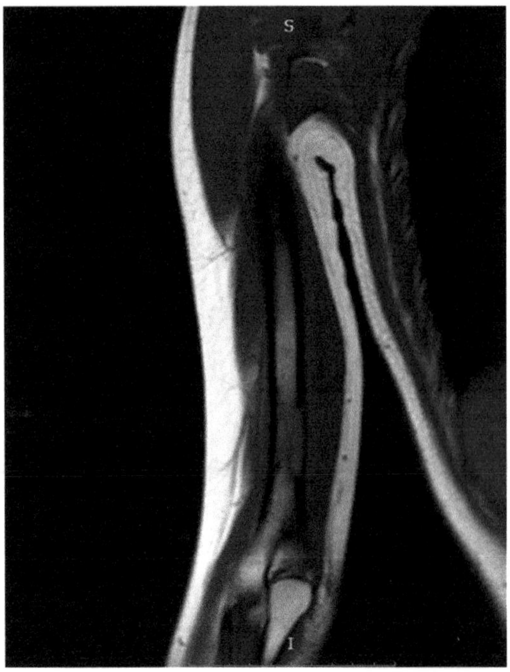

Fig. 29.7 Coronal T1-weighted MR image of the right humerus

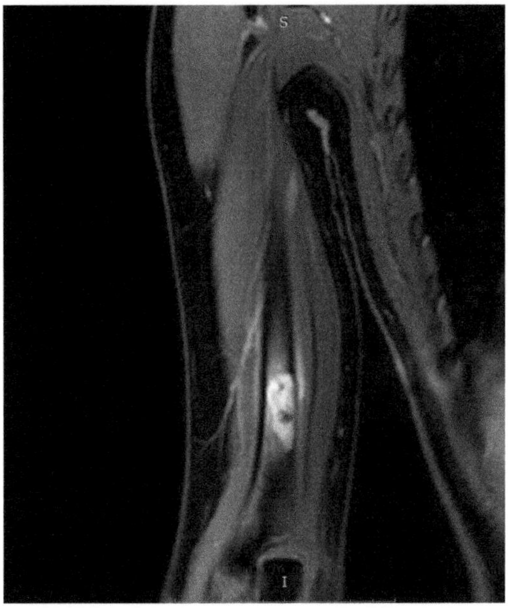

Fig. 29.8 Coronal post-contrast fat-suppressed T1-weighted MR image of the right humerus

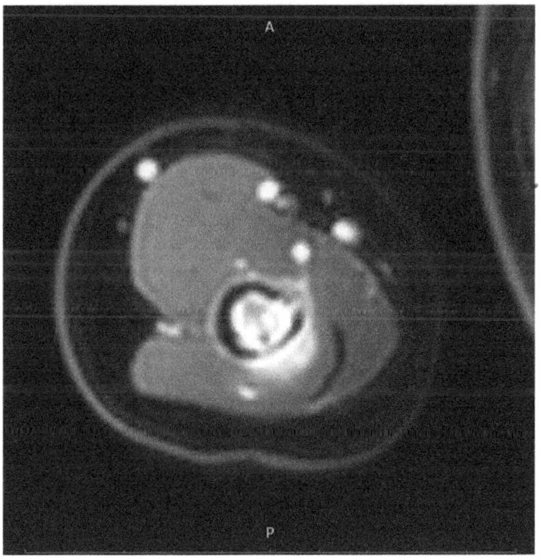

Fig. 29.9 Axial post-contrast fat-suppressed T1-weighted MR image of the right humerus

MR images of the right humerus demonstrate the lesion at the distal humerus with iso-intense T1 signal and heterogeneous high T2 signal. There is focal thinning of the cortex with marrow cdcma. Heterogeneous enhancement is noted.

29.4 Description and Discussion from Residents

The patient is an adolescent. Radiograph shows focal osseous destruction of the distal right humerus with the long axis parallel to the humerus and thinning of the cortex without periosteal reaction. On the CT images, there is no soft tissue mass or peripheral sclerosis. Focal enhancement is noted. This could be eosinophilic granuloma; however, neoplasm could not be excluded. On the MR images, there is marrow edema of the lesion with linear edema along the cortex, again suggestive of eosinophilic granuloma. Osteomyelitis should be excluded. Usually, with osteomyelitis, the clinical symptom is severe, not consistent with the current case.

29.5 Analysis and Comments from Professor Xiaoguang Cheng

The patient is an adolescent. Radiographs demonstrate the lesion at the shaft of the distal right humerus with clear margin and focal cortical thinning, the top consideration is eosinophilic granuloma. No soft tissue mass is seen on the CT scan, Ewing sarcoma can be excluded. MR images show surrounding soft tissue edema with enhancement, which could be an eosinophilic granuloma.

29.6 Diagnosis

Langerhans cell histiocytosis (Eosinophilic granuloma).

Suggested Reading

Samet J, Weinstein J, Fayad LM. MRI and clinical features of Langerhans cell histiocytosis (LCH) in the pelvis and extremities: can LCH really look like anything? Skeletal Radiol. 2016 May;45(5):607–13.

Zaveri J, La Q, Yarmish G, et al. More than just Langerhans cell histiocytosis: a radiologic review of histiocytic disorders. Radiographics. 2014 Nov–Dec;34(7):2008–24.

Clear Cell Sarcoma: Case 5

30

30.1 Medical History

The patient is a 20-year-old male. He presented with right elbow mass about 6 years ago without inciting event. The mass increased in size about 1 year ago and became painful. The patient had history of biopsy with chemotherapy and radiation.

30.2 Physical Examination

There was a 4 cm × 3 cm palpable mass at the lateral aspect of the right elbow, hard, non-mobile with focal point tenderness.

30.3 Imaging Findings

30.3.1 Radiograph

X. Cheng et al., *Imaging of Bone Tumors in Shoulder and Elbow*,
https://doi.org/10.1007/978-981-33-6150-8_30

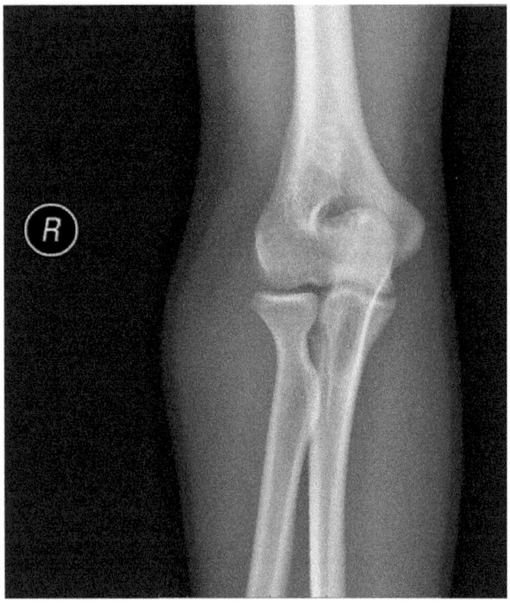

Fig. 30.1 Frontal view of the right elbow

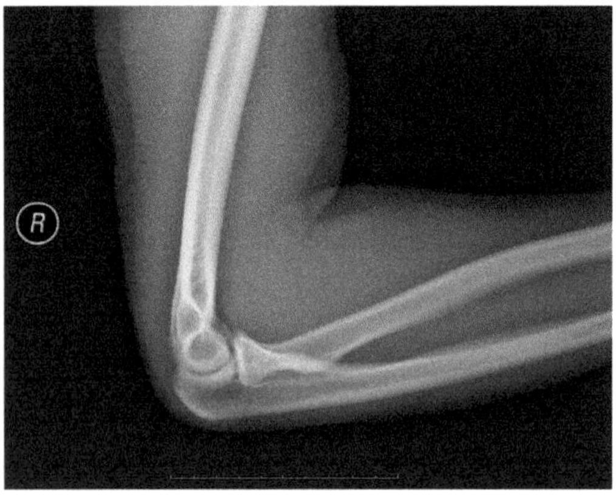

Fig. 30.2 Lateral view of the right elbow

Radiographs of the right elbow demonstrate lateral soft tissue swelling of the right elbow. No abnormality is noted in the osseous structures.

30.3.2 CT Imaging

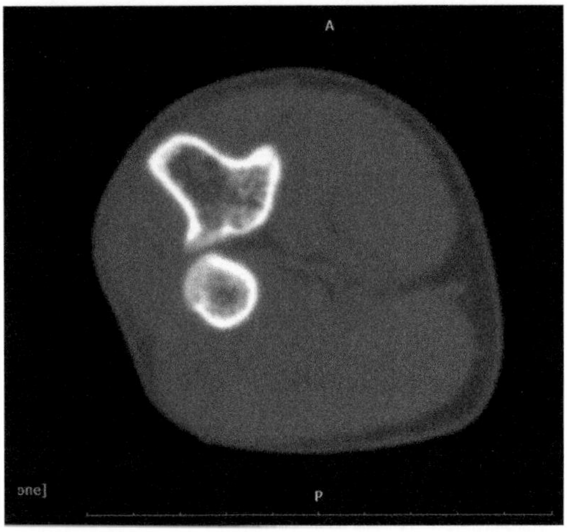

Fig. 30.3 Axial CT image of the right elbow in bone window

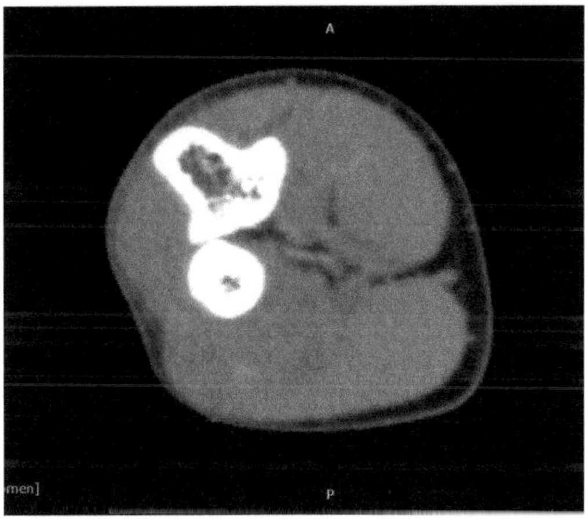

Fig. 30.4 Axial CT image of the right elbow in soft tissue window

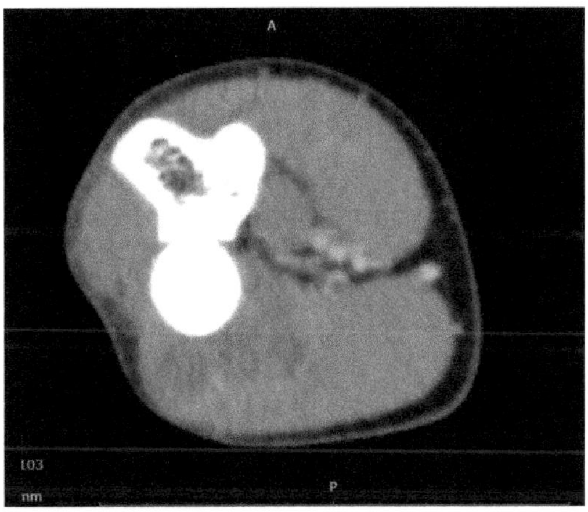

Fig. 30.5 Axial post-contrast CT image of the right elbow in soft tissue window

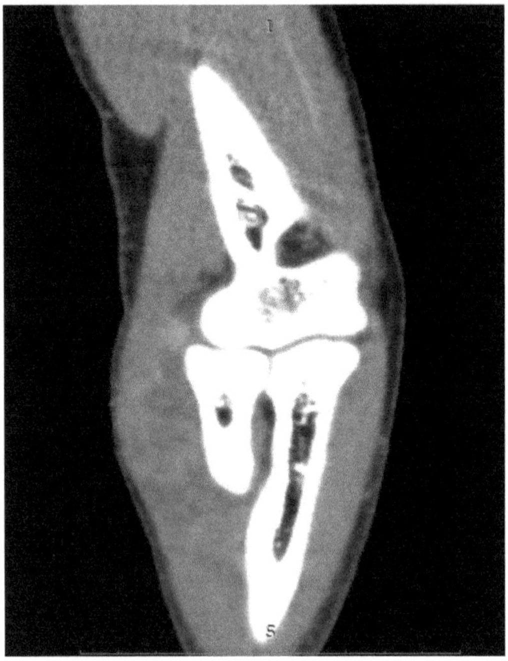

Fig. 30.6 Coronal post-contrast CT image of the right elbow in soft tissue window

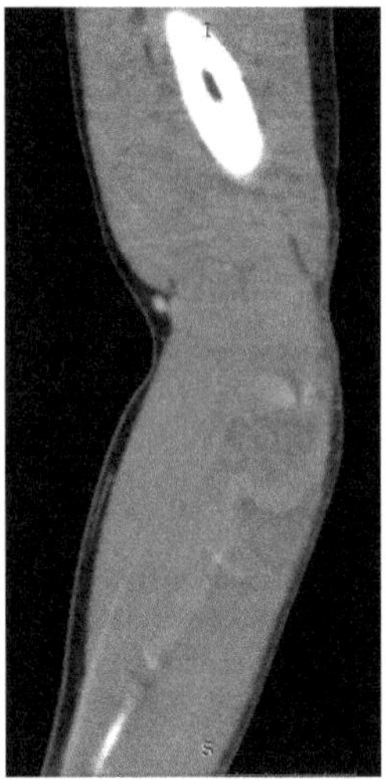

Fig. 30.7 Sagittal post-contrast CT image of the right elbow in soft tissue window

CT images of the right elbow demonstrate soft tissue mass around the right elbow with homogeneous densities but no clear margin. There is irregular enhancement. No abnormality is noted in the osseous structures.

30.3.3 MR Imaging

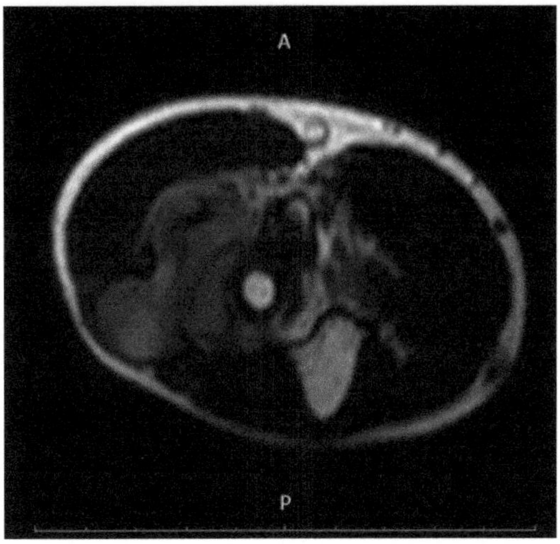

Fig. 30.8 Axial T2-weighted MR image of the right elbow

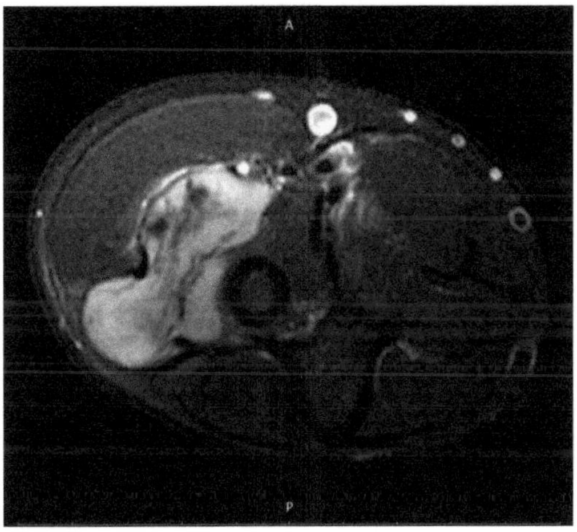

Fig. 30.9 Axial fat-suppressed T2-weighted MR image of the right elbow

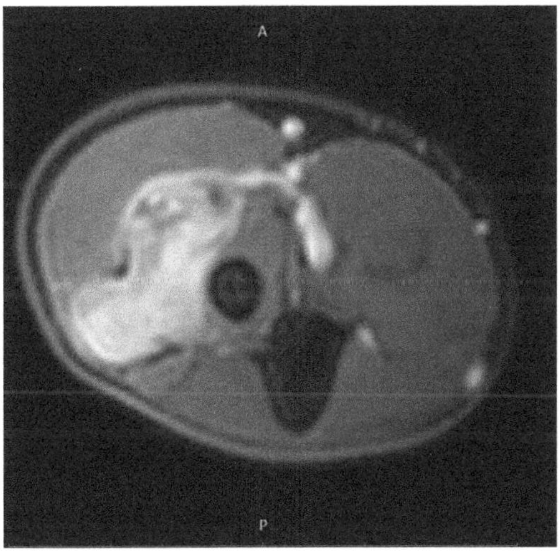

Fig. 30.10 Axial post-contrast fat-suppressed T1-weighted MR image of the right elbow

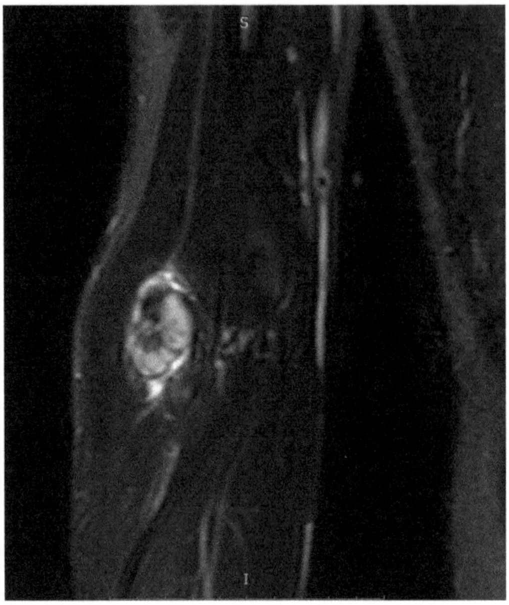

Fig. 30.11 Coronal fat-suppressed T2-weighted MR image of the right elbow

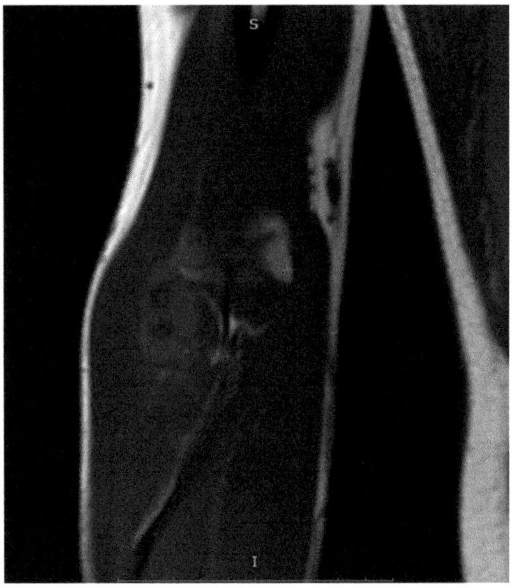

Fig. 30.12 Coronal T1-weighted MR image of the right elbow

MR images of the right elbow demonstrate the soft tissue mass around the radial aspect of the right elbow. The mass is of iso-intense T1 signal to muscle, mixed heterogeneous high T2 signal on fat-suppressed sequence and heterogeneous enhancement.

30.4 Description and Discussion from Residents

The patient is a young male. There is soft tissue swelling at the lateral aspect of the right elbow on radiographs without osseous abnormality. On CT images, the soft tissue mass around the right elbow is noted surrounding the proximal radius and ulna with inhomogeneous density and no clear margin. Avid enhancement is noted with circular morphology and internal patchy low density. The adjacent osseous structures are intact. Given the relatively long history, this is likely of a benign process. The lesion is noted to be lateral to the proximal radius, elliptical in shape. Low signal is noted on T1 and fat-suppressed T2 weighted sequences, likely representing desmoid-type fibromatosis. Nerve sheath tumor and synovial sarcoma are in the differential diagnosis.

30.5 Analysis and Comments from Professor Xiaoguang Cheng

Based on radiographs alone, it is extremely hard to be certain if there is a soft tissue mass along the radial aspect of the right elbow. On the CT images, there is soft tissue mass along the radial head with low density and no clear margin with avid enhancement. The adjacent osseous structures are intact. MR images demonstrate soft tissue mass at the radial aspect of the elbow without a clear margin with avid enhancement. The top consideration is desmoid-type fibromatosis with synovial sarcoma in the differential diagnosis.

30.6 Diagnosis

Clear cell sarcoma.

Suggested Reading

De Beuckeleer LH, De Schepper AM, Vandevenne JE, et al. MR imaging of clear cell sarcoma (malignant melanoma of the soft parts): a multicenter correlative MRI-pathology study of 21 cases and literature review. Skeletal Radiol. 2000 Apr;29(4):187–95.

Isoda H, Kuroda M, Saitoh M, et al. MR findings of clear cell sarcoma: two case reports. Clin Imaging. 2003 Jul-Aug;27(4):229–32.

31 Chondrosarcoma: Case 6

31.1 Medical History

The patient is a 22-year-old male. He presented with right anterior arm pain for 5 years and worsening pain with restriction of extension of the elbow joint for 3 years. He had a history of biopsy.

31.2 Physical Examination

There is a flexion deformity of the right elbow with an anterior protruding mass, hard.

31.3 Imaging Findings

31.3.1 Radiograph

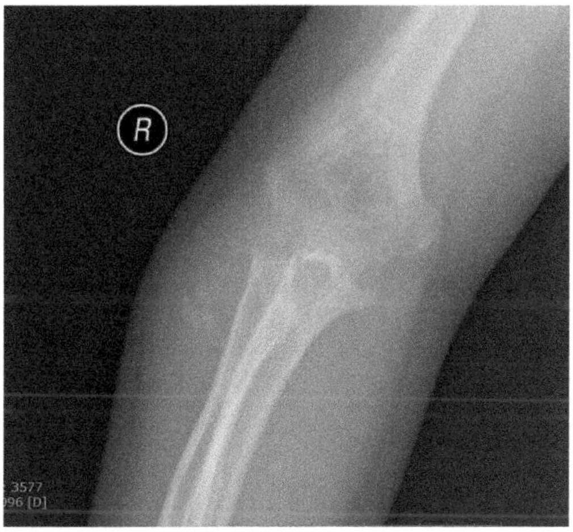

Fig. 31.1 Frontal view of the right elbow

X. Cheng et al., *Imaging of Bone Tumors in Shoulder and Elbow*,
https://doi.org/10.1007/978-981-33-6150-8_31

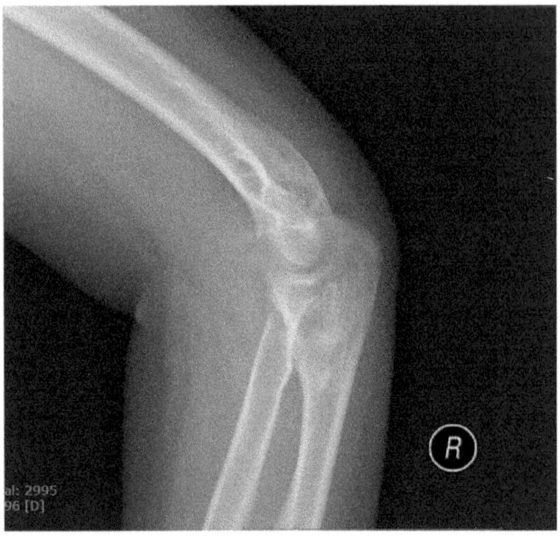

Fig. 31.2 Lateral view of the right elbow

Radiographs of the right elbow demonstrate osseous destruction around the elbow with adjacent soft tissue mass and internal linear high densities.

31.3.2 CT Imaging

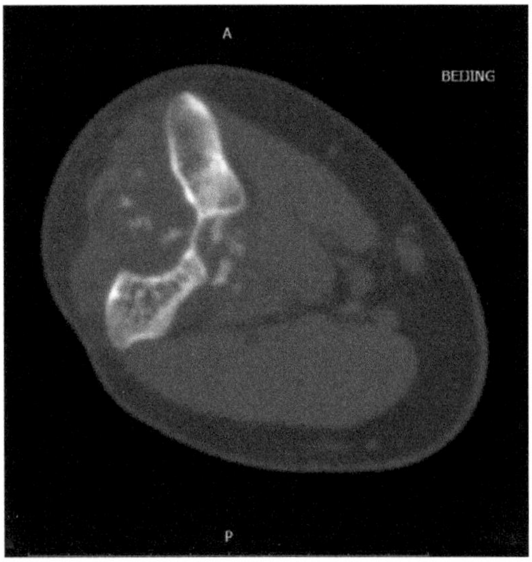

Fig. 31.3 Axial CT image of the right elbow in bone window

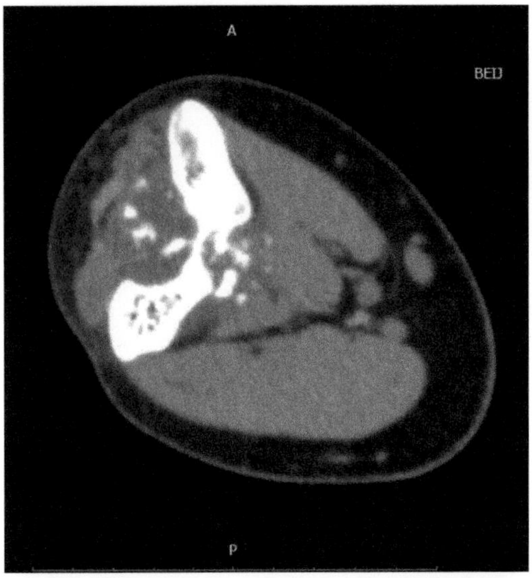

Fig. 31.4 Axial CT image of the right elbow in soft tissue window

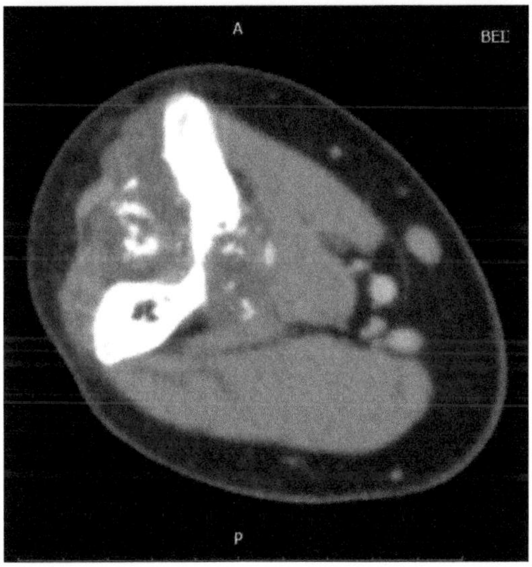

Fig. 31.5 Axial post-contrast CT image of the right elbow in soft tissue window

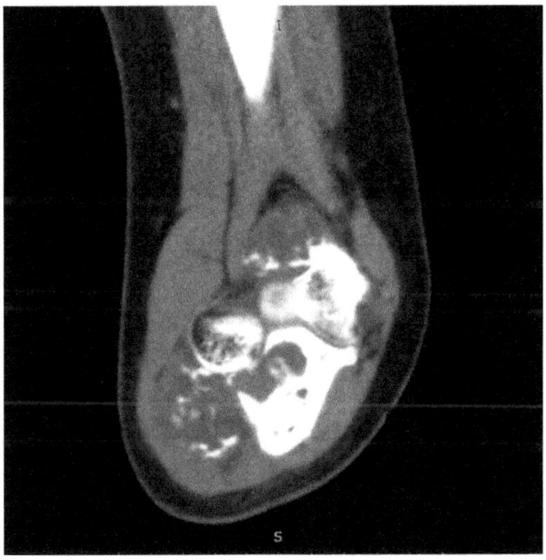

Fig. 31.6 Coronal CT image of the right elbow in soft tissue window

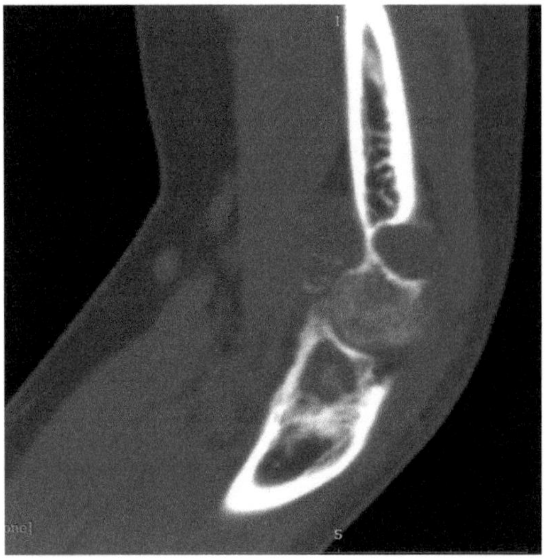

Fig. 31.7 Sagittal CT image of the right elbow in bone window

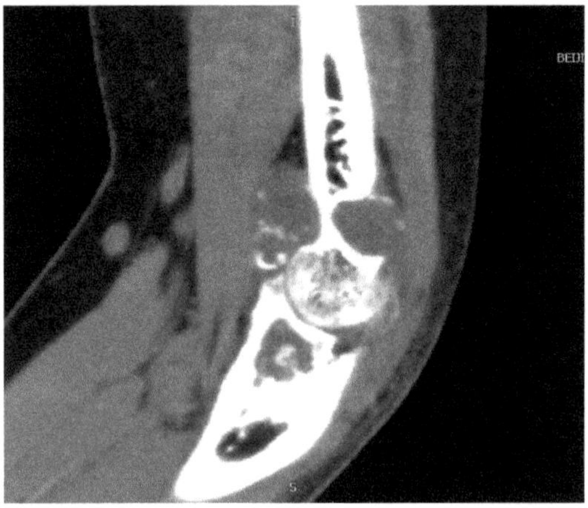

Fig. 31.8 Sagittal CT image of the right elbow in soft tissue window

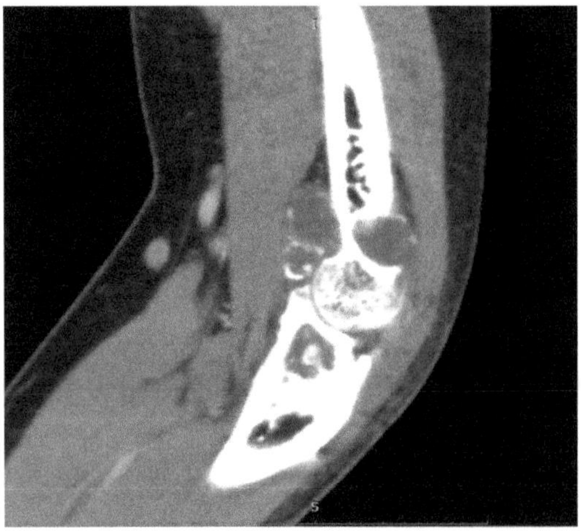

Fig. 31.9 Sagittal post-contrast CT image of the right elbow in soft tissue window

CT images of the right elbow demonstrate osseous destruction around the proximal radius and ulna with indistinct margin. There is irregular soft tissue mass in the elbow joint with internal multiple septations and scattered high densities. Mild peripheral enhancement is noted.

31.3.3 MR Imaging

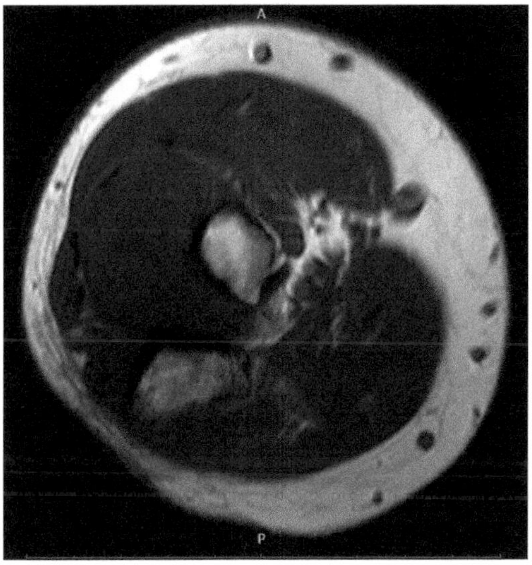

Fig. 31.10 Axial T1-weighted MR image of the right elbow

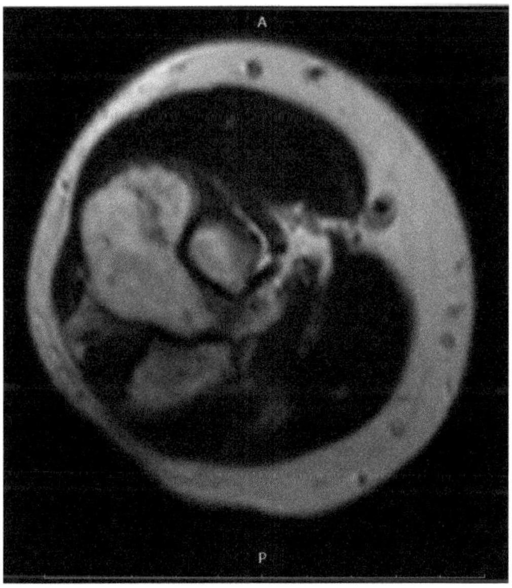

Fig. 31.11 Axial T2-weighted MR image of the right elbow

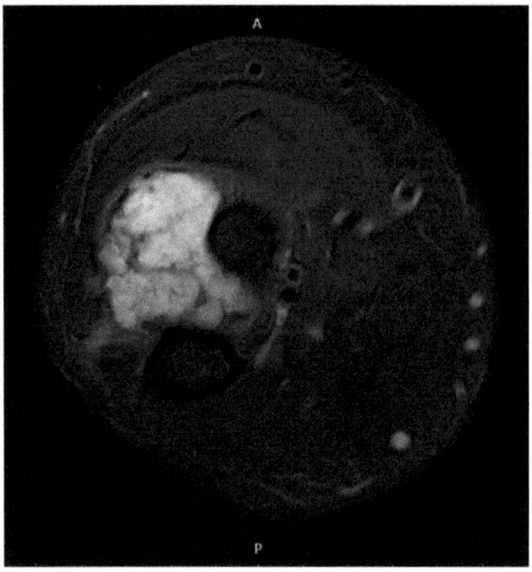

Fig. 31.12 Axial fat-suppressed T2-weighted MR image of the right elbow

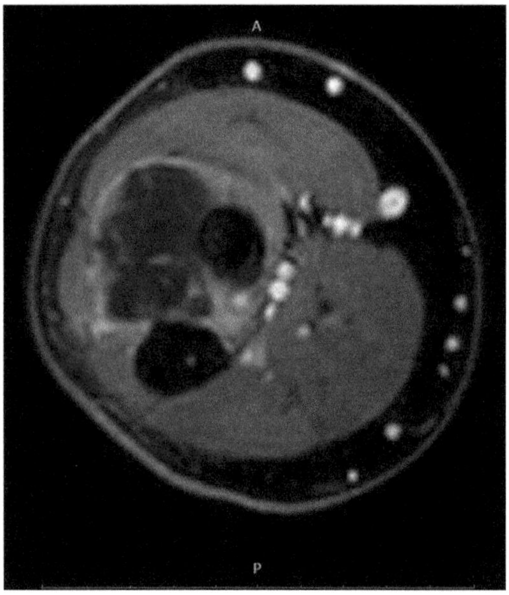

Fig. 31.13 Axial post-contrast fat-suppressed T1-weighted MR image of the right elbow

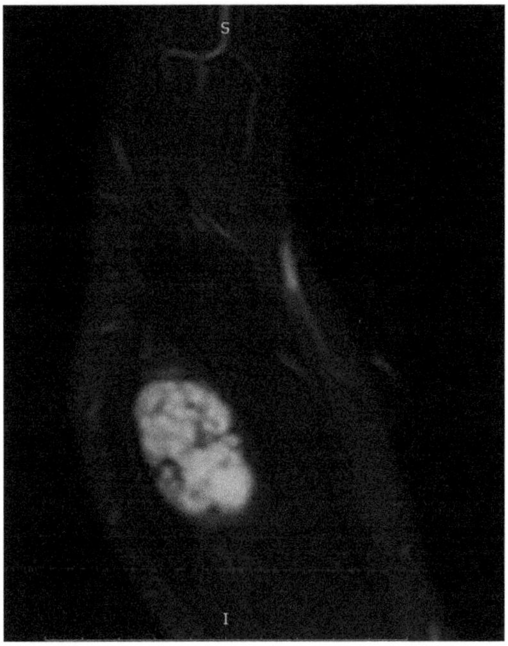

Fig. 31.14 Sagittal fat-suppressed T2-weighted MR image of the right elbow

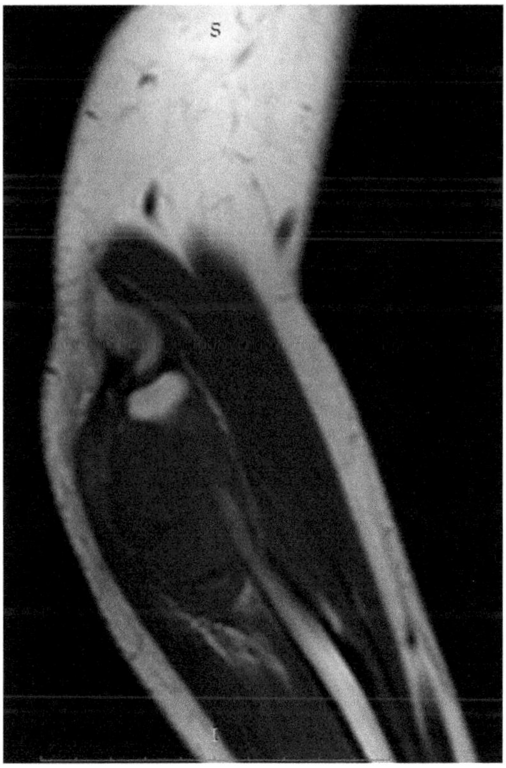

Fig. 31.15 Sagittal T1-weighted MR image of the right elbow

MR images of the right elbow demonstrate the soft tissue mass around the proximal radius and ulna with iso-intense T1 signal to muscle and high T2 signal. There are small septations in the mass with peripheral enhancement and enhancement around the septations.

31.4 Description and Discussion from Residents

The patient is a young male. Radiographs demonstrate osseous destruction around the right elbow joint with internal heterogeneous densities. There is adjacent soft tissue mass with internal linear high densities. The above findings support arthropathy, such as synovial osteochondromatosis. On the CT images, there are calcifications along the septations of the soft tissue mass around the right elbow with mild peripheral enhancement and enhancement along the septations. These findings are suggestive of a chondrogenic tumor. MR images demonstrate chondroid matrix in the lesion, support chondrogenic tumor. However, chondrogenic tumor rarely grows along the joint, differential diagnosis should include synovial osteochondromatosis.

31.5 Analysis and Comments from Professor Xiaoguang Cheng

The radiographs demonstrate a forced position of the right elbow. There are internal calcifications within the soft tissue mass around the proximal radius without joint space compromise. On the CT images, multiple tiny calcifications are noted within the joint with relatively preserved joint space, thus, inflammatory arthropathy and tuberculosis can be excluded. No avid enhancement is noted, the first consideration is synovial osteochondromatosis. However, there are imaging features that do not support this diagnosis: synovial osteochondromatosis rarely causes such a large extent of osseous destruction. The next consideration is chondrosarcoma; however, there is usually tumor-centric expansion and it rarely affects the joint. On the MR images, there is a significant amount of chondroid matrix in the joint without significant enhancement. Overall, synovial osteochondromatosis is the favored diagnosis, while chondrosarcoma is in the differential diagnosis.

31.6 Diagnosis

Chondrosarcoma.

Suggested Reading

Douis H, Saifuddin A. The imaging of cartilaginous bone tumours. II. Chondrosarcoma. Skeletal Radiol. 2013 May;42(5):611–26.

Murphey MD, Walker EA, Wilson AJ, et al. From the archives of the AFIP: imaging of primary chondrosarcoma: radiologic-pathologic correlation. Radiographics. 2003 Sep-Oct;23(5):1245–78.

Pigmented Villonodular Synovitis (PVNS): Case 7

32

32.1 Medical History

The patient is a 47-year-old female. She presented with left elbow pain for 8 months. She had a history of biopsy.

32.2 Physical Examination

There was a deep mass around the left elbow with clear margin, rubbery, smooth, and mobile, without point tenderness.

32.3 Imaging Findings

32.3.1 Radiograph

X. Cheng et al., *Imaging of Bone Tumors in Shoulder and Elbow*,
https://doi.org/10.1007/978-981-33-6150-8_32

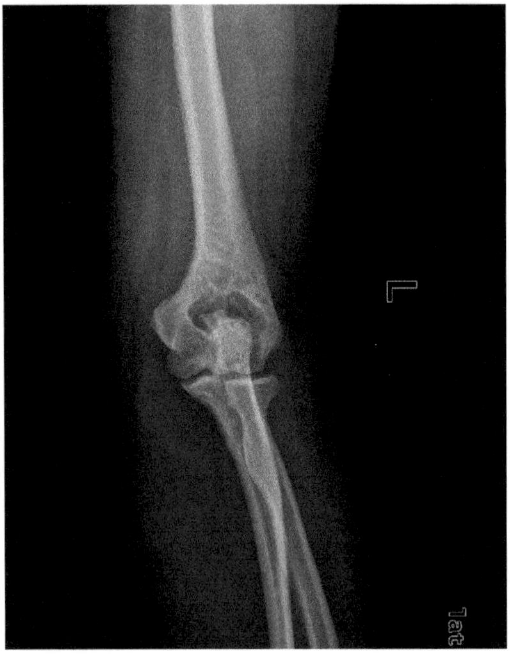

Fig. 32.1 Frontal view of the left elbow

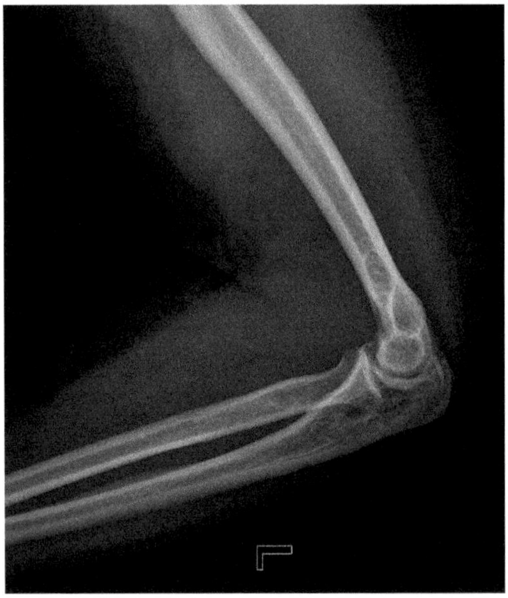

Fig. 32.2 Lateral view of the left elbow

Radiographs of the left elbow demonstrate osseous destruction around the distal humerus, and around the coronoid process of the ulna with clear margin and surrounding soft tissue swelling. There is a relatively preserved joint space.

32.3.2 CT Imaging

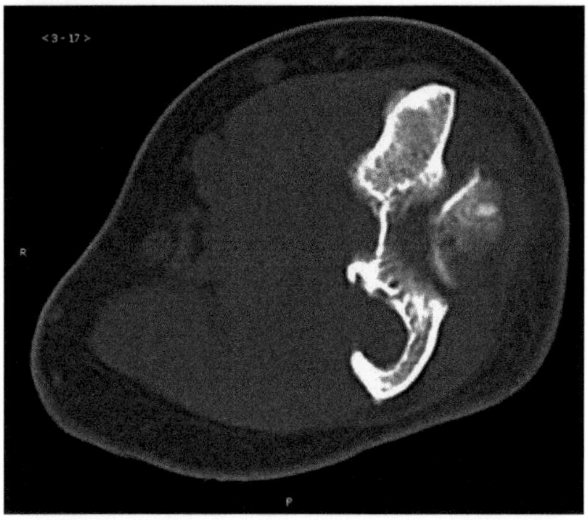

Fig. 32.3 Axial CT image of the left elbow in bone window

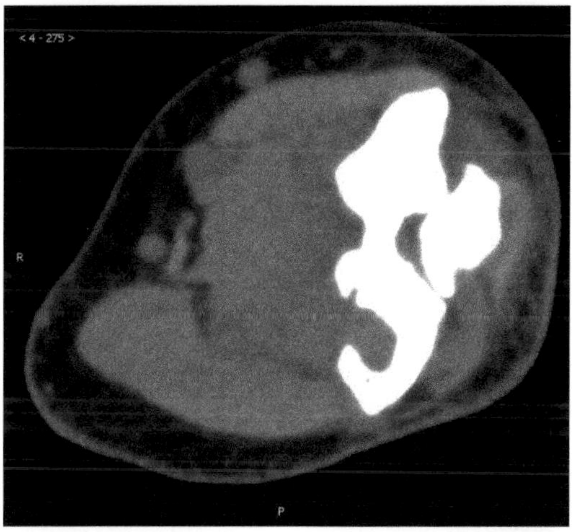

Fig. 32.4 Axial CT image of the left elbow in soft tissue window

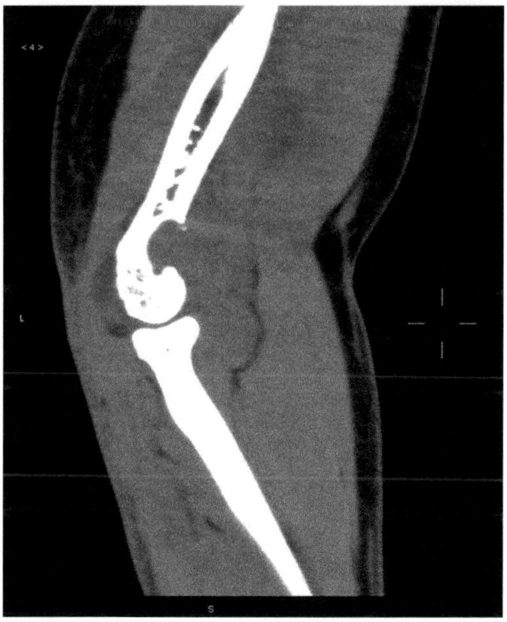

Fig. 32.5 Sagittal CT image of the left elbow in soft tissue window

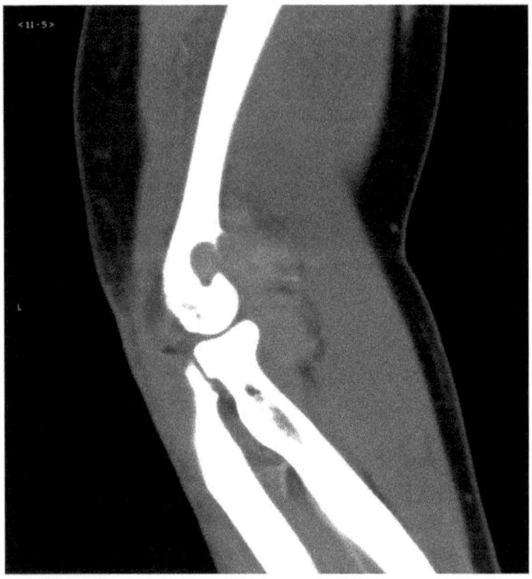

Fig. 32.6 Sagittal post-contrast CT image of the left elbow in soft tissue window

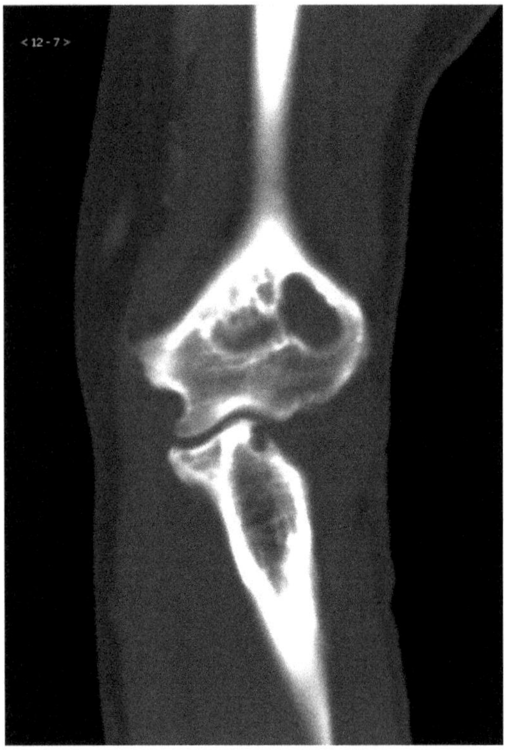

Fig. 32.7 Coronal CT image of the left elbow in bone window

CT images of the left elbow demonstrate osseous destruction around the distal humerus and coronoid process of the ulna with thickening of the elbow joint capsule. There is a soft tissue mass around the left elbow. Avid enhancement is noted around the soft tissue mass.

32.3.3 MR Imaging

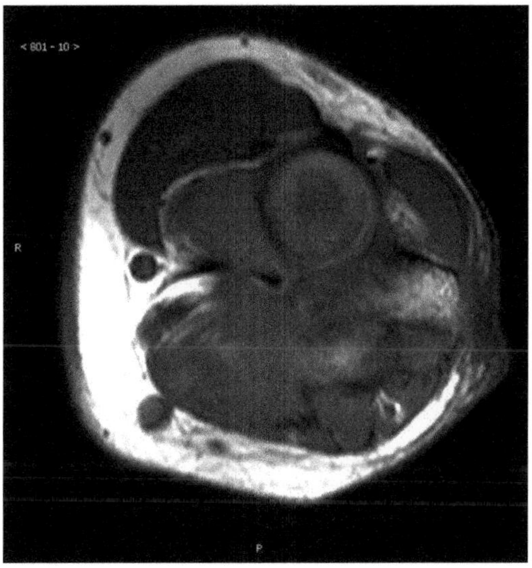

Fig. 32.8 Axial T1-weighted MR image of the left elbow

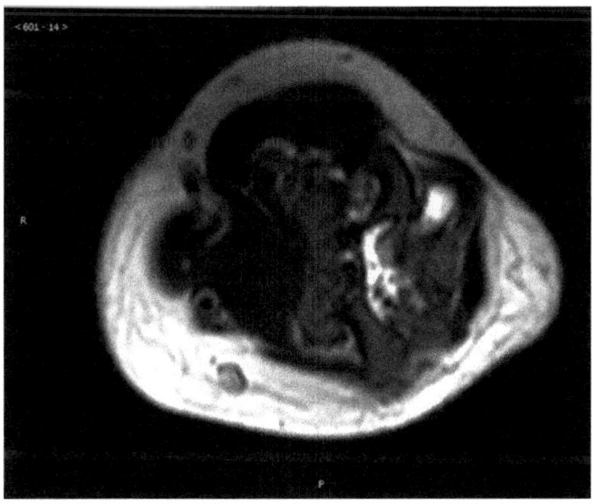

Fig. 32.9 Axial T2-weighted MR image of the left elbow

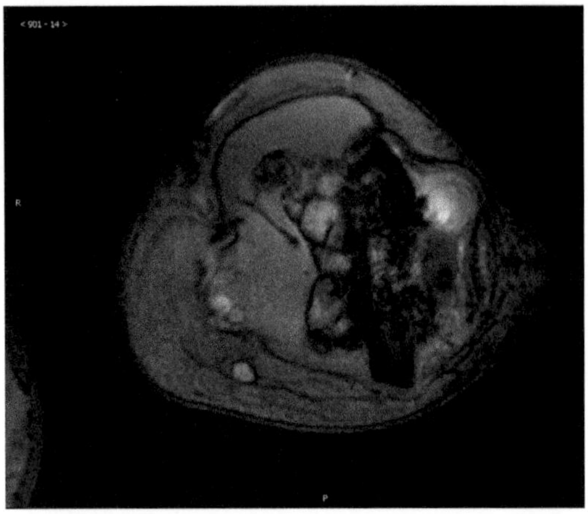

Fig. 32.10 Axial GRE (gradient echo) sequence MR image of the left elbow

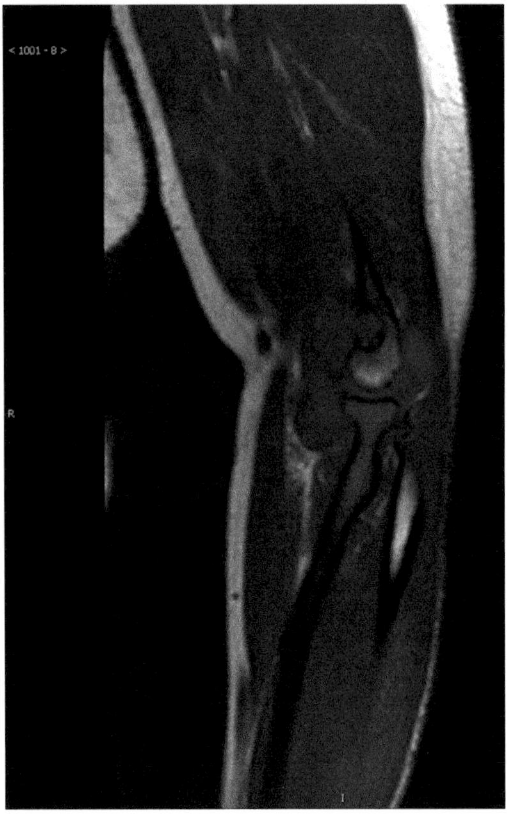

Fig. 32.11 Sagittal T1-weighted MR image of the left elbow

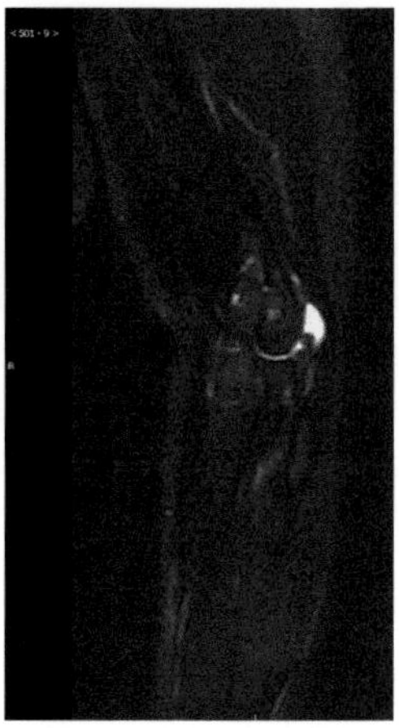

Fig. 32.12 Sagittal fat-suppressed T2-weighted MR image of the left elbow

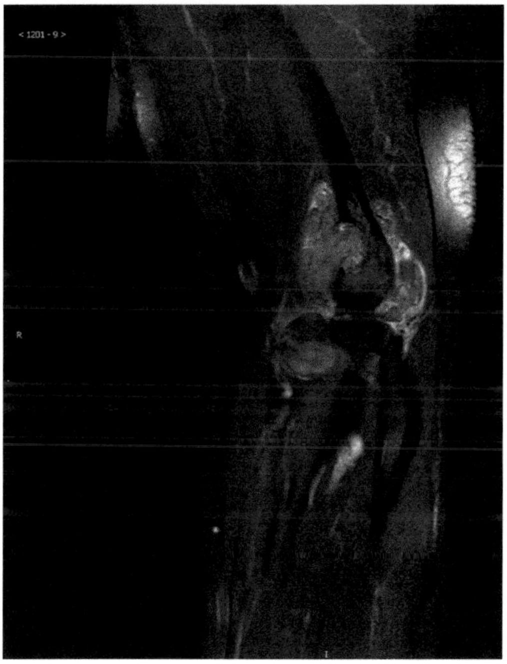

Fig. 32.13 Sagittal post-contrast fat-suppressed T1-weighted MR image of the left elbow

MR images of the left elbow demonstrate marked nodular thickening of the synovium around the elbow. There is related destruction of the distal humerus and the coronoid process of the ulna with blooming artifacts on the GRE sequence. Heterogenous enhancement is also noted.

32.4 Description and Discussion from Residents

The patient is a middle-aged female. Radiographs demonstrate osseous destruction around the left distal humerus and the coronoid process of the ulna with associated soft tissue mass and relatively preserved joint spaces. On the CT images, there are cyst-like erosions around the bones of the elbow with a clear margin, communicating with the joint. The associated soft tissue mass extends along the joint capsule, suggesting the synovial origin of the lesion. The osseous erosions appear to be caused by the thickened synovium, typical for pigmented villonodular synovitis (PVNS). There are nodular and lobular enhancements along the hypertrophied synovium on the post-contrast images. Low signal is noted in all sequences on the MR images, compatible with hemosiderin deposition. Overall, the diagnosis favors PVNS.

32.5 Analysis and Comments from Professor Xiaoguang Cheng

The radiographs demonstrate preserved joint space of the left elbow without decreased bone density, indicating a joint centric process. CT images demonstrate osseous erosions caused by hypertrophied synovium. MR images demonstrate characteristic hemosiderin deposition. Thus, this is a typical case of PVNS. Differential diagnoses should include idiopathic synovitis, hemophilia, and deposition disorder such as gout. The key characteristics of PVNS include: (1) Imaging findings out of proportion with the clinical symptoms; (2) no decreased bone density around the joint; and (3) relatively preserved joint space.

32.6 Diagnosis

Pigmented villonodular synovitis (PVNS).

Suggested Reading

Cheng XG, You YH, Liu W, et al. MRI features of pigmented villonodular synovitis (PVNS). Clin Rheumatol. 2004 Feb;23(1):31–34. Epub 2004 Jan 9.

Murphey MD, Rhee JH, Lewis RB, et al. Pigmented villonodular synovitis: radiologic-pathologic correlation. Radiographics. 2008 Sep-Oct;28(5):1493–518.

33 Polyostotic Fibrous Dysplasia: Case 8

33.1 Medical History

The patient is a 28-year-old male. He presented with right upper arm pain and discomfort for 1 month, worsening at night. The symptoms can resolve on their own.

33.2 Physical Examination

There was a hard mass around the right elbow without point tenderness. Secondary restriction of right elbow extension was noted.

33.3 Imaging Findings

33.3.1 Radiograph

X. Cheng et al., *Imaging of Bone Tumors in Shoulder and Elbow*,
https://doi.org/10.1007/978-981-33-6150-8_33

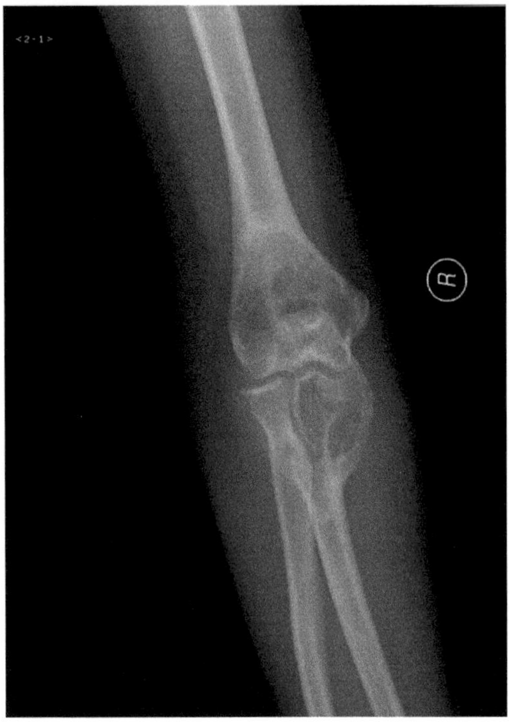

Fig. 33.1 Frontal view of the right elbow

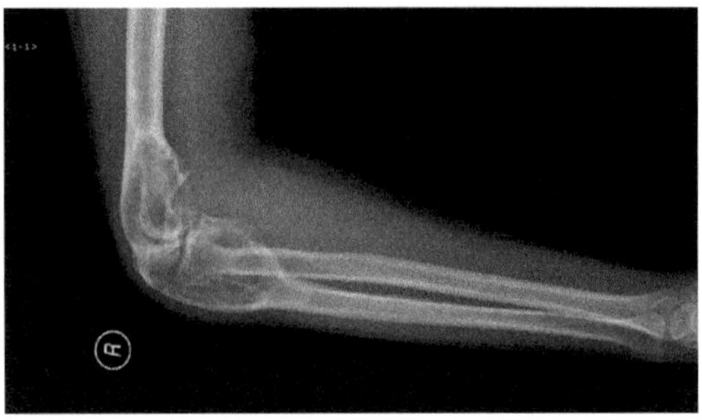

Fig. 33.2 Lateral view of the right elbow

Radiographs of the right elbow demonstrate osseous expansion of the distal humerus and proximal ulna with clear margin and peripheral sclerosis. There are internal septations. The joint spaces are relatively preserved.

33.3.2 CT Imaging

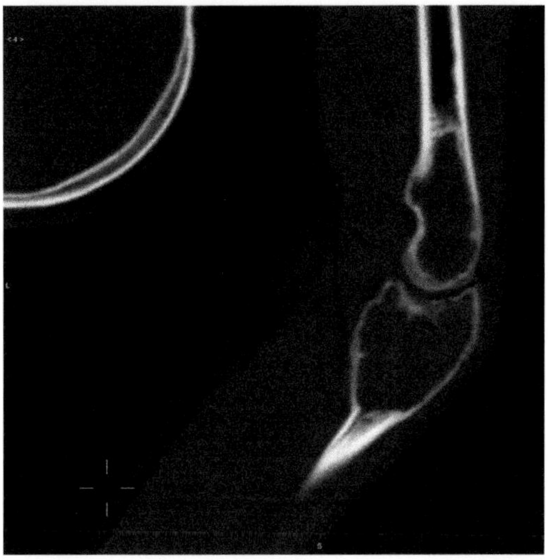

Fig. 33.3 Sagittal CT image of the right elbow in bone window

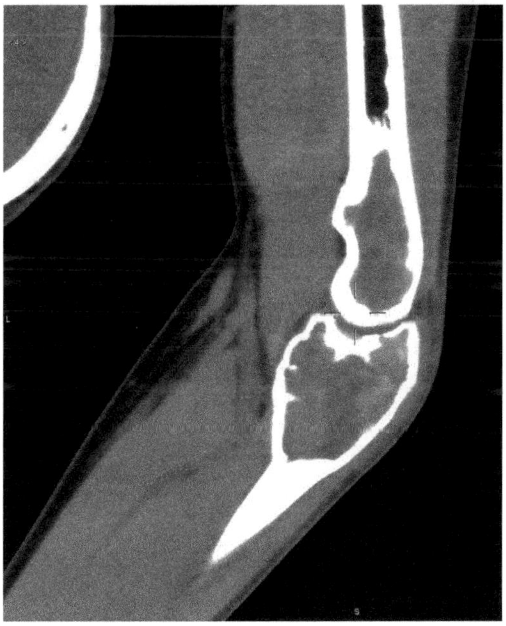

Fig. 33.4 Sagittal CT image of the right elbow in soft tissue window

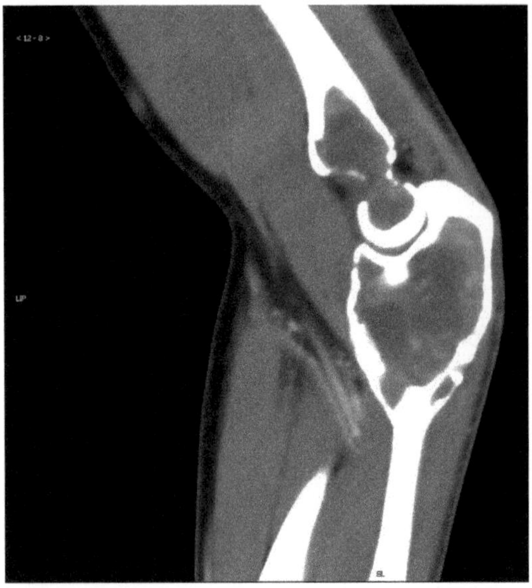

Fig. 33.5 Sagittal post-contrast CT image of the right elbow in soft tissue window

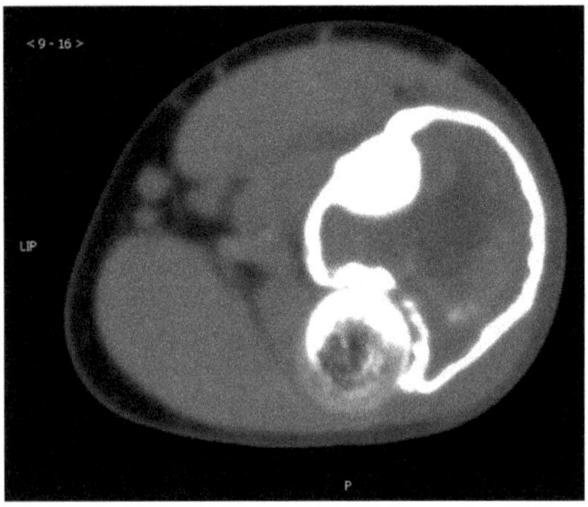

Fig. 33.6 Axial CT image of the right elbow in soft tissue window

CT images of the right elbow demonstrate osseous expansion of the distal humerus and proximal ulna with thinning of the cortex. There are heterogeneous densities of the intramedullary cavity of the affected areas with few high densities like osteoid matrix within. There are some focal cortical disruptions. No associated soft tissue mass is noted. Mild to moderate enhancement is seen of the lesion.

33.4 Description and Discussion from Residents

The patient is a young male. Radiographs demonstrate expansile osseous destructions of the right distal humerus and proximal ulna. CT images demonstrate the lesion with outer shell and peripheral sclerosis and no associated soft tissue mass. Heterogeneous density with focal ground-glass appearance is typical of fibrous dysplasia. Main differential diagnoses include multicentric giant cell tumor of bone and brown tumor from hyperparathyroidism. Focal discontinuity of the cortex likely reflects pathological fracture. Mild to moderate heterogeneous enhancement within the lesion, suggesting an active phase of the lesion.

33.5 Analysis and Comments from Professor Xiaoguang Cheng

The patient is a young male. Radiographs show multifocal expansile osseous destruction around the right elbow without decreased bone density or joint space loss, most likely a benign process. CT images demonstrate multifocal expansile osseous destruction and heterogeneous density of the intramedullary cavity with patchy ground-glass appearances, most suggestive of polyostotic fibrous dysplasia. Differential diagnosis includes multicentric giant cell tumor of bone. Multicentric giant cell tumor of bone is exceedingly rare with different enhancement patterns.

33.6 Diagnosis

Polyostotic fibrous dysplasia.

Suggested Reading

Jee WH, Choi KH, Choe BY, et al. Fibrous dysplasia: MR imaging characteristics with radiopathologic correlation. AJR Am J Roentgenol. 1996 Dec;167(6):1523–7.

Kransdorf MJ, Moser RP Jr, Gilkey FW. Fibrous dysplasia. Radiographics. 1990 May;10(3):519–37.

34 Angiolipoma: Case 9

34.1 Medical History

The patient is a 77-year-old female. She presented with a mass around the anterior and medial aspect of the left elbow for 4 years. The mass measured 4 cm × 3 cm. She noticed rapid growth with enlargement of the mass in the last half-year.

34.2 Physical Examination

There was a palpable, hard mass around the left elbow, measuring 6 cm × 3 cm × 3 cm with a clear margin and no point tenderness.

34.3 Imaging Findings

34.3.1 Radiograph

X. Cheng et al., *Imaging of Bone Tumors in Shoulder and Elbow*,
https://doi.org/10.1007/978-981-33-6150-8_34

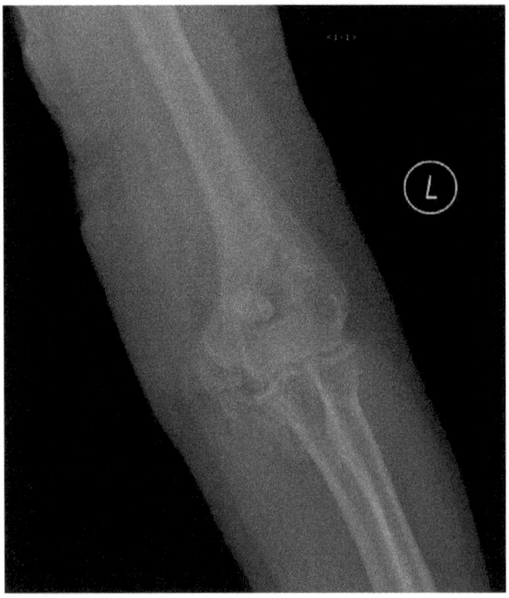

Fig. 34.1 Frontal view of the left elbow

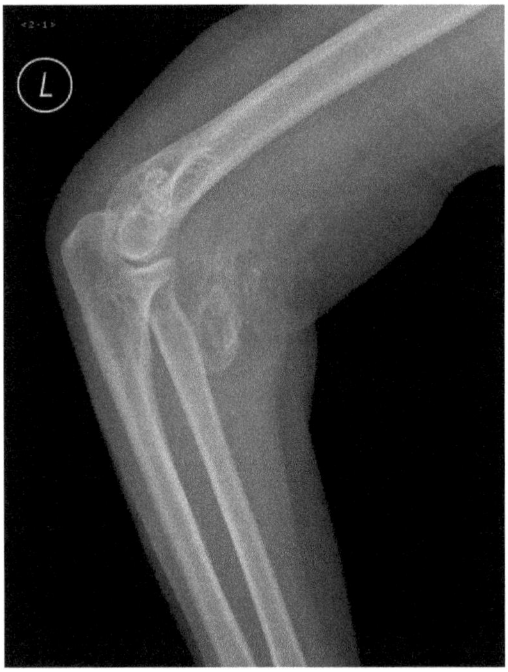

Fig. 34.2 Lateral view of the left elbow

Radiographs of the left elbow demonstrate a soft tissue mass in the ventral aspect with internal heterogeneous high densities. There is no osseous destruction around the elbow.

34.3.2 CT Imaging

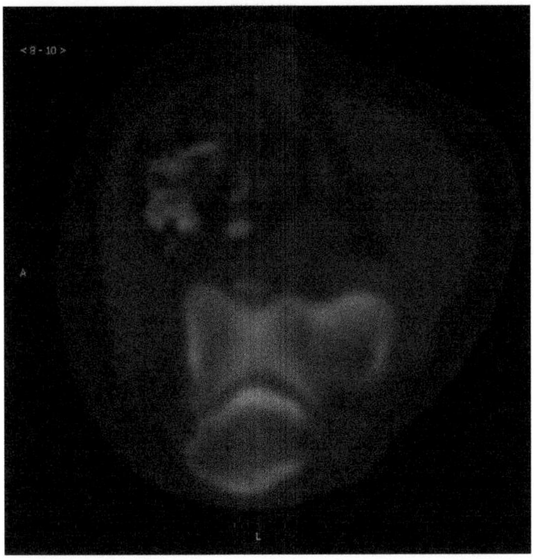

Fig. 34.3 Axial CT image of the left elbow in bone window

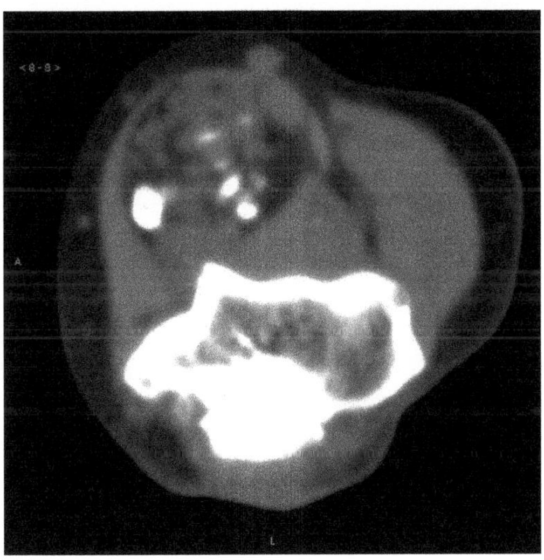

Fig. 34.4 Axial CT image of the left elbow in soft tissue window

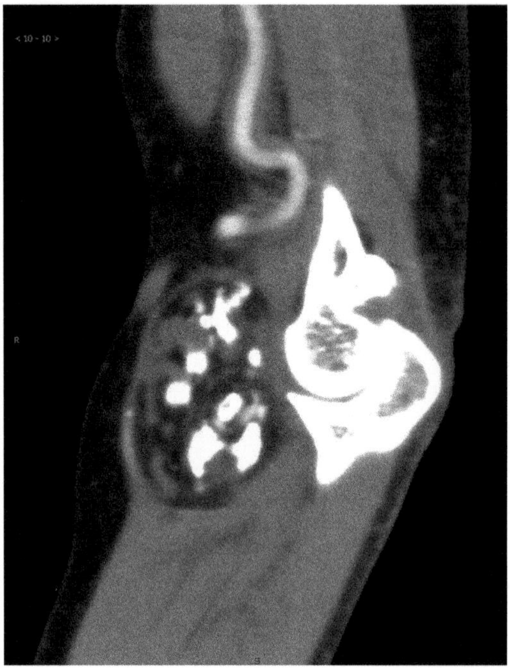

Fig. 34.5 Sagittal post-contrast CT image of the left elbow in soft tissue window

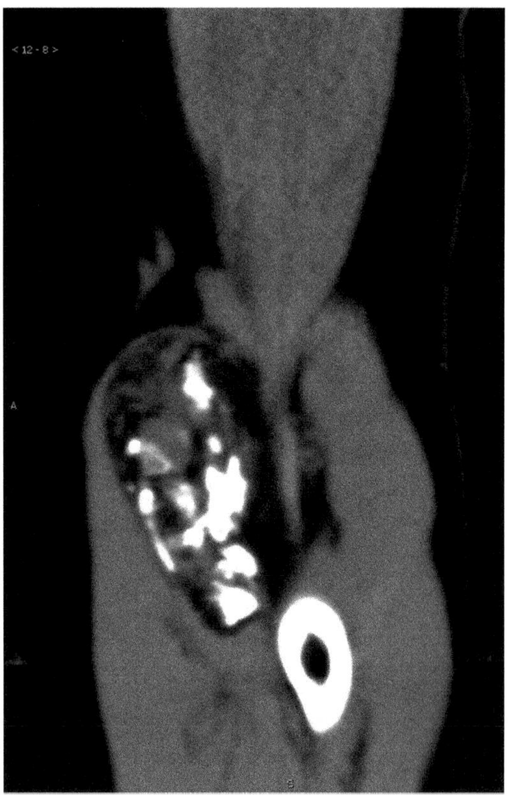

Fig. 34.6 Coronal post-contrast CT image of the left elbow in soft tissue window

CT images of the left elbow demonstrate a mass around the intermuscular space at the ventral aspect of the elbow. There are soft tissue densities, calcifications, and fatty densities within the mass. The mass is well circumscribed without enhancement. High densities are also seen around the olecranon fossa.

34.3.3 MR Imaging

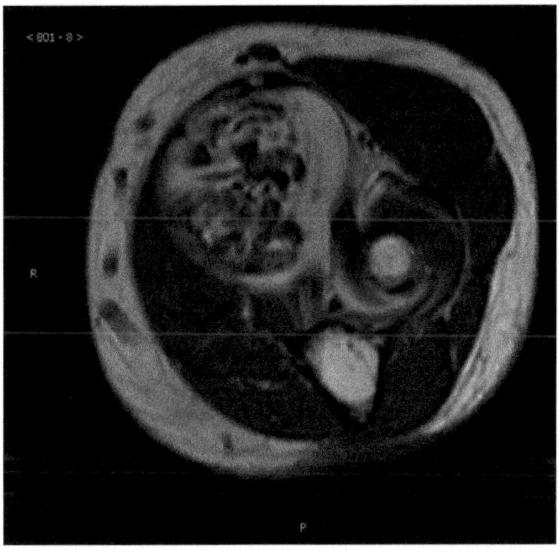

Fig. 34.7 Axial T1-weighted MR image of the left elbow

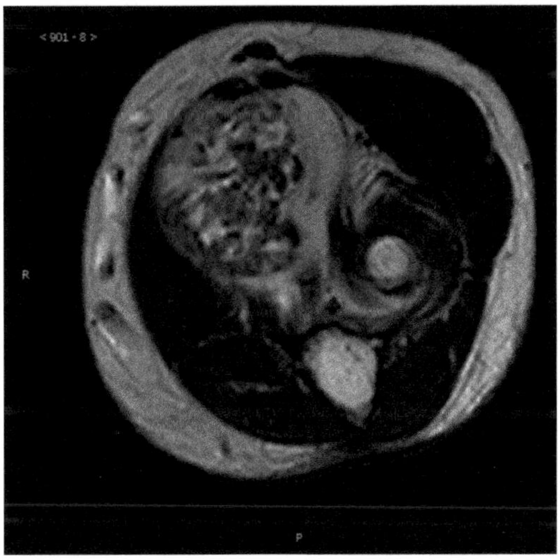

Fig. 34.8 Axial T2-weighted MR image of the left elbow

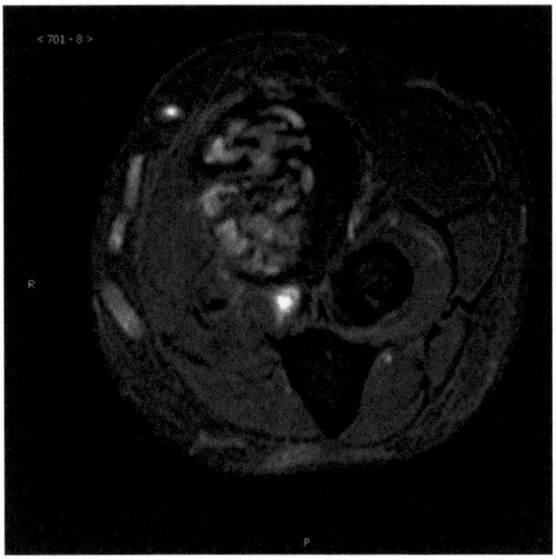

Fig. 34.9 Axial fat-suppressed T2-weighted MR image of the left elbow

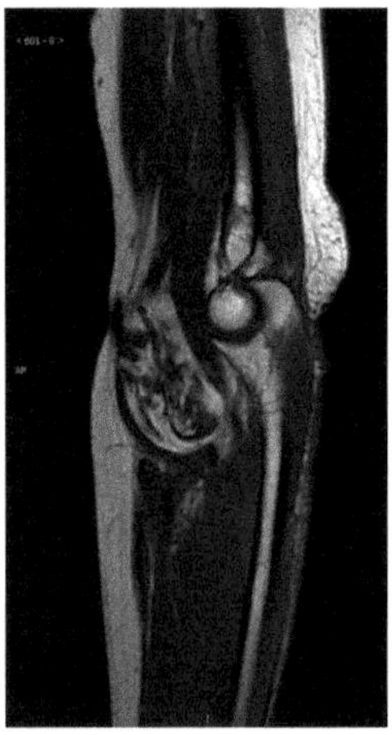

Fig. 34.10 Sagittal T1-weighted MR image of the left elbow

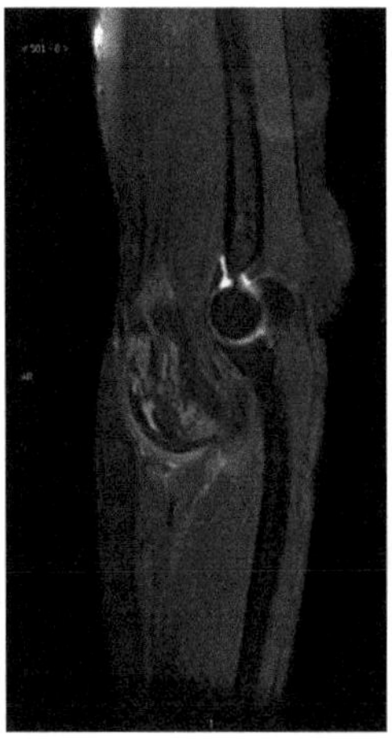

Fig. 34.11 Sagittal fat-suppressed T2-weighted MR image of the left elbow

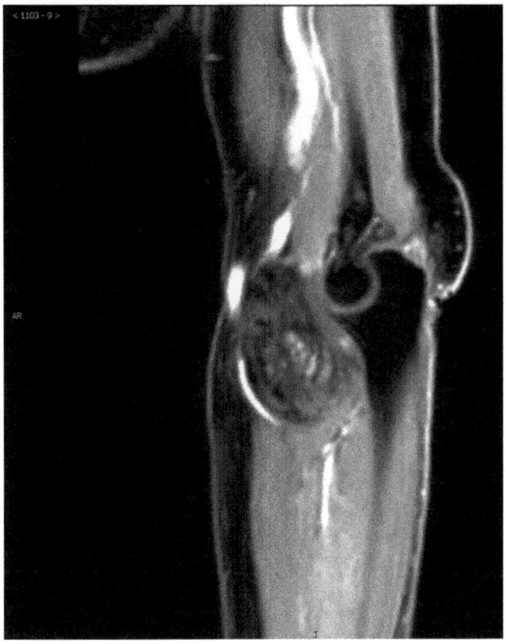

Fig. 34.12 Sagittal post-contrast fat-suppressed T1-weighted MR image of the left elbow

MR images of the left elbow demonstrate a mass at the ventral aspect with heterogeneous signals and no enhancement. Mass effect upon the vessels in the left elbow is noted.

34.4 Description and Discussion from Residents

The patient is an older female with a relatively long history. Radiographs demonstrate soft tissue mass at the ventral aspect of the left elbow with internal heterogeneous high densities, no osseous involvement, and relatively preserved joint space with subchondral sclerosis. CT and MR images demonstrate the ventral mass away from the osseous structures of the left elbow and no clear relationship with the joint space. There are soft tissue densities, fat and calcifications within the lesion, and curvilinear densities, suggestive of vascular lesion. Given the lack of enhancement, this is likely a more mature vascular lesion with differential diagnoses include lipoma and liposarcoma. Also, high densities are noted in the olecranon fossa, which could represent intra-articular body versus synovial osteochondromatosis, favoring the first one.

34.5 Analysis and Comments from Professor Xiaoguang Cheng

The radiographs demonstrate no osseous destruction around the left elbow with preserved joint space, suggesting the lesion is outside of the joint, likely a soft tissue tumor. Heterogeneous components of soft tissue, fat and calcifications are noted on both CT and MR images within the lesion. There is no clear relationship with the joint of the lesion and no enhancement is noted. The findings support teratoma-like lesion. High densities are noted in the olecranon fossa, favoring synovial osteochondromatosis.

34.6 Diagnosis

Likely Angiolipoma (pathology from biopsy).

Suggested Reading

Gupta P, Potti TA, Wuertzer SD, et al. Spectrum of fat-containing soft-tissue masses at MR imaging: the common, the uncommon, the characteristic, and the sometimes confusing. Radiographics. 2016 May–Jun;36(3):753–66.

Sheybani EF, Eutsler EP, Navarro OM. Fat-containing soft-tissue masses in children. Pediatr Radiol. 2016 Dec;46(13):1760–73.

35 Osteosarcoma: Case 10

35.1 Medical History

The patient is a 14-year-old adolescent girl. She presents with left elbow pain for 2 months and worsening with swelling in the past half month. She has a history of repeated radial head subluxation of the left elbow in the past.

35.2 Physical Examination

There is point tenderness around the left elbow with focal swelling.

35.3 Imaging Findings

35.3.1 Radiograph

X. Cheng et al., *Imaging of Bone Tumors in Shoulder and Elbow*,
https://doi.org/10.1007/978-981-33-6150-8_35

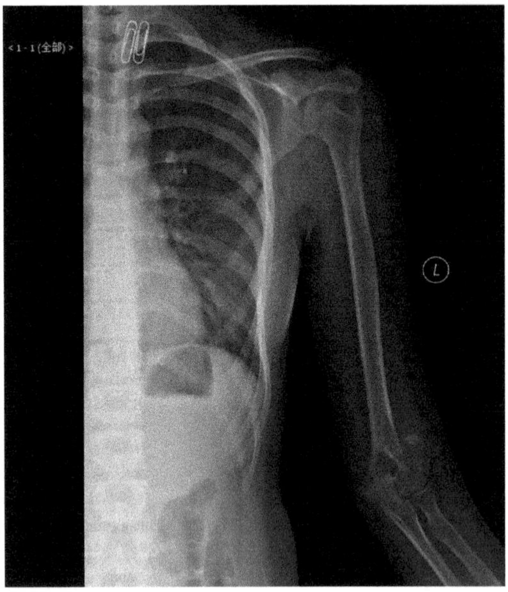

Fig. 35.1 Frontal view of the left elbow

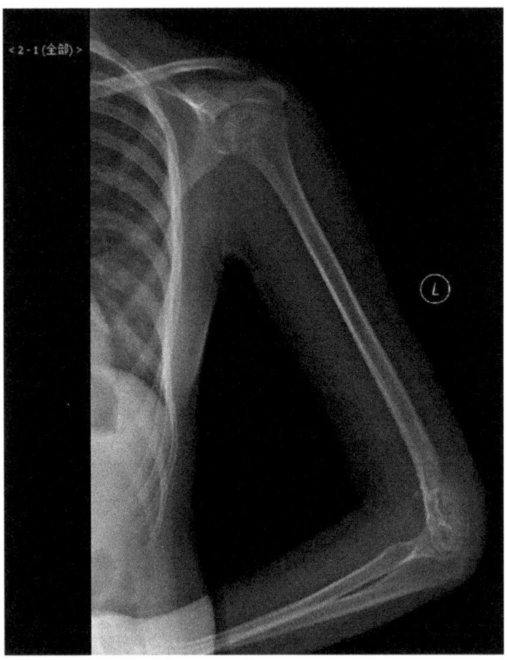

Fig. 35.2 Lateral view of the left elbow

Radiographs of the left elbow demonstrate mixed osseous destructiona around the lateral humeral condyle with cortical disruption and periosteal reaction. Soft tissue mass is noted without a clear margin.

35.3.2 CT Imaging

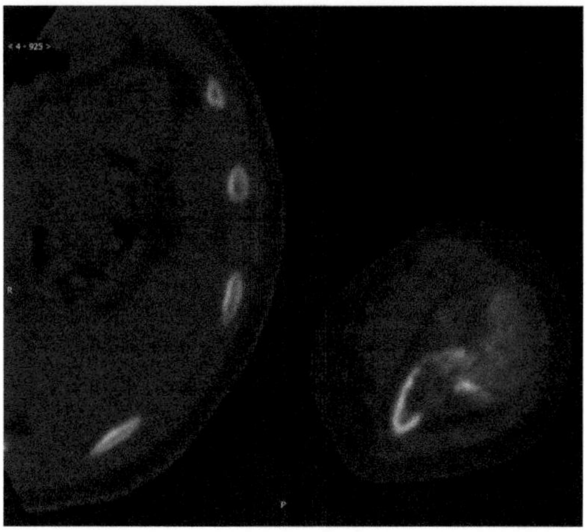

Fig. 35.3 Axial CT image of the left elbow in bone window

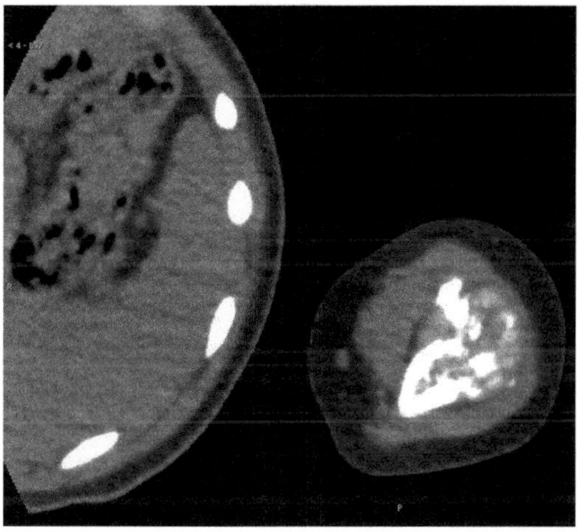

Fig. 35.4 Axial CT image of the left elbow in soft tissue window

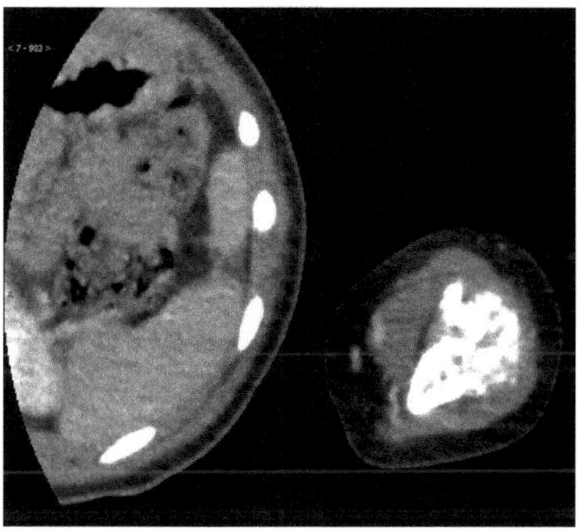

Fig. 35.5 Axial post-contrast CT image of the left elbow in soft tissue window

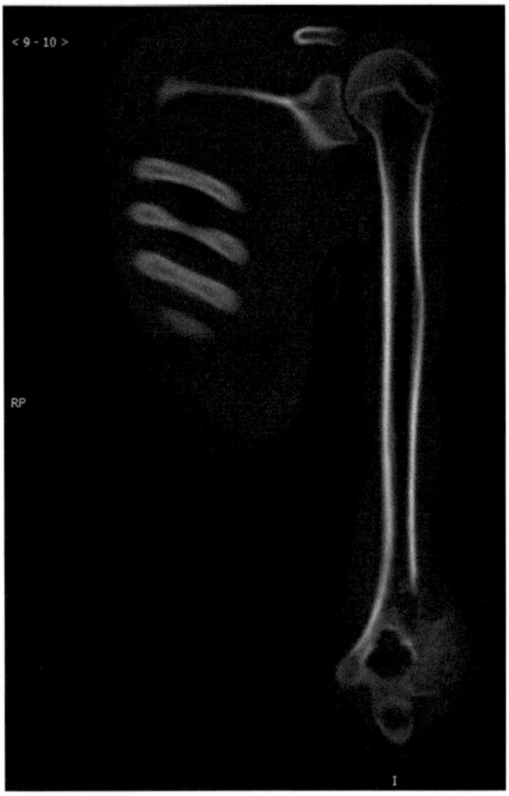

Fig. 35.6 Coronal CT image of the left elbow in bone window

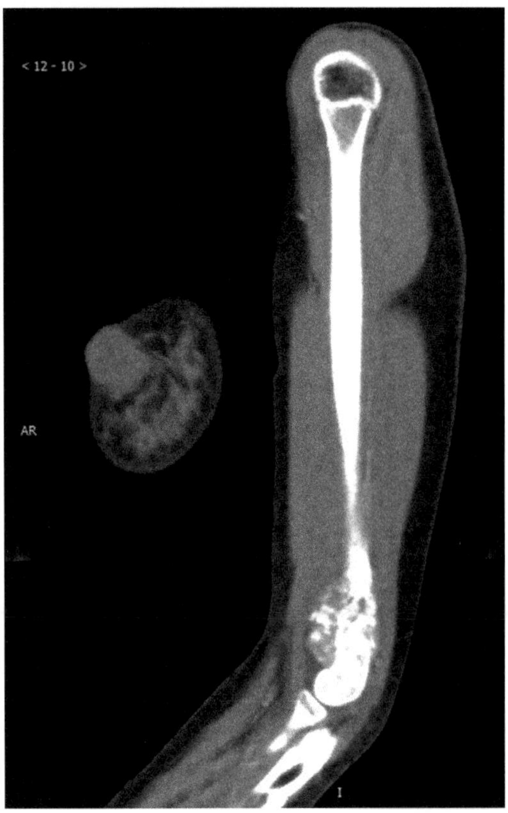

Fig. 35.7 Sagittal post-contrast CT image of the left elbow in soft tissue window

CT images of the left elbow demonstrate lytic osseous destruction around the lateral humeral condyle with soft tissue mass. There are internal ivory-like densities. Heterogeneous enhancement is noted with focal avid enhancement.

35.3.3 MR Imaging

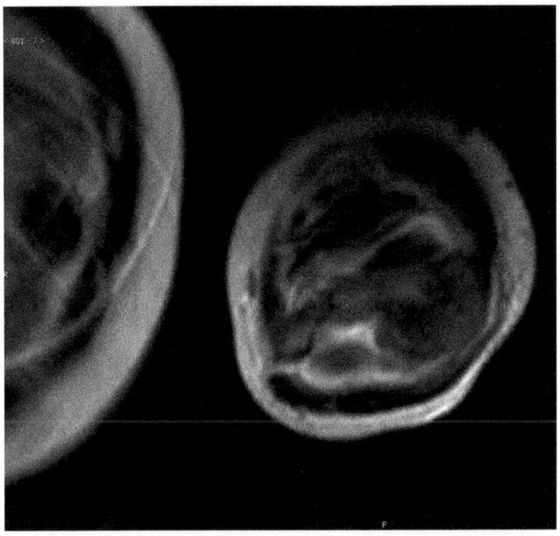

Fig. 35.8 Axial T2-weighted MR image of the left elbow

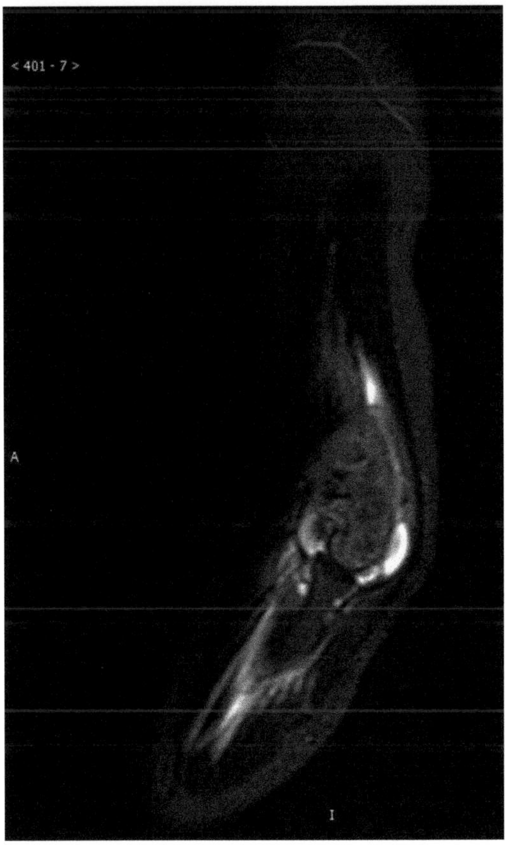

Fig. 35.9 Sagittal fat-suppressed T2-weighted MR image of the left elbow

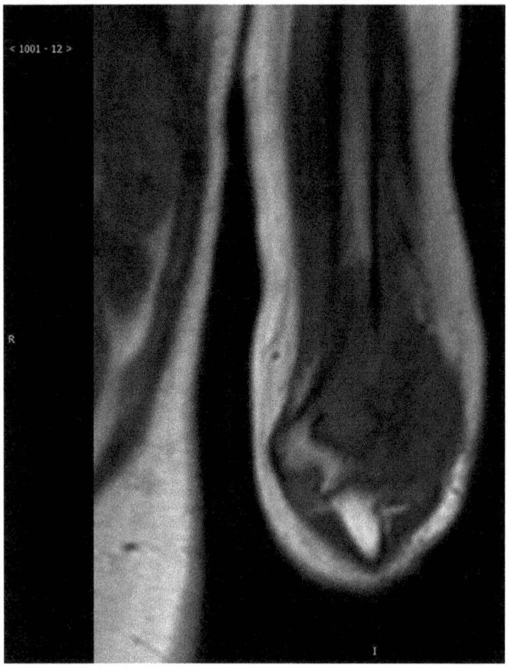

Fig. 35.10 Coronal T1-weighted MR image of the left elbow

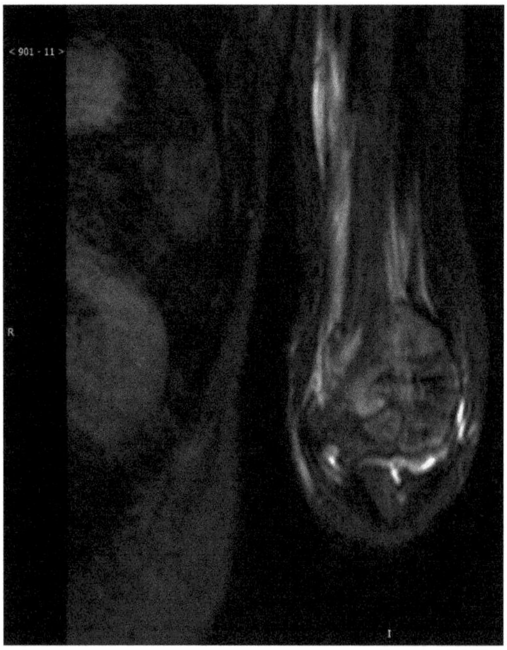

Fig. 35.11 Coronal fat-suppressed T2-weighted MR image of the left elbow

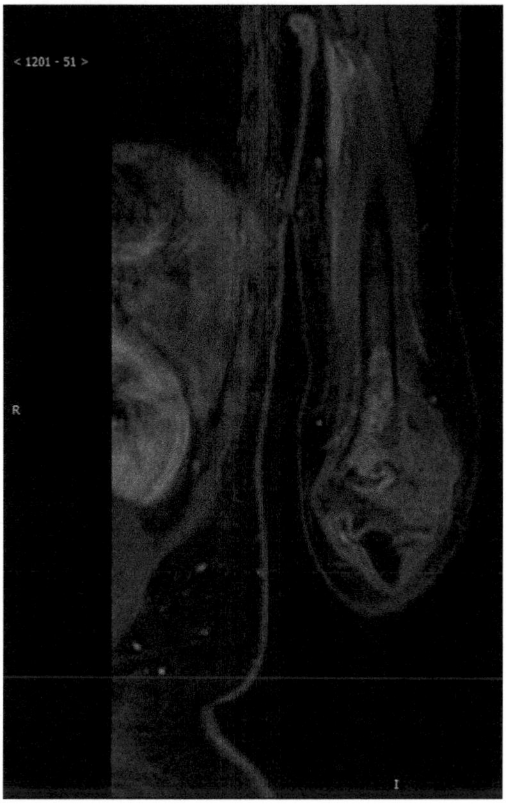

Fig. 35.12 Coronal post-contrast fat-suppressed T1-weighted MR image of the left elbow

MR images of the left elbow demonstrate a lesion at the lateral humeral condyle with soft tissue mass. The lesion demonstrates heterogenous low T1 and T2 signals with heterogeneous enhancement.

35.4 Description and Discussion from Residents

The patient is an adolescent. Radiographs demonstrate mixed osseous destruction around the left lateral humeral condyle with internal patchy osteoid matrix and focal cortical disruption. There is an irregular margin of the lesion with soft tissue mass. The articular surface of the lateral humeral condyle is preserved. The above imaging findings favor the malignant process. CT images demonstrate mixed osseous destruction, soft tissue mass, and ivory-like osteoid matrix with interrupted periosteal reaction and heterogeneous enhancement, all consistent with typical osteosarcoma. Ewing sarcoma is in the differential diagnosis. MR images better depict the extent of the involvement and the presence of joint effusion.

35.5 Analysis and Comments from Professor Xiaoguang Cheng

The patient is an adolescent. Radiographs and CT images both demonstrate osseous destruction at the left distal humerus, around the metaphysis with soft tissue mass. The lesion is ill-defined with an osteoid matrix. Given the patient's age, the top consideration is osteosarcoma. Ewing sarcoma is in the differential diagnosis. Usually, there is no osteoid matrix within the lesion with Ewing sarcoma, not consistent with the current case. MRI can better demonstrate the extent of the involvement of the tumor.

35.6 Diagnosis

Osteosarcoma.

Suggested Reading

Fox MG, Trotta BM. Osteosarcoma: review of the various types with emphasis on recent advancements in imaging. Semin Musculoskelet Radiol. 2013 Apr;17(2):123–36.

Murphey MD, Robbin MR, McRae GA, et al. The many faces of osteosarcoma. Radiographics. 1997 Sep–Oct;17(5):1205–31.

Charcot Arthropathy: Case 11

36

36.1 Medical History

The patient was seen at an outpatient clinic.

36.2 Imaging Findings

36.2.1 Radiograph

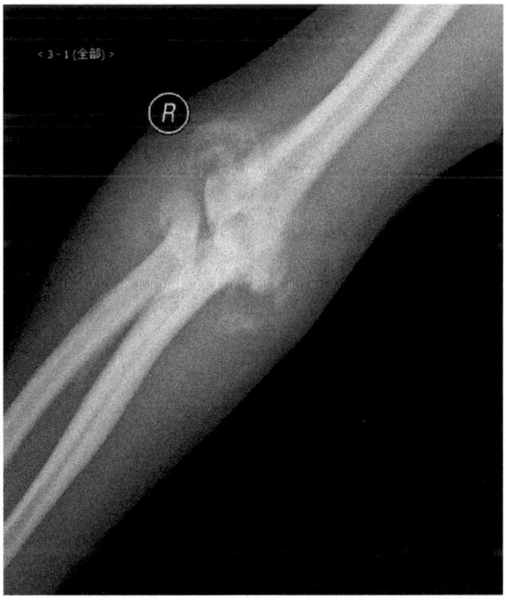

Fig. 36.1 Frontal view of the right elbow

X. Cheng et al., *Imaging of Bone Tumors in Shoulder and Elbow*,
https://doi.org/10.1007/978-981-33-6150-8_36

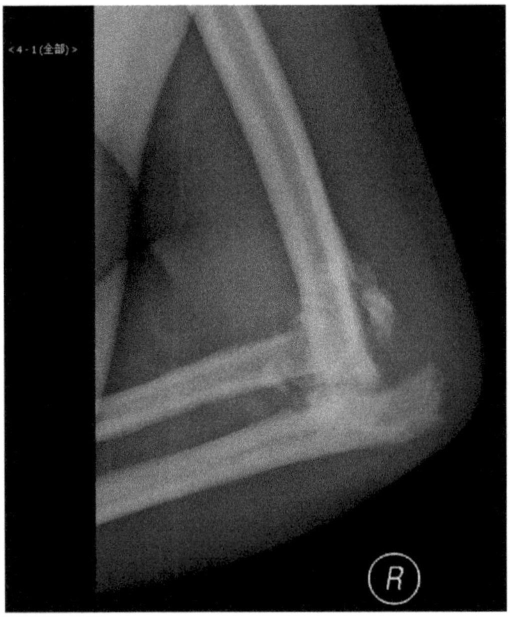

Fig. 36.2 Lateral view of the right elbow

Radiographs of the right elbow demonstrate disorganization around the elbow with dislocation and multiple fragments around the joint. Osseous destructive changes are noted around the joint with soft tissue swelling.

36.2.2 CT Imaging

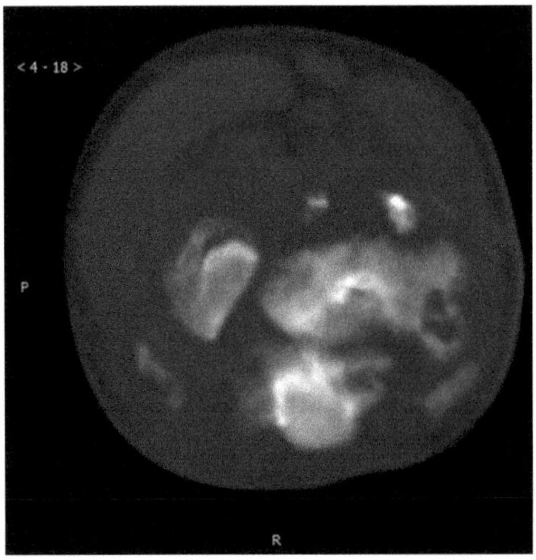

Fig. 36.3 Axial CT image of the right elbow in bone window

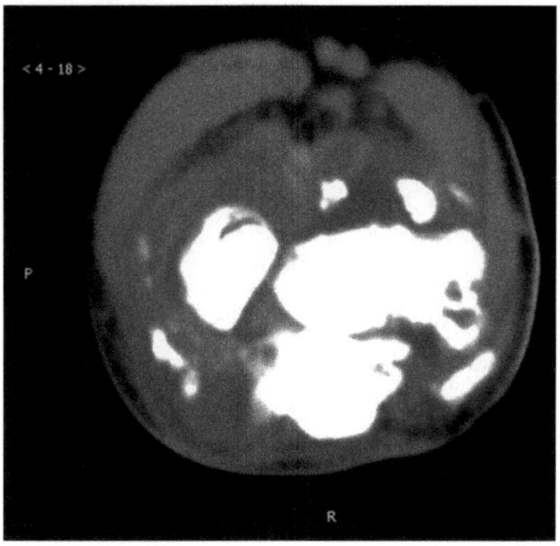

Fig. 36.4 Axial CT image of the right elbow in soft tissue window

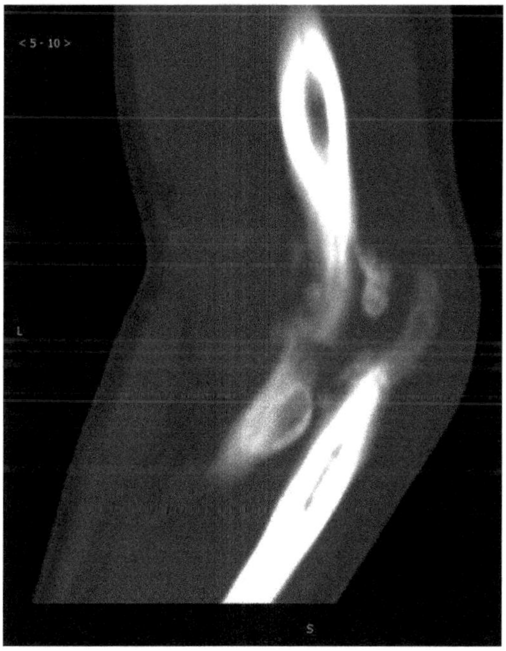

Fig. 36.5 Sagittal CT image of the right elbow in bone window

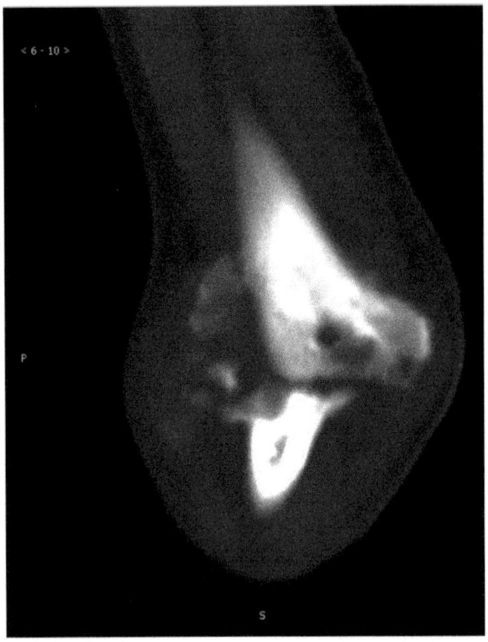

Fig. 36.6 Coronal CT image of the right elbow in bone window

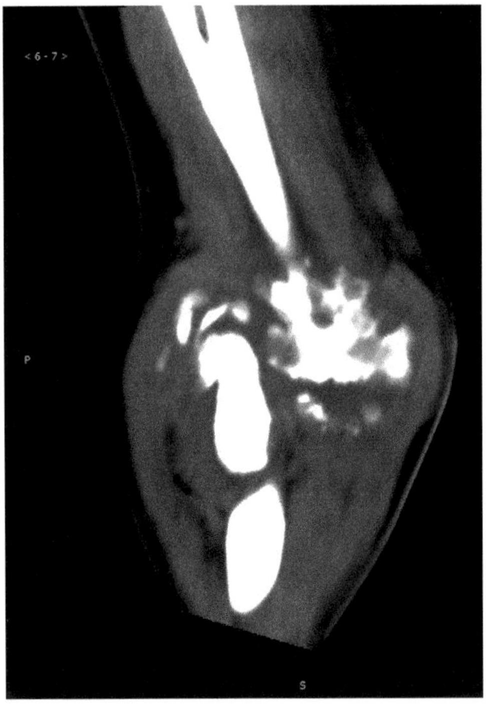

Fig. 36.7 Coronal CT image of the right elbow in soft tissue window

CT images demonstrate dislocation at the right elbow with extensive osseous destructive changes. The osseous structures appear sclerotic with destruction around the articular surface. There is swelling about the joint capsule, containing multiple fragments.

36.2.3 MR Imaging

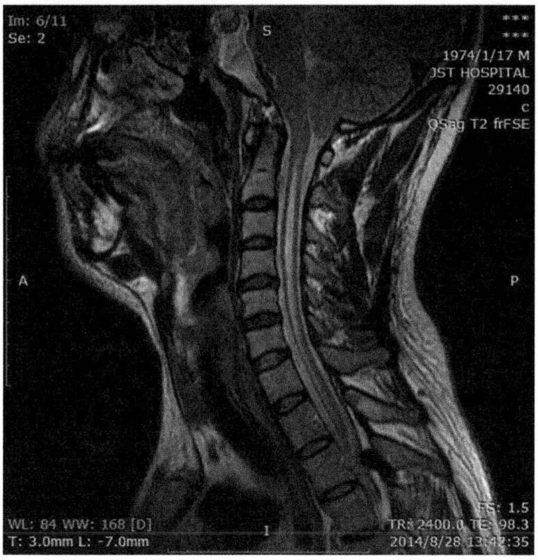

Fig. 36.8 Sagittal T2-weighted MR image of the cervical spine

MR image of the cervical spine demonstrates herniation of the cerebellar tonsil and syrinx in the cervical spinal cord.

36.3 Description and Discussion from Residents

Radiographs demonstrate osseous destruction around the right elbow with dislocation, destruction around the articular surface, and fragments/debris in the joint. There is an extension of the joint capsule with an internal high density of synovial calcification and joint effusion. With the presence of Chiari malformation and cervical spinal cord syrinx, this is most consistent with Charcot arthropathy.

36.4 Analysis and Comments from Professor Xiaoguang Cheng

This is a classic case presentation. Dislocation of the right elbow joint with joint capsule extension and knife-like appearance of the distal humerus are noted. CT images demonstrate right elbow osseous destruction, disorganization, joint effusion, typical for Charcot arthropathy. Examination for cervical spine abnormality should be performed. Charcot arthropathy is usually seen in patients with diabetes in adults and in patients with congenital insensitivity to pain in pediatric patients. Differential diagnoses include tuberculosis (usually with osteopenia) and synovial osteochondromatosis (usually without joint dislocation).

36.5 Diagnosis

Charcot arthropathy (neuropathic arthropathy).

Suggested Reading

Aliabadi P, Nikpoor N, Alparslan L. Imaging of neuropathic arthropathy. Semin Musculoskelet Radiol. 2003 Sep;7(3):217–25.

Jones EA, Manaster BJ, May DA, et al. Neuropathic osteoarthropathy: diagnostic dilemmas and differential diagnosis. Radiographics. 2000 Oct;20:S279–93.

37 Melorheostosis: Case 12

37.1 Medical History

The patient is a 45-year-old female. She presented with right elbow mass for 13 years and pain for 6 months.

37.2 Physical Examination

There was swelling around the right proximal ulna. Focal mass was noted with irregular margin, hard and with point tenderness.

37.3 Imaging Findings

37.3.1 Radiograph

X. Cheng et al., *Imaging of Bone Tumors in Shoulder and Elbow*,
https://doi.org/10.1007/978-981-33-6150-8_37

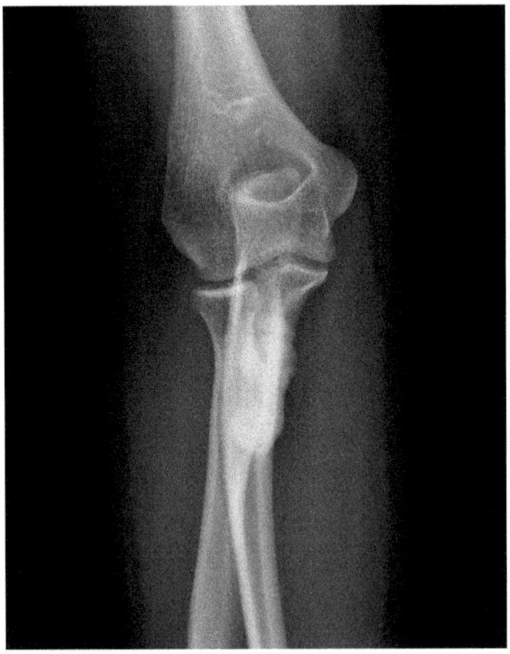

Fig. 37.1 Frontal view of the right elbow

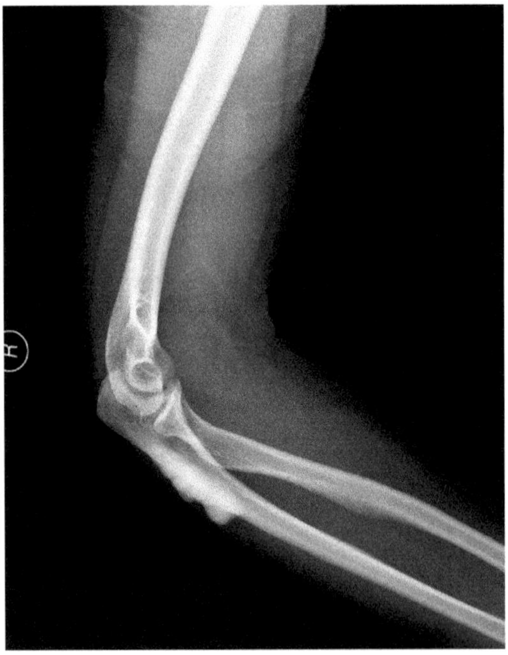

Fig. 37.2 Lateral view of the right elbow

Radiographs of the right elbow demonstrate cortical thickening around the proximal ulna with sclerosis. There is no involvement of the intramedullary cavity.

37.3.2 CT Imaging

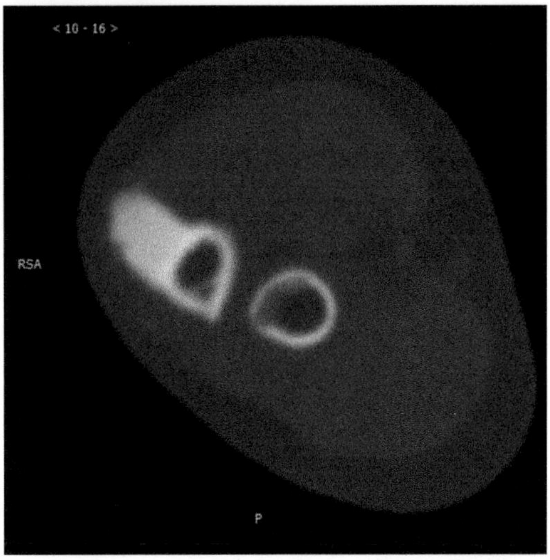

Fig. 37.3 Axial CT image of the right elbow in bone window

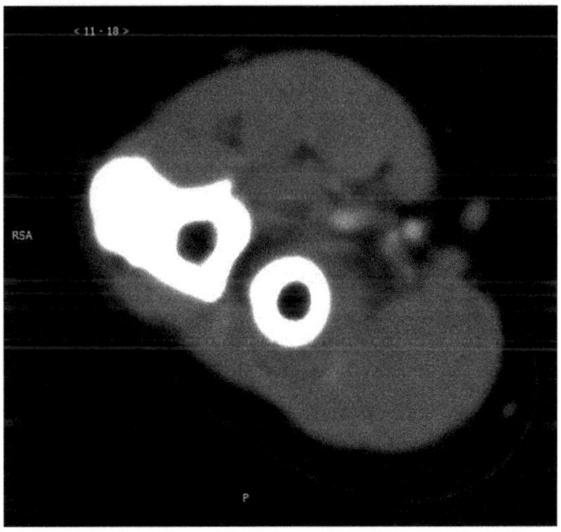

Fig. 37.4 Axial post-contrast CT image of the right elbow in soft tissue window

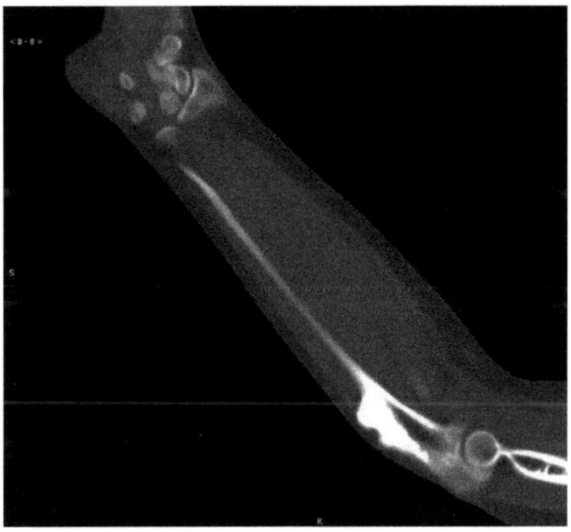

Fig. 37.5 Sagittal CT image of the right elbow in bone window

CT images of the right elbow demonstrate cortical thickening with protuberance along the proximal ulna. The lesion is well-circumscribed with homogeneous density and no associated soft tissue mass.

37.4 Description and Discussion from Residents

The patient is a middle-aged female with a long course of the symptoms. There is focal cortical thickening along the proximal right ulna with smooth margin and well-circumscribed, without associated soft tissue mass. This is most likely a benign process of hyperplasia of focal periosteum, such as melorheostosis and osteoma. Parosteal osteosarcoma can be seen in middle-aged patients and need to be excluded. Additionally, cortical vascular lesions can also incite a reactive thickening of the cortex.

37.5 Analysis and Comments from Professor Xiaoguang Cheng

There is focal sclerosis of the right proximal ulna, just affecting the cortex with a clear margin, typical for melorheostosis. Differential diagnoses include parosteal osteosarcoma, osteoid osteoma, and vascular lesion. This is a "do not touch" lesion; no biopsy should be attempted; only follow-up observation is necessary.

37.6 Diagnosis

Melorheostosis.

Suggested Reading

Fick CN, Fratzl-Zelman N, Roschger P, et al. Melorheostosis: a clinical, pathologic, and radiologic case series. Am J Surg Pathol. 2019 Nov;43(11):1554–9.

Freyschmidt J. Melorheostosis: a review of 23 cases. Eur Radiol. 2001;11(3):474–9.

Jha S, Laucis N, Kim L, et al. CT analysis of anatomical distribution of melorheostosis challenges the sclerotome hypothesis. Bone. 2018 Dec;117:31–6.

38 Tuberculosis: Case 13

38.1 Medical History

A 20-year-old male with elbow pain.

38.2 Imaging Findings

38.2.1 Radiograph

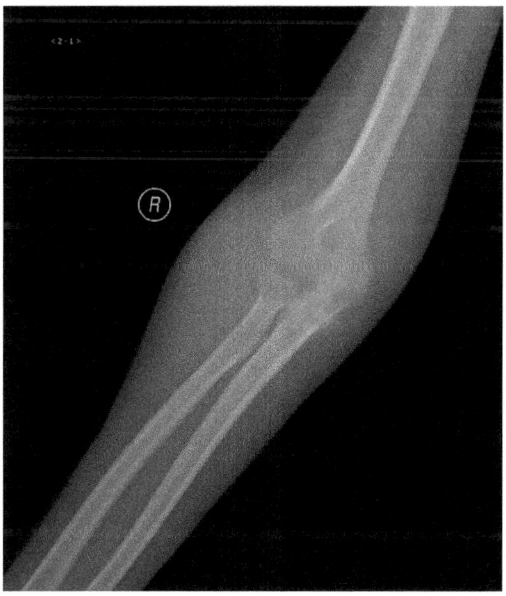

Fig. 38.1 Frontal view of the right elbow

X. Cheng et al., *Imaging of Bone Tumors in Shoulder and Elbow*,
https://doi.org/10.1007/978-981-33-6150-8_38

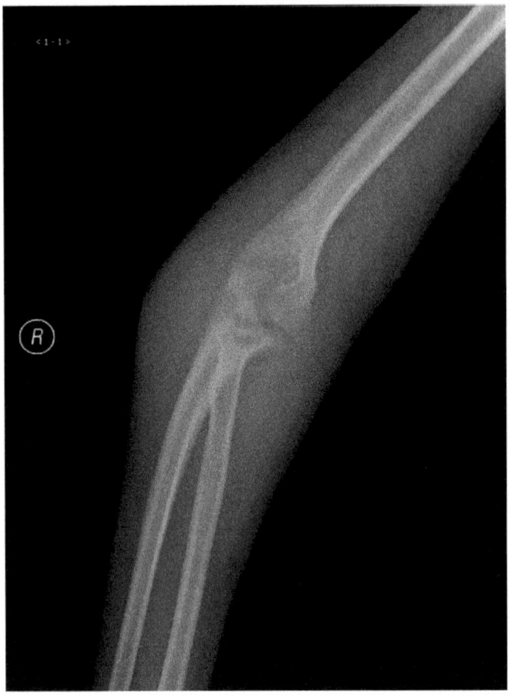

Fig. 38.2 Lateral view of the right elbow

Radiographs demonstrate decreased bone density around the distal right humerus and proximal radius and ulna. Focal osseous destruction is noted around the proximal ulna. Periosteal reaction is seen around the proximal ulna and radius. There is soft tissue swelling about the right elbow in the radial aspect.

38.2.2 CT Imaging

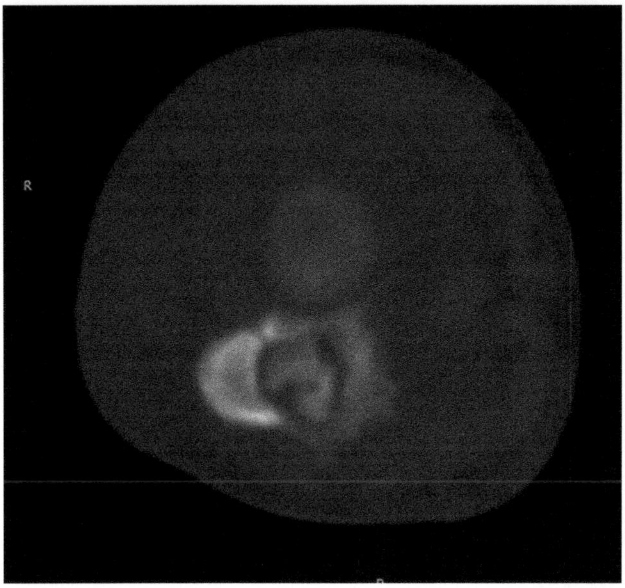

Fig. 38.3 Axial CT image of the right elbow in bone window

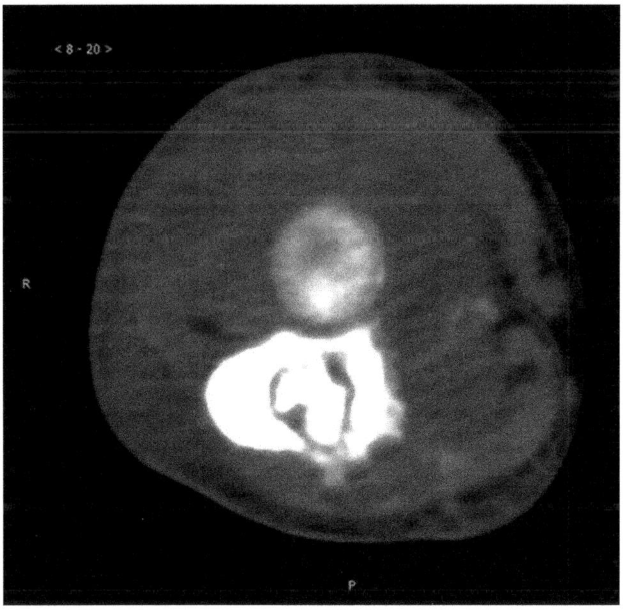

Fig. 38.4 Axial CT image of the right elbow in soft tissue window

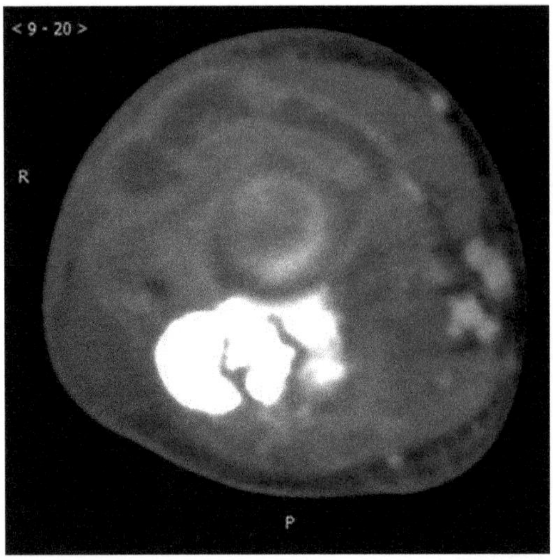

Fig. 38.5 Axial post-contrast CT image of the right elbow in soft tissue window

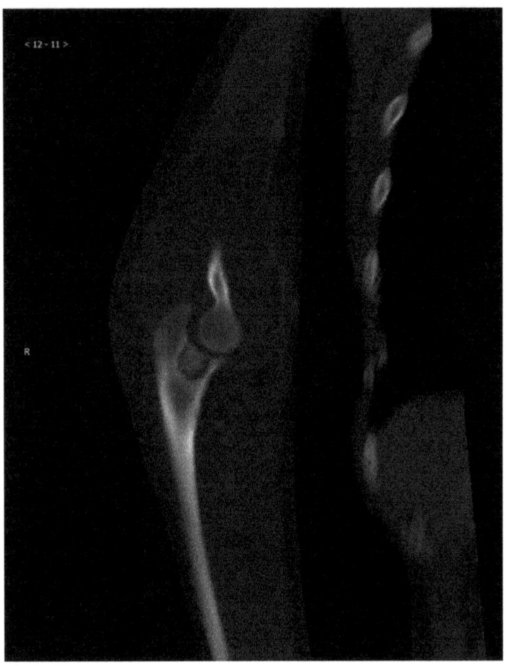

Fig. 38.6 Sagittal CT image of the right elbow in bone window

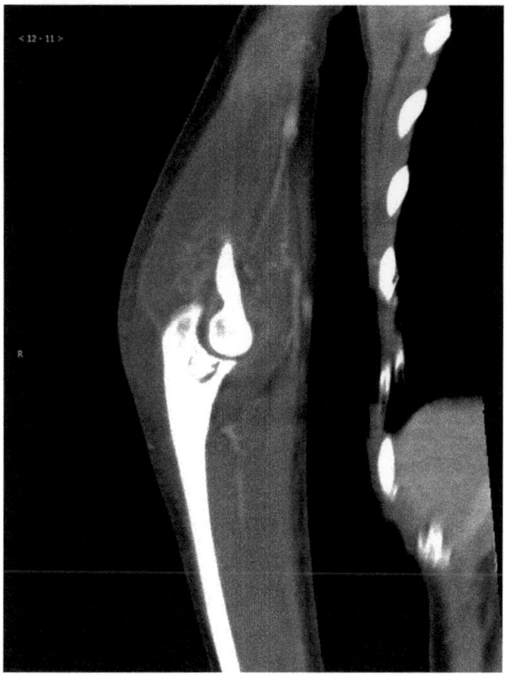

Fig. 38.7 Sagittal post-contrast CT image of the right elbow in soft tissue window

CT scan demonstrates focal osseous destruction around the proximal ulna with internal high density. Periosteal reaction is noted along the proximal ulna and radius. There is soft tissue swelling around the right elbow joint. There is synovial enhancement around the joint.

38.2.3 MR Imaging

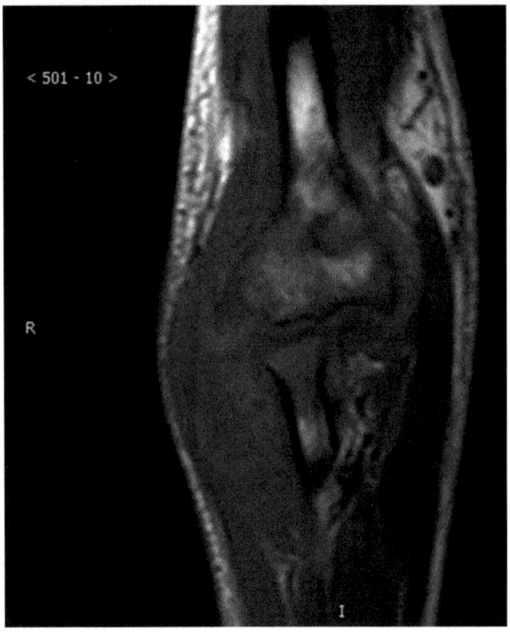

Fig. 38.8 Coronal T1-weighted MR image of the right elbow

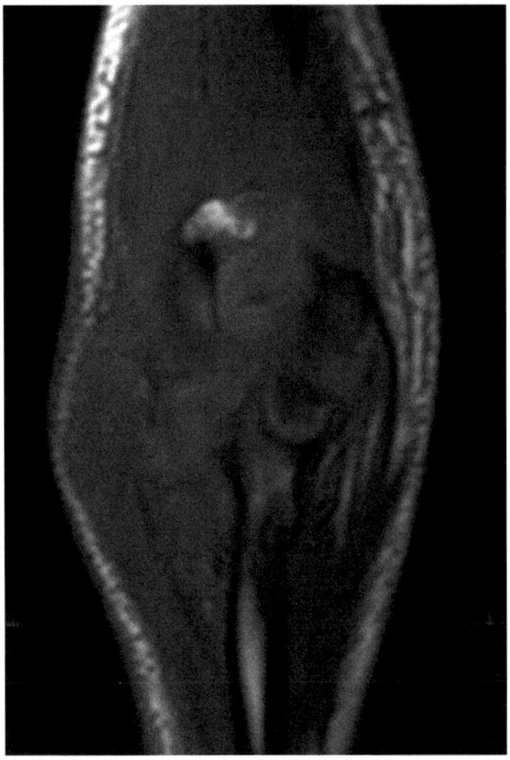

Fig. 38.9 Coronal T1-weighted MR image of the right elbow

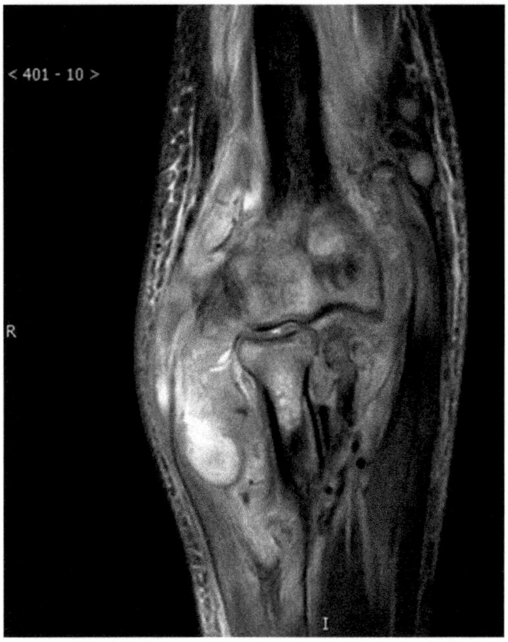

Fig. 38.10 Coronal fat-suppressed T2-weighted MR image of the right elbow

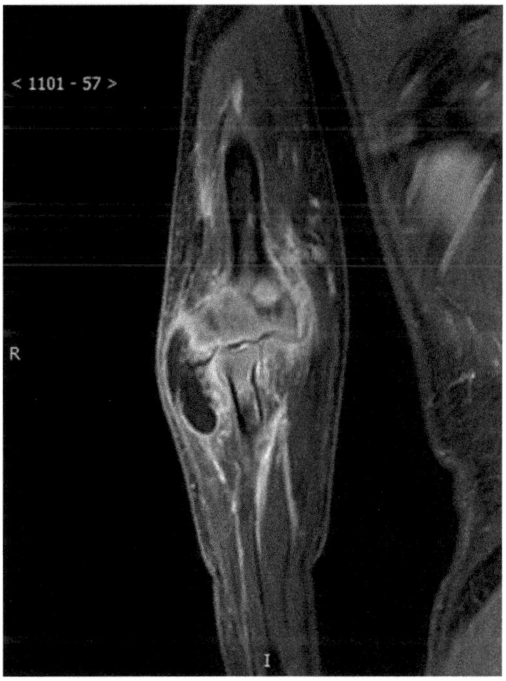

Fig. 38.11 Coronal post-contrast fat-suppressed T1-weighted MR image of the right elbow

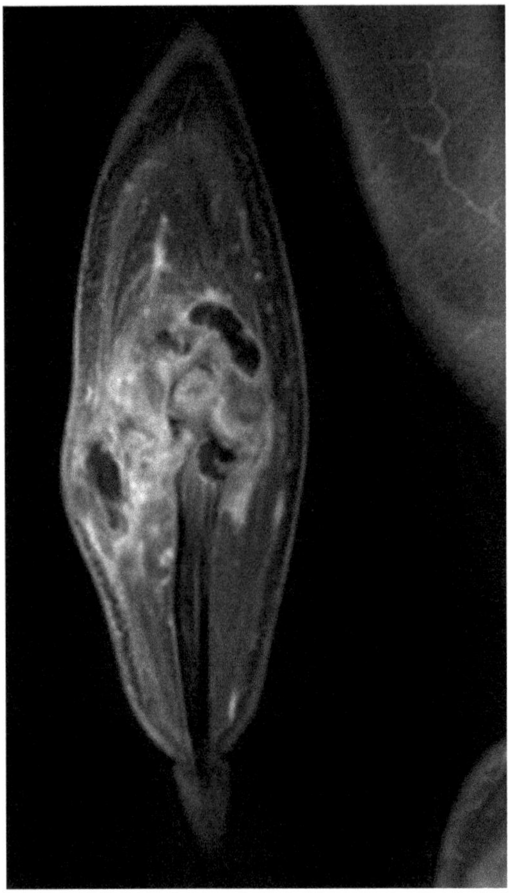

Fig. 38.12 Coronal post-contrast fat-suppressed T1-weighted MR image of the right elbow

MRI scan demonstrates low T1 signal and high T2 signal of distal humerus and proximal ulna and radius. There is significant joint distension of the right elbow with avid enhancement around the synovium with focal circular morphology. Extensive soft tissue edema around the joint is noted.

38.3 Description and Discussion from Residents

Radiographs demonstrate decreased bone density of the distal right humerus and proximal ulna and radius with peripheral periosteal reaction. Focal osseous destruction is noted around the semilunar notch of the ulna with internal patchy high bone density on CT images and raising concern for sequestrum. However, calcification inside an osteoid osteoma or osteoblastoma could not be entirely excluded. Extensive marrow edema of the distal humerus and proximal ulna and radius is noted on MR images with extensive soft tissue swelling around the joint. There is subcutaneous soft tissue edema, with joint effusion, distention, and enhancement, indicating infectious process, likely tuberculosis.

38.4 Analysis and Comments from Professor Xiaoguang Cheng

The patient is a young male with osseous destruction around the right olecranon with clear margin and internal high density and joint distention of the right elbow, raising concern for tuberculosis. However, the current case is with extensive osseous destruction and relative preservation of the joint space and articular surface, not that consistent with tuberculosis. So, nonaggressive tumors cannot be excluded, such as chondroblastoma or osteoblastoma.

38.5 Diagnosis

Tuberculosis.

Suggested Reading

De Backer AI, Mortelé KJ, Vanhoenacker FM, et al. Imaging of extraspinal musculoskeletal tuberculosis. Eur J Radiol. 2006 Jan;57(1):119–30.

Prasad A, Manchanda S, Sachdev N, et al. Imaging features of pediatric musculoskeletal tuberculosis. Pediatr Radiol. 2012 Oct;42(10):1235–49.

Chondrosarcoma: Case 14

39

39.1 Medical History

The patient is a 63-year-old female. She presented with mass around the left elbow for 2 months with a history of surgical biopsy.

39.2 Imaging Findings

39.2.1 Radiograph

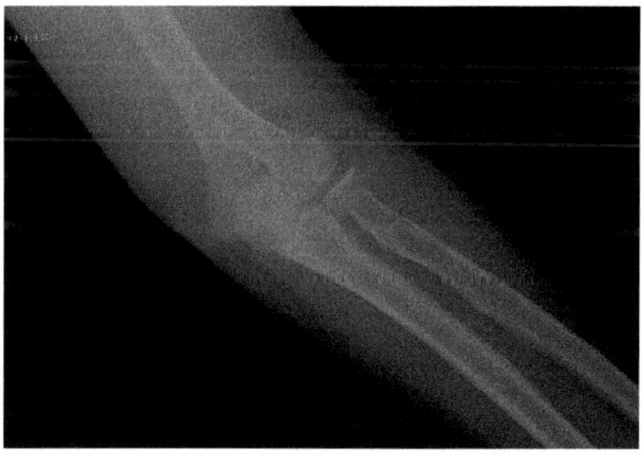

Fig. 39.1 Frontal view of the left elbow

Radiograph of the left elbow demonstrates osseous irregularity around the medial humeral condyle and proximal ulna with adjacent soft tissue swelling.

X. Cheng et al., *Imaging of Bone Tumors in Shoulder and Elbow*,
https://doi.org/10.1007/978-981-33-6150-8_39

39.2.2 CT Imaging

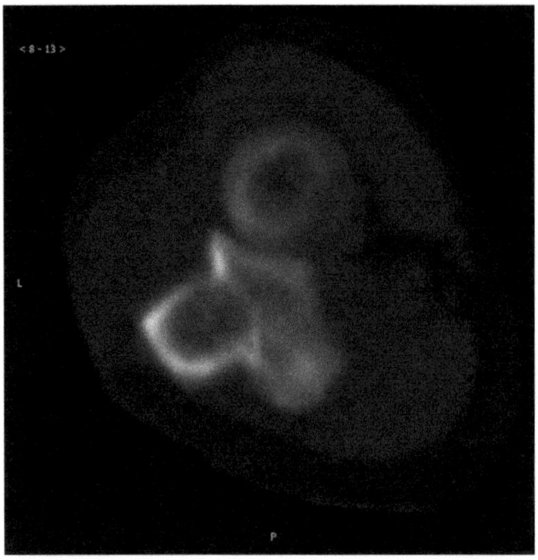

Fig. 39.2 Axial CT image of the left elbow in bone window

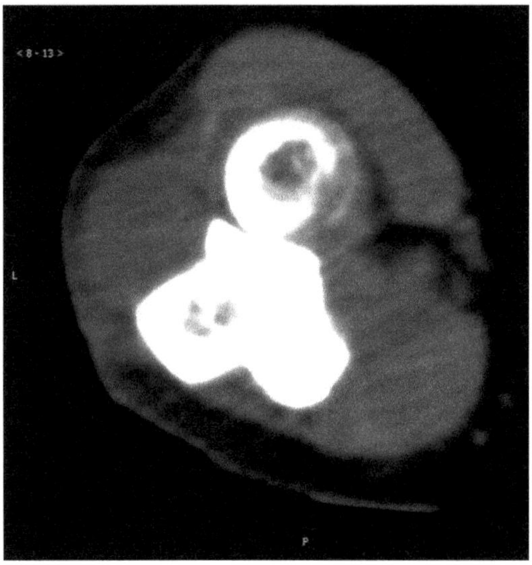

Fig. 39.3 Axial CT image of the left elbow in soft tissue window

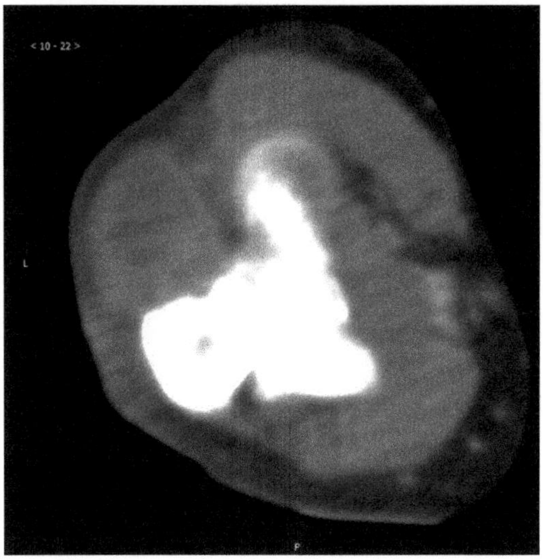

Fig. 39.4 Axial post-contrast CT image of the left elbow in soft tissue window

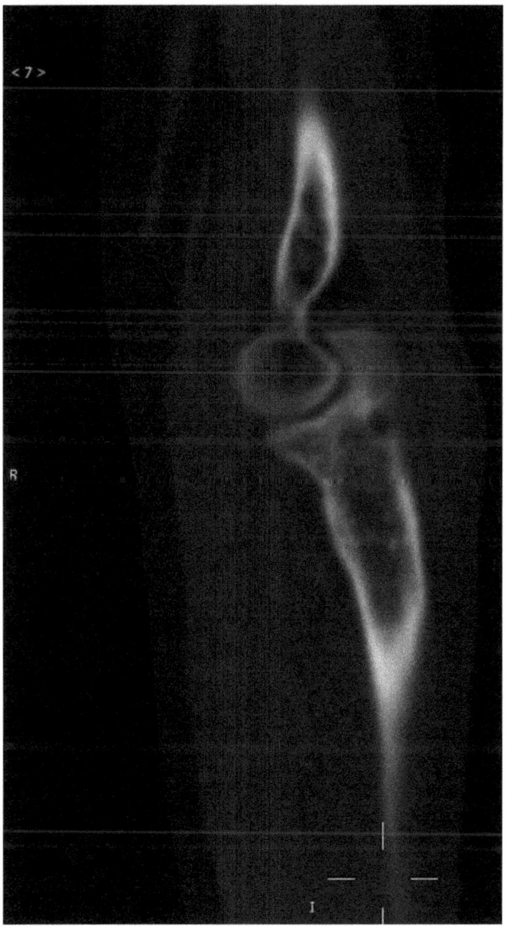

Fig. 39.5 Sagittal CT image of the left elbow in bone window

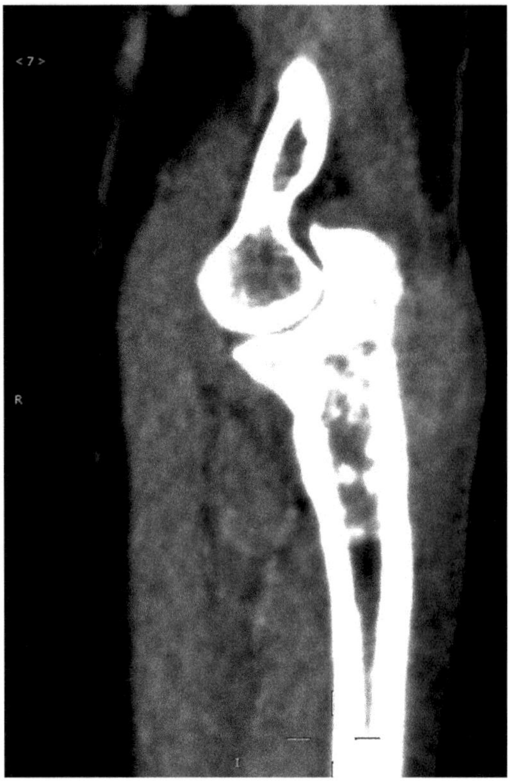

Fig. 39.6 Sagittal post-contrast CT image of the left elbow in soft tissue window

CT images of the left elbow demonstrate soft tissue mass at the posterior aspect of the elbow joint with internal heterogeneous densities and osseous destruction around the adjacent olecranon. Peripheral enhancement around the soft tissue mass is also noted.

39.3 Description and Discussion from Residents

Radiograph demonstrates cortical irregularity around the medial humeral condyle and proximal ulna with adjacent soft tissue swelling. CT images demonstrate fusiform soft tissue mass at the posterior left elbow with irregular margin and heterogeneous density. Defect is noted around the olecranon, likely destruction from the soft tissue mass. Peripheral enhancement is noted. This is likely a soft tissue tumor, with fusiform shape and peripheral enhancement, top consideration is nerve sheath tumor.

39.4 Analysis and Comments from Professor Xiaoguang Cheng

There is destruction around the olecranon with increased density within the intramedullary cavity and scattered calcifications and peripheral enhancement, and adjacent multiple soft tissue masses. For the patient's age, the top consideration is chondrosarcoma. Given the lesion is in proximity to the tendon insertions, related diseases should be excluded, such as gout. However, the presentation is not consistent with gout.

39.5 Diagnosis

Chondrosarcoma.

Suggested Reading

Douis H, Saifuddin A. The imaging of cartilaginous bone tumours. II. Chondrosarcoma. Skelet Radiol. 2013 May;42(5):611–26.

Murphey MD, Walker EA, Wilson AJ, et al. From the archives of the AFIP: imaging of primary chondrosarcoma: radiologic-pathologic correlation. Radiographics. 2003 Sep-Oct;23(5):1245–78.

40 Hemangioma: Case 15

40.1 Medical History

The patient is a 15-year-old female who presented with right forearm pain for 2 years and worsening with palpable mass for 1 year.

40.2 Physical Examination

There is a deep-seated mass at the right forearm posteriorly, measuring 3 cm × 2 cm with a clear margin, rubbery, smooth, mobile with point tenderness. A vascular murmur is noted.

40.3 Imaging Findings

40.3.1 Radiograph

X. Cheng et al., *Imaging of Bone Tumors in Shoulder and Elbow*,
https://doi.org/10.1007/978-981-33-6150-8_40

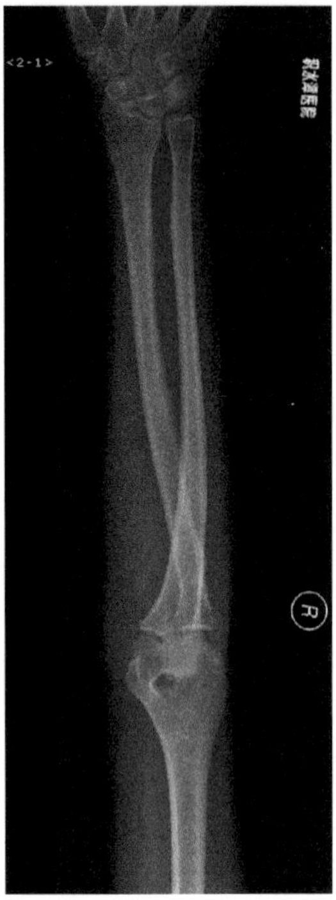

Fig. 40.1 Frontal view of the right forearm

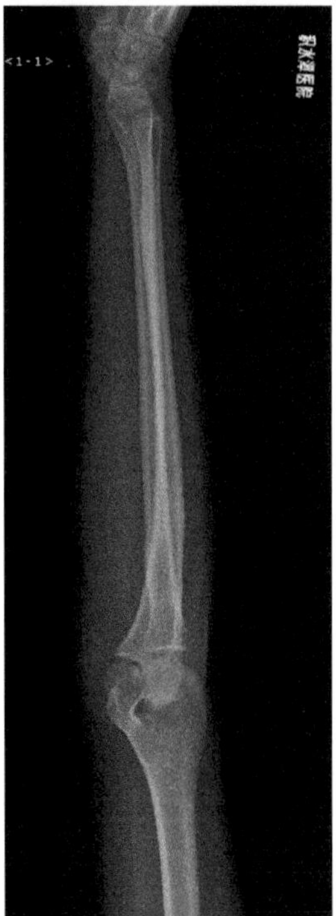

Fig. 40.2 Lateral view of the right forearm

Radiographs of the right forearm demonstrate no cortical abnormality and no obvious soft tissue mass.

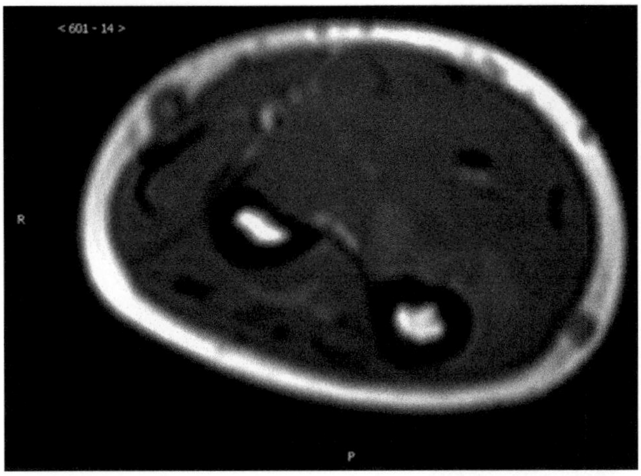

Fig. 40.3 Axial T1-weighted MR image of the right forearm

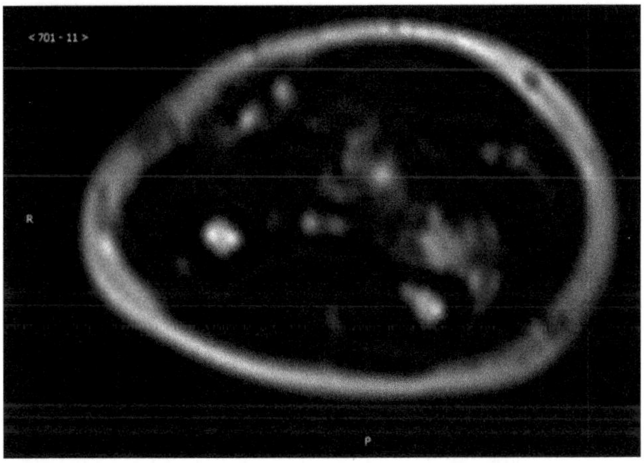

Fig. 40.4 Axial T2-weighted MR image of the right forearm

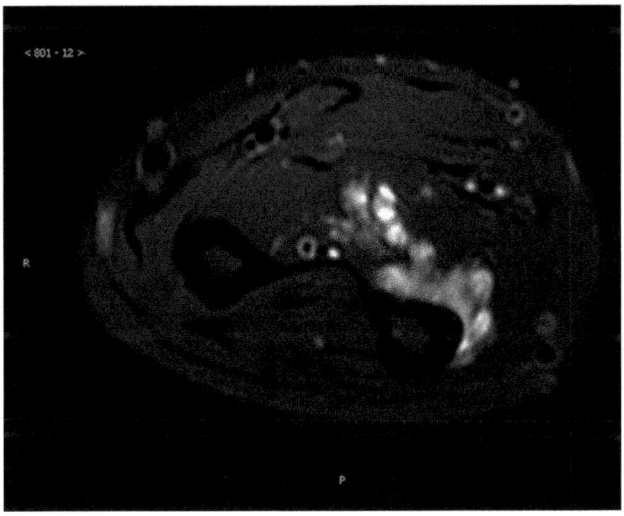

Fig. 40.5 Axial fat-suppressed T2-weighted MR image of the right forearm

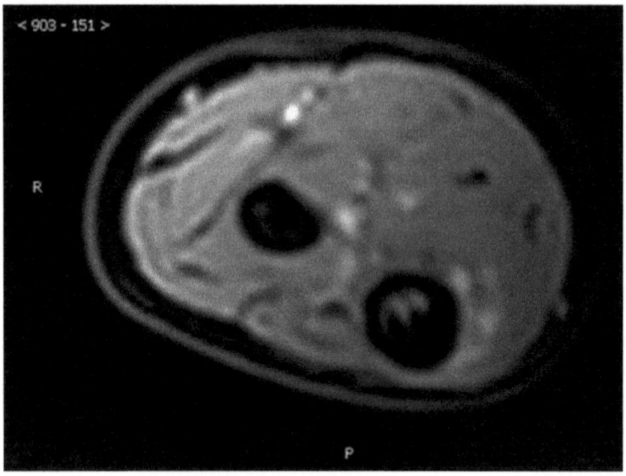

Fig. 40.6 Axial post-contrast fat-suppressed T1-weighted MR image of the right forearm

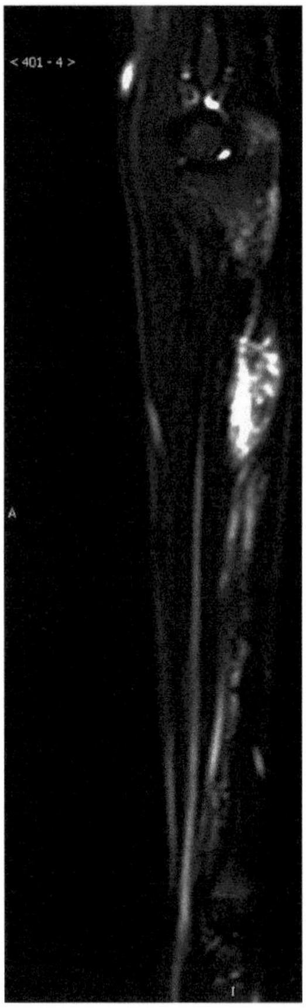

Fig. 40.7 Sagittal fat-suppressed T2-weighted MR image of the right forearm

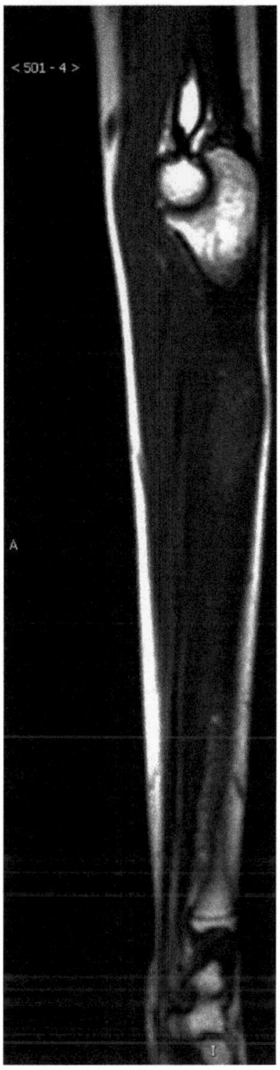

Fig. 40.8 Sagittal T1-weighted MR image of the right forearm

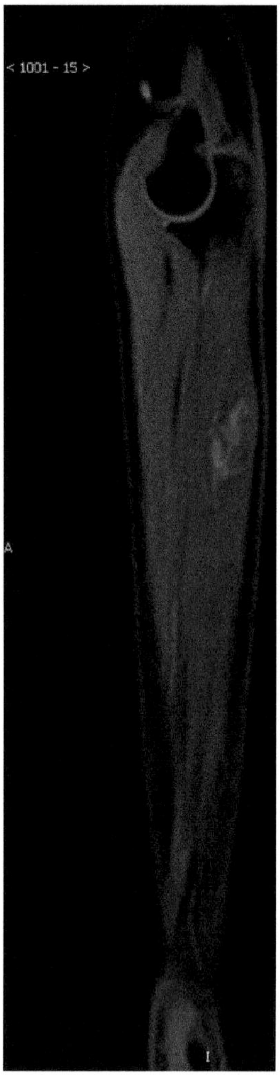

Fig. 40.9 Sagittal post-contrast fat-suppressed T1-weighted MR image of the right forearm

40.3.2 MR Imaging

MR images of the right forearm demonstrate an irregular shaped soft tissue mass around the right proximal ulna. The lesion demonstrates high T1, heterogenous high T2 signal with irregular margin and patchy, linear enhancement.

40.4 Description and Discussion from Residents

The patient is an adolescent female. No abnormality is noted on radiographs. Soft tissue mass around the proximal right ulna is demonstrated on MR images with inhomogeneous signal and no clear margin. Patchy, linear avid enhancement is noted. The osseous structures are intact. The above findings are most suggestive of hemangioma, differential diagnosis is nerve sheath tumor.

40.5 Analysis and Comments from Professor Xiaoguang Cheng

There is a soft tissue mass at the right proximal ulna with an irregular shape and indistinct margin. The lesion demonstrates a high T1 signal and heterogeneous T2 signal with a high T2 signal on fat-suppressed sequence. There is no clear margin of the mass with some abnormal marrow signal noted of the adjacent ulna, likely reactive. Overall, this is most suggestive of hemangioma. The differential diagnosis includes lymphangioma, which usually presents with skin thickening.

40.6 Diagnosis

Hemangioma.

Suggested Reading

Cohen EK, Kressel HY, Perosio T, et al. MR imaging of soft-tissue hemangiomas: correlation with pathologic findings. AJR Am J Roentgenol. 1988 May;150(5):1079–81.

Yilmaz S, Kozakewich HP, Alomari AI, et al. Intramuscular capillary-type hemangioma: radiologic-pathologic correlation. Pediatr Radiol. 2014 May;44(5):558–65.

41 Epithelioid Angiosarcoma: Case 16

41.1 Medical History

The patient is a 39-year-old male. He presented with an enlarged left forearm from birth. About 1 year ago, he noticed a 1 cm mass at the left forearm with pain and enlarging. He underwent surgical resection. However, there was a recurrence, and the mass is now about 7 cm in size. Surface ulceration was noted about 5 days ago.

41.2 Physical Examination

There was significant enlargement of the left forearm. An 8-cm mass was noted at the ulnar side with ulceration and bleeding.

41.3 Imaging Findings

41.3.1 Radiograph

X. Cheng et al., *Imaging of Bone Tumors in Shoulder and Elbow*,
https://doi.org/10.1007/978-981-33-6150-8_41

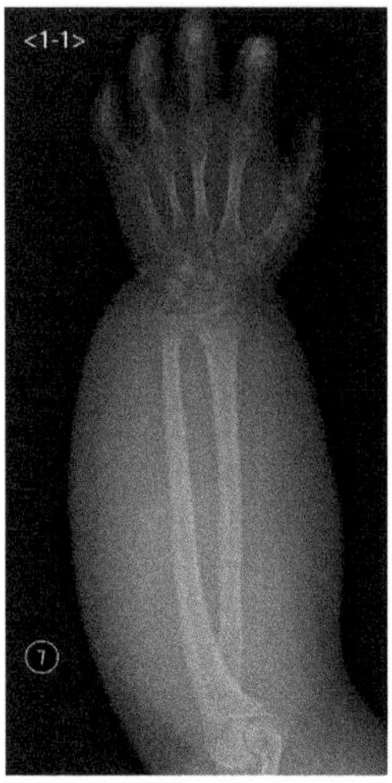

Fig. 41.1 Frontal view of the left forearm

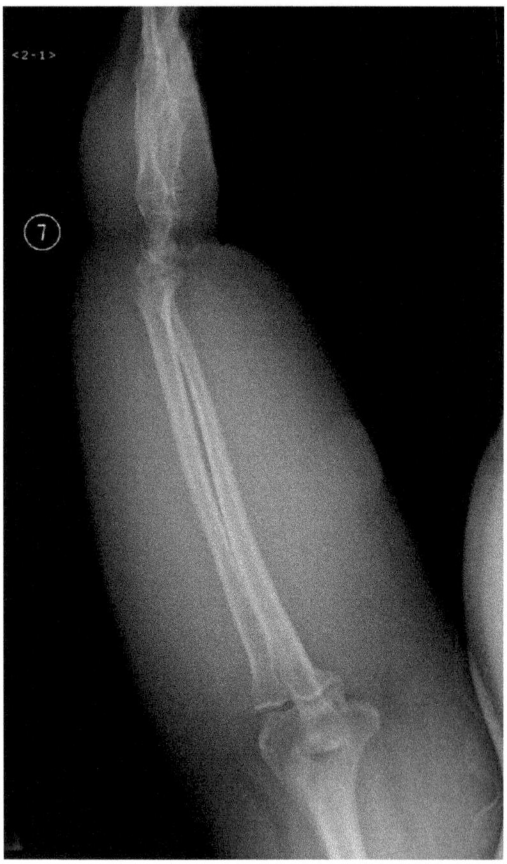

Fig. 41.2 Lateral view of the left forearm

Radiographs of the left forearm demonstrate soft tissue swelling with a mass. The left radius and ulna appear unremarkable.

41.3.2 CT Imaging

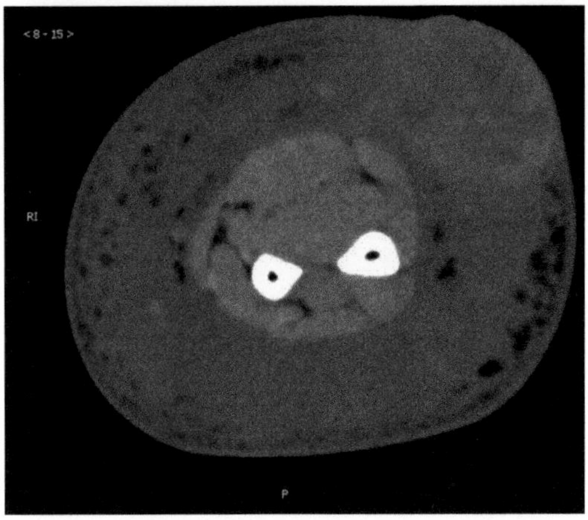

Fig. 41.3 Axial CT image of the left forearm in soft window

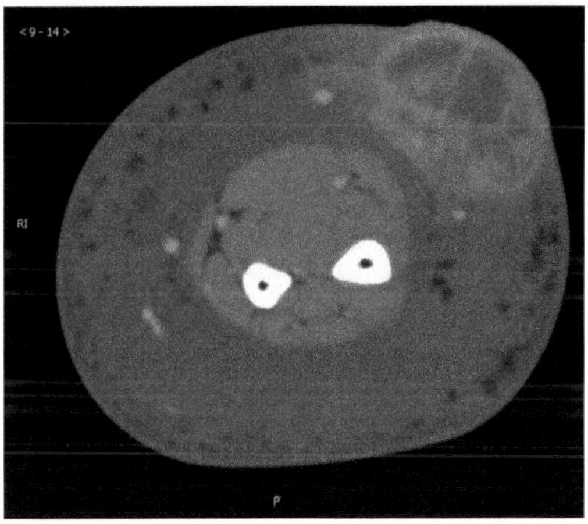

Fig. 41.4 Axial post-contrast CT image of the left forearm in soft tissue window

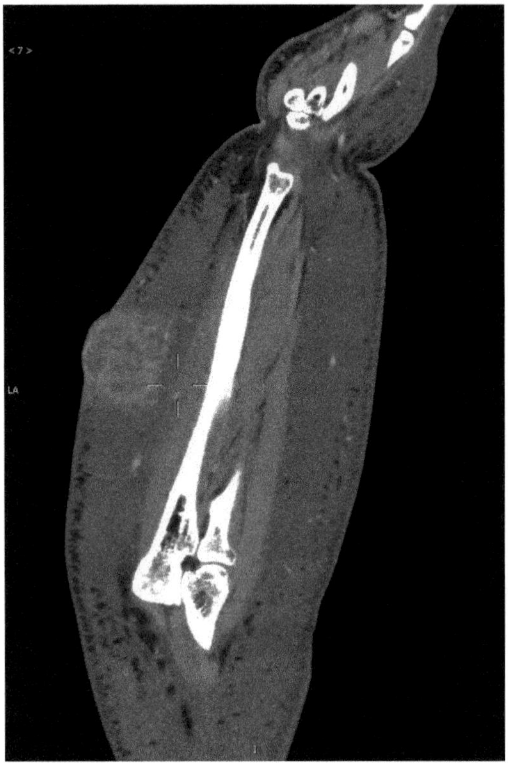

Fig. 41.5 Sagittal post-contrast CT image of the left forearm in soft tissue window

CT images of the left forearm demonstrate soft tissue swelling. There is a subcutaneous mass around the mid-forearm. Heterogeneous enhancement is noted with focal avid enhancement. The left radius and ulna are unremarkable.

41.3.3 MR Imaging

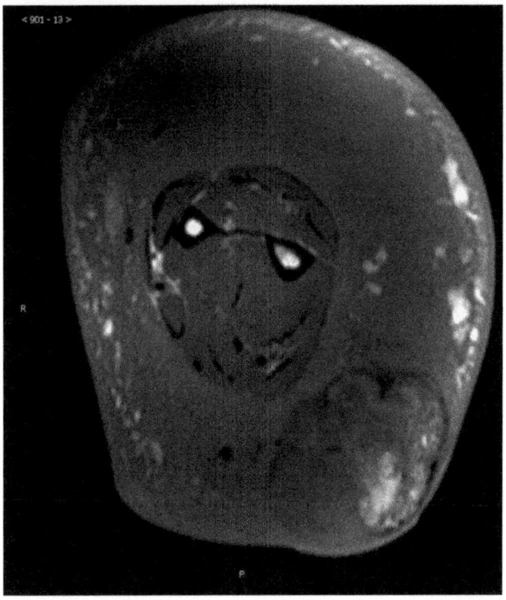

Fig. 41.6 Axial T1-weighted MR image of the left forearm

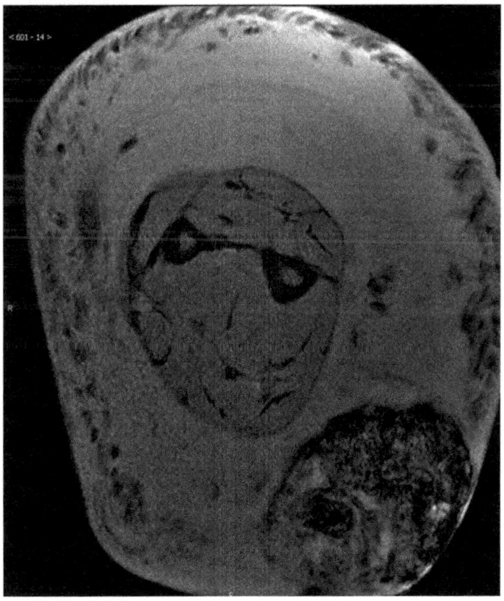

Fig. 41.7 Axial gradient echo sequence MR image of the left forearm

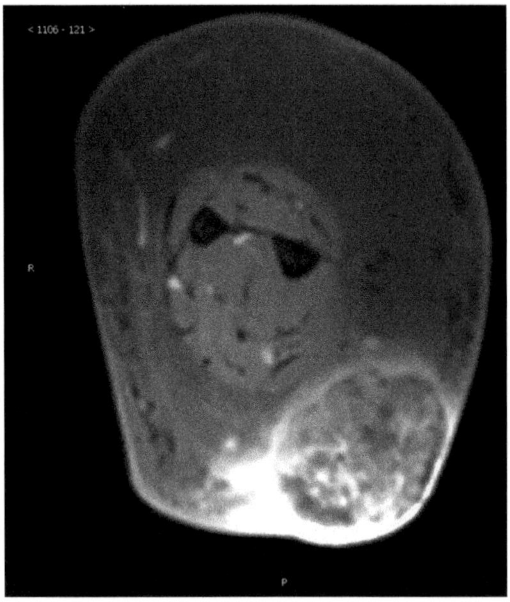

Fig. 41.8 Axial post-contrast fat-suppressed T1-weighted MR image of the left forearm

MR images of the left forearm demonstrate soft tissue swelling with subcutaneous mass in the mid-section. The mass shows heterogeneous T1 and T2 signal with heterogeneous enhancement.

41.4 Description and Discussion from Residents

Radiographs demonstrate left forearm soft tissue swelling with subcutaneous soft tissue mass in the mid-section and intact radius and ulna. On the CT images, there is soft tissue swelling of the left forearm with a normal density of the musculature. Subcutaneous mass is noted in the mid-left forearm with heterogeneous increased density. There is peripheral lobulation with an indistinct margin. Heterogeneous enhancement is noted. The left radius and ulna are not affected. Give the above findings, the malignant process is favored. On the MR images, there is soft tissue swelling of the left forearm with preserved signal in the musculature. Subcutaneous mass shows heterogeneous T1, T2 signal with lobulation and indistinct margin and heterogeneous enhancement, most suggestive of a malignant process, such as soft tissue sarcoma.

41.5 Analysis and Comments from Professor Xiaoguang Cheng

The patient has a history of congenital developmental anomaly of the left upper extremity, with significant swelling of the subcutaneous soft tissue of the left forearm and normal bones and muscles. The soft tissue mass shows avid heterogeneous enhancement. Clinically, there is ulceration with bleeding. However, the imaging features of the mass are nonspecific, favoring soft tissue sarcoma. The mass may not be related to the underlying congenital developmental anomaly of the left upper extremity. Usually, with segmental overgrowth, there is enlargement of all structures, not consistent with the current case.

41.6 Diagnosis

Epithelioid angiosarcoma.

Suggested Reading

Rosenberg A, Agulnik M. Epithelioid hemangioendothelioma: update on diagnosis and treatment. Curr Treat Options Oncol. 2018;19(4):19.

Suchak R, Thway K, Zelger B, et al. Primary cutaneous epithelioid angiosarcoma: a clinicopathologic study of 13 cases of a rare neoplasm occurring outside the setting of conventional angiosarcomas and with predilection for the limbs. Am J Surg Pathol. 2011;35(1):60–9.

Aneurysmal Bone Cyst: Case 17

42

42.1 Medical History

The patient is a 14-year-old girl. She fell from a chair and bumped on the table with focal pain around the left elbow about 2 months ago. She noticed a mass in the region about 1 month ago.

42.2 Physical Examination

There was a mass around the proximal left forearm with an indistinct margin, hard with point tenderness.

42.3 Imaging Findings

42.3.1 Radiograph

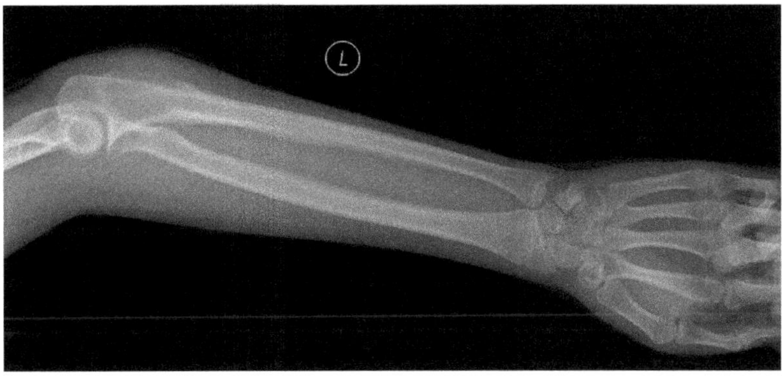

Fig. 42.1 Lateral view of the left elbow

X. Cheng et al., *Imaging of Bone Tumors in Shoulder and Elbow*,
https://doi.org/10.1007/978-981-33-6150-8_42

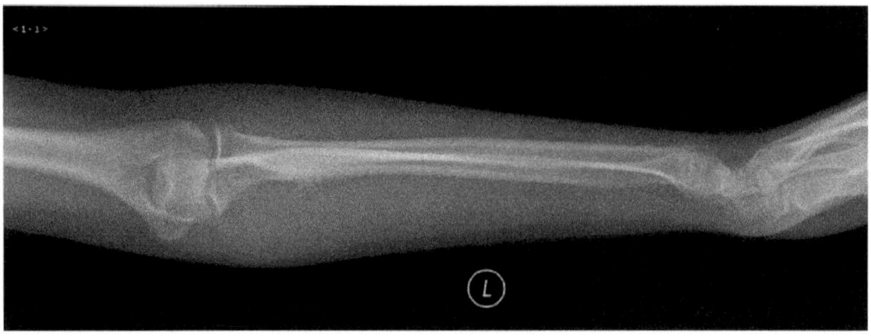

Fig. 42.2 Frontal view of the left elbow

Radiographs of the left elbow demonstrate asymmetric lytic osseous destruction about the proximal ulna with peripheral thin shell and mild adjacent soft tissue swelling.

42.3.2 CT Imaging

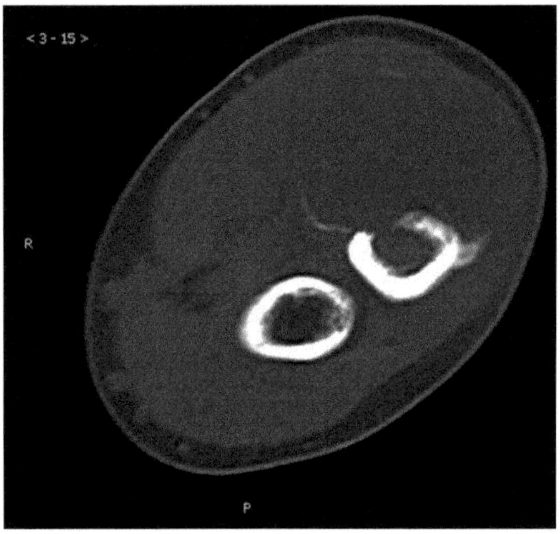

Fig. 42.3 Axial CT image of the left elbow in bone window

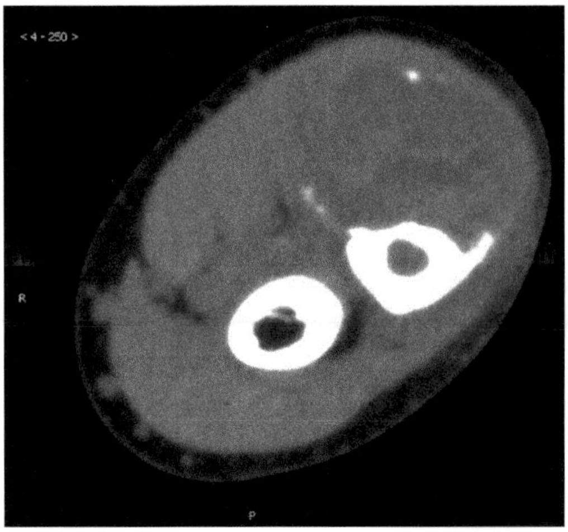

Fig. 42.4 Axial CT image of the left elbow in soft tissue window

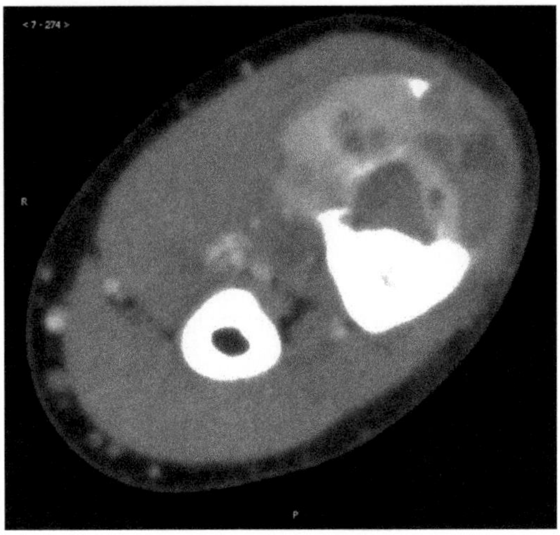

Fig. 42.5 Axial post-contrast CT image of the left elbow in soft tissue window

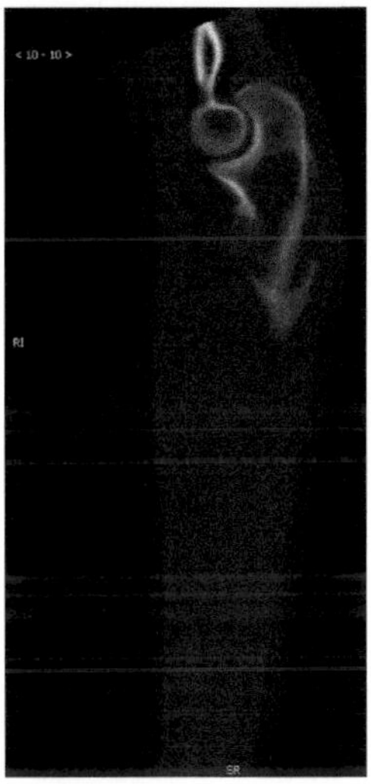

Fig. 42.6 Sagittal CT image of the left elbow in bone window

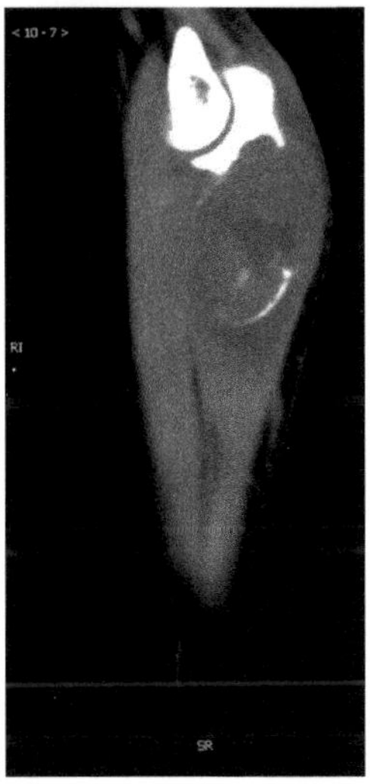

Fig. 42.7 Sagittal CT image of the left elbow in soft tissue window

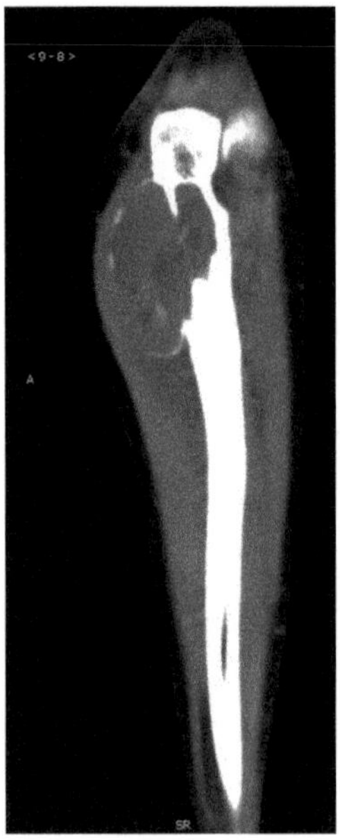

Fig. 42.8 Coronal CT image of the left elbow in soft tissue window

CT images of the left elbow demonstrate asymmetric proximal ulna lytic osseous change with expansile appearance. Septations are noted within the lesion. Adjacent soft tissue demonstrates mild swelling. Solid portion of the lesion shows avid enhancement.

42.3.3 MR Imaging

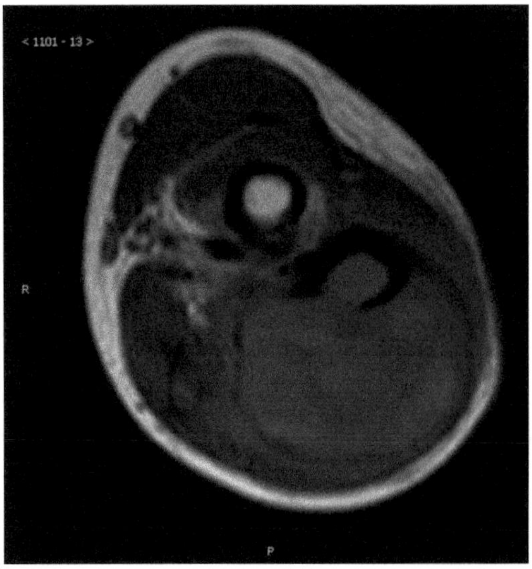

Fig. 42.9 Axial T1-weighted MR image of the left forearm

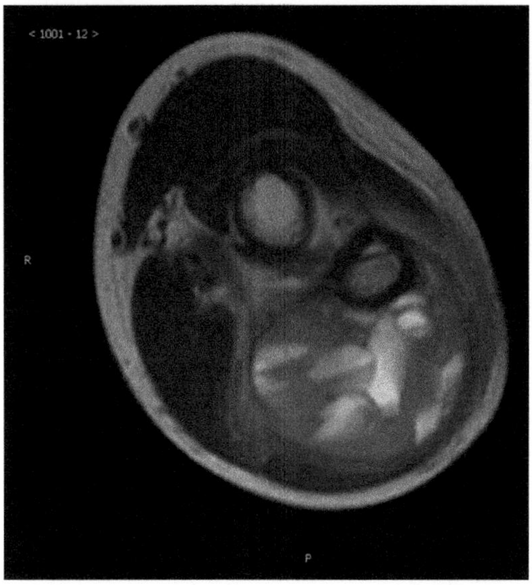

Fig. 42.10 Axial T2-weighted MR image of the left forearm

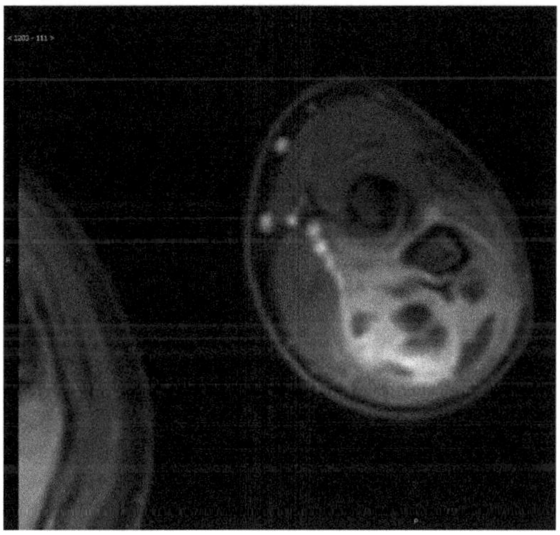

Fig. 42.11 Axial post-contrast fat-suppressed T1-weighted MR image of the left forearm

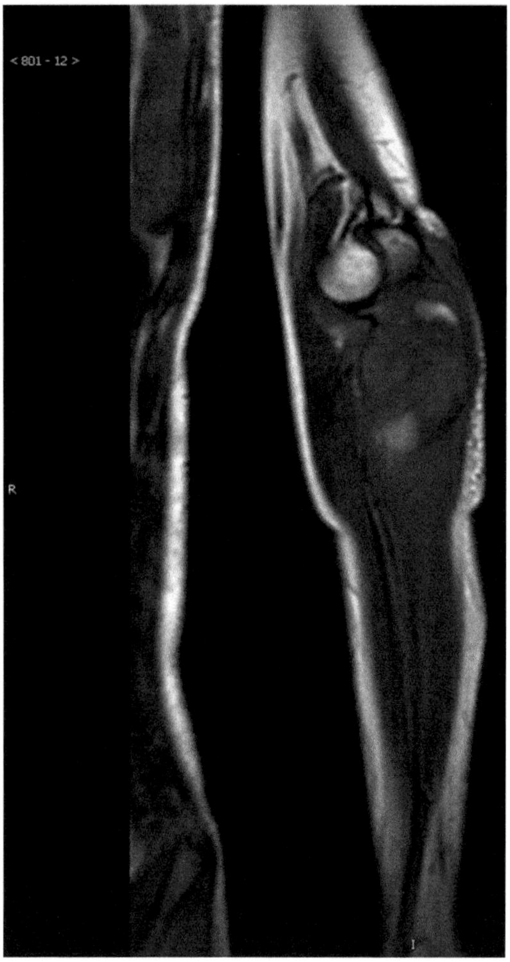

Fig. 42.12 Sagittal T1-weighted MR image of the left elbow

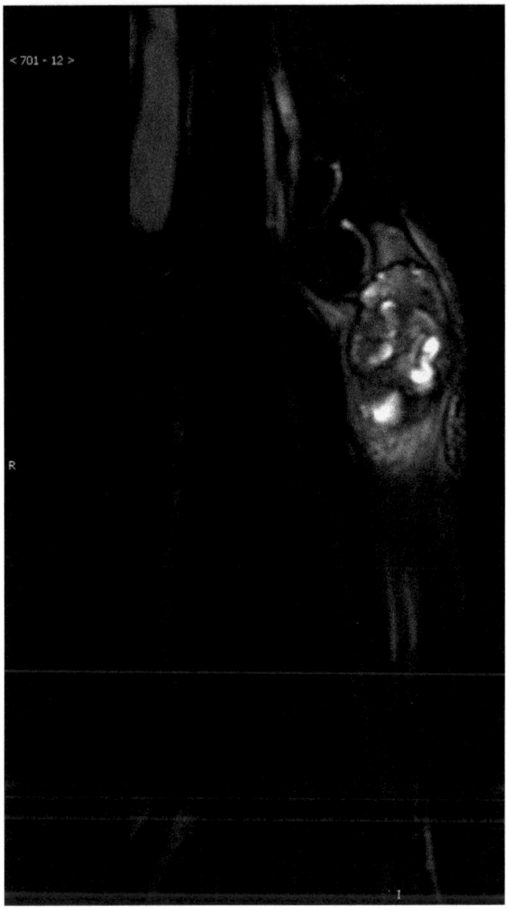

Fig. 42.13 Sagittal fat-suppressed T2 weighted MR image of the left forearm

MR images of the left forearm demonstrate asymmetric lytic osseous destruction of the proximal ulna with heterogeneous T1 and T2 signal and internal septations with fluid–fluid levels. Enhancement is noted at the solid portion of the lesion.

42.4 Description and Discussion from Residents

The patient is an adolescent. Radiographs demonstrate the asymmetric lytic osseous destruction around the proximal ulna with peripheral thin shell, without periosteal reaction. Mild adjacent soft tissue swelling is noted. CT and MRI scans both show the asymmetric lytic destruction of the proximal ulna with heterogeneous densities and signals with internal septations and multiple fluid–fluid levels and peripheral thin shell. No periosteal reaction is noted. Mild adjacent soft tissue swelling is seen. The solid component of the lesion demonstrates avid enhancement. Overall, this is most likely a benign process, such as giant cell tumor with secondary aneurysmal bone cyst (ABC), telangiectatic osteosarcoma is in the differential diagnosis. However, no cluster of fluid–fluid levels of various sizes are noted, which are characteristics for telangiectatic osteosarcoma.

42.5 Analysis and Comments from Professor Xiaoguang Cheng

The patient is an adolescent. With asymmetric lytic destruction of the proximal left ulna, internal septations with fluid–fluid levels, and avid enhancement of the solid portion of the lesion, the top consideration is osseous pathology with ABC. However, the osseous pathology is nonspecific. Given the patient's young age, the possibility of a malignant process cannot be excluded. As for the diagnose of giant cell tumors with ABC, only the enhancement pattern supports giant cell tumors. There are many signs that are not supportive of it, such as the lesion is not at end of the bone, the lesion mostly involves the cortex and the patient's age is young. The characteristics for telangiectatic osteosarcoma are a cluster of fluid–fluid levels of various sizes and osteogenic matrix, not seen in the current case, can be excluded.

42.6 Diagnosis

Aneurysmal bone cyst.

Suggested Reading

Kransdorf MJ, Sweet DE. Aneurysmal bone cyst: concept, controversy, clinical presentation, and imaging. AJR Am J Roentgenol. 1995;164(3):573–80.

Mascard E, Gomez-Brouchet A, Lambot K. Bone cysts: unicameral and aneurysmal bone cyst. Orthop Traumatol Surg Res. 2015;101(1 Suppl):S119–27.

Van Dyck P, Vanhoenacker FM, Vogel J, et al. Prevalence, extension and characteristics of fluid-fluid levels in bone and soft tissue tumors. Eur Radiol. 2006;16(12):2644–51.

43 Osteoid Osteoma: Case 18

43.1 Medical History

The patient is a 9-year-old girl. She presented with left elbow pain, restricted motion around the joint for 1 year.

43.2 Physical Examination

There was soft tissue swelling about the left elbow with restricted motion.

43.3 Imaging Findings

43.3.1 Radiograph

X. Cheng et al., *Imaging of Bone Tumors in Shoulder and Elbow*,
https://doi.org/10.1007/978-981-33-6150-8_43

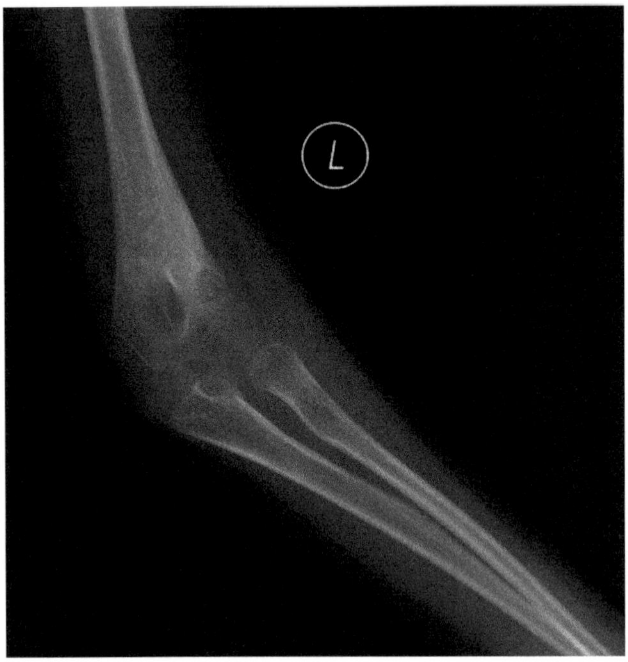

Fig. 43.1 Frontal view of the left elbow

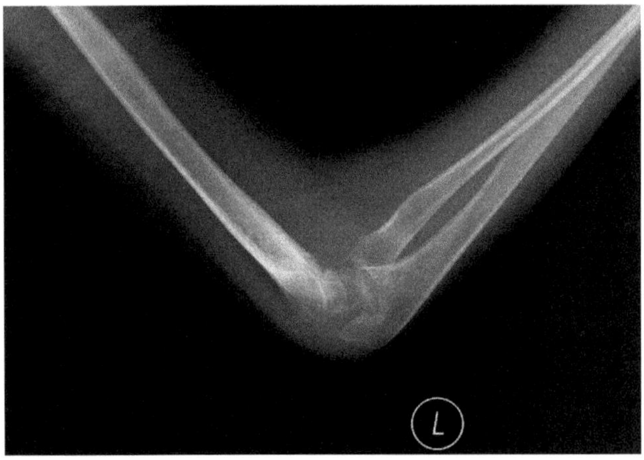

Fig. 43.2 Lateral view of the left elbow

Radiographs of the left elbow demonstrate destruction around the distal lateral humeral epicondyle with peripheral sclerosis and periosteal reaction and soft tissue edema.

43.3.2 CT Imaging

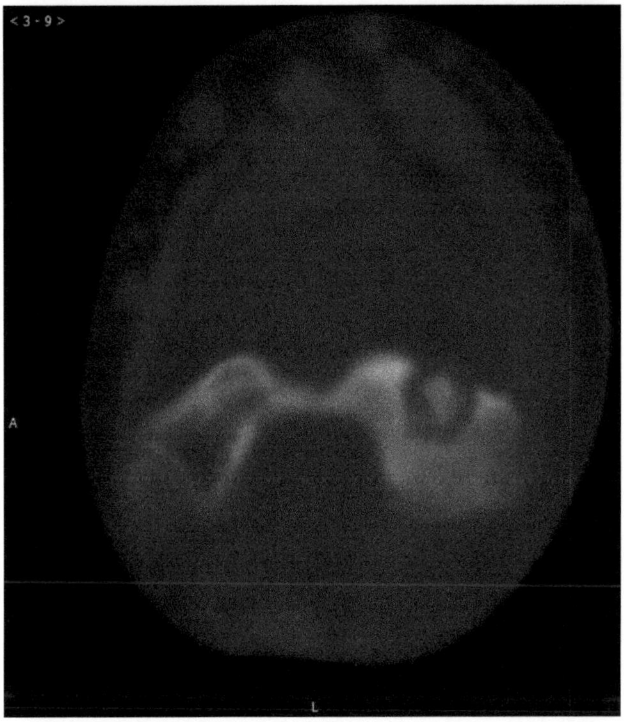

Fig. 43.3 Axial CT image of the left elbow in bone window

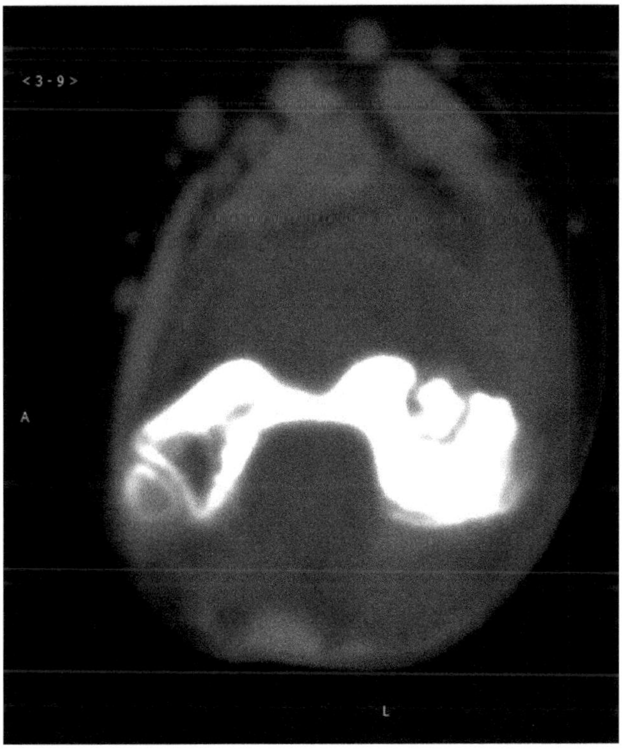

Fig. 43.4 Axial CT image of the left elbow in soft tissue window

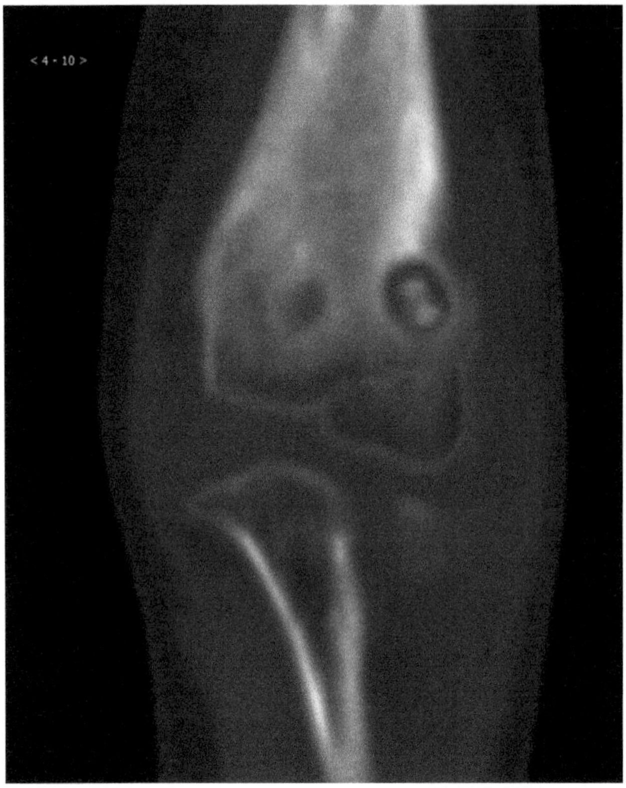

Fig. 43.5 Coronal CT image of the left elbow in bone window

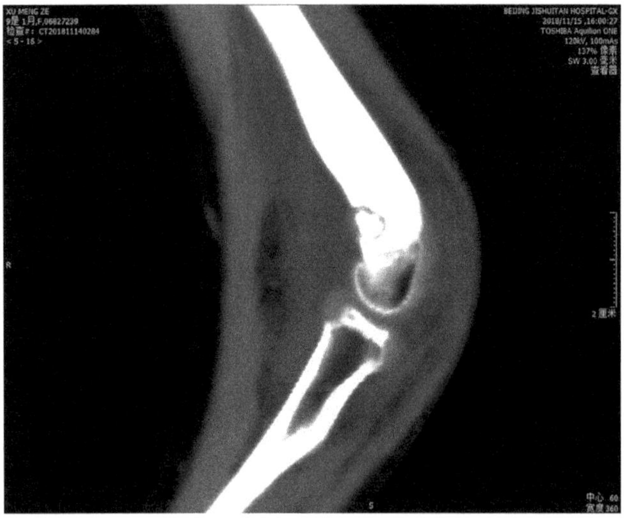

Fig. 43.6 Sagittal CT image of the left elbow in soft tissue window

CT images of the left elbow demonstrate circular lytic destruction around the distal lateral epicondyle with internal high density and clear margin. Periosteal reactions are noted in the surrounding osseous structures. There is soft tissue swelling with joint effusion.

43.3.3 MR Imaging

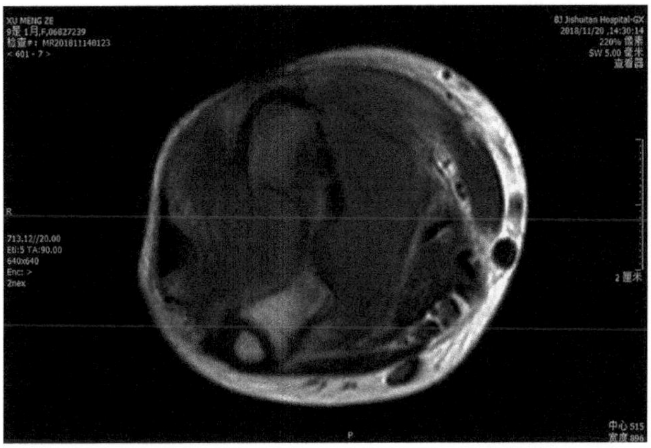

Fig. 43.7 Axial T1-weighted MR image of the left elbow

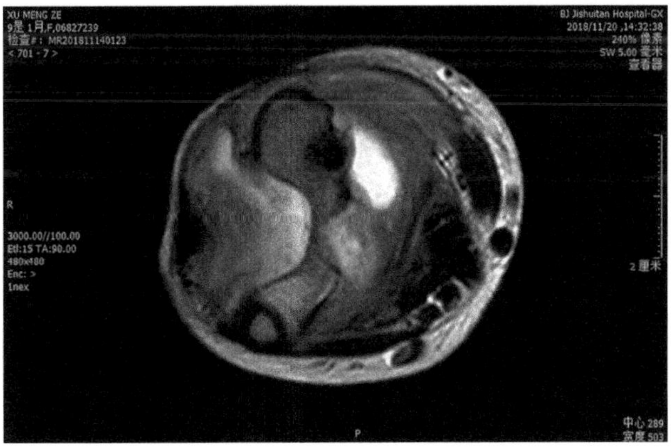

Fig. 43.8 Axial T2-weighted MR image of the left elbow

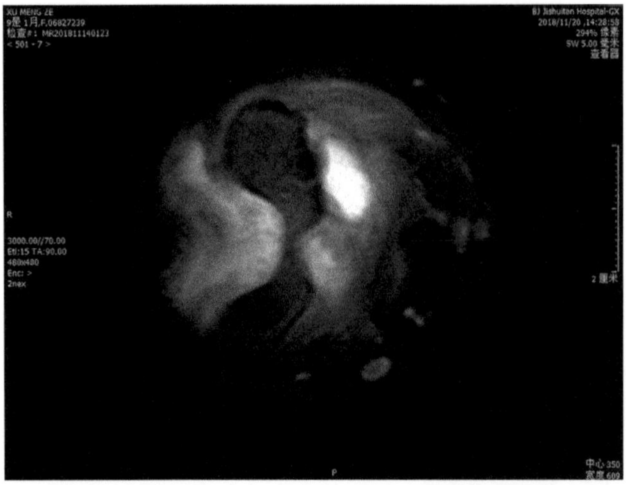

Fig. 43.9 Axial fat-suppressed T2-weighted MR image of the left elbow

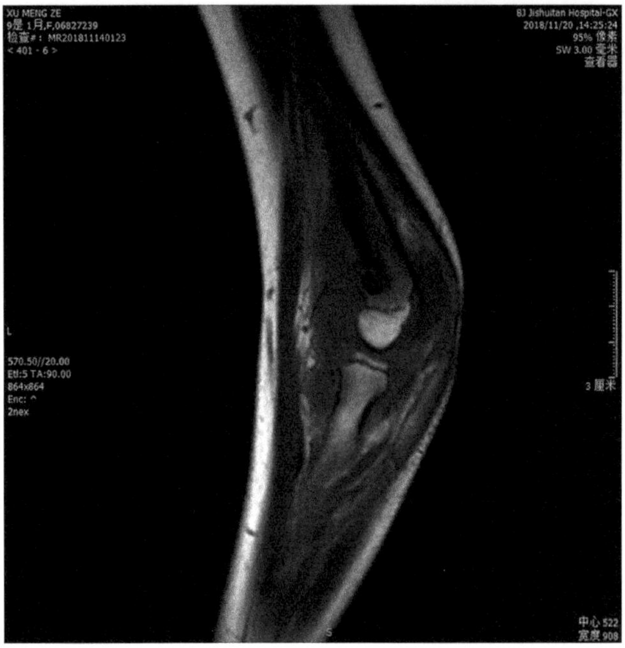

Fig. 43.10 Sagittal T1-weighted MR image of the left elbow

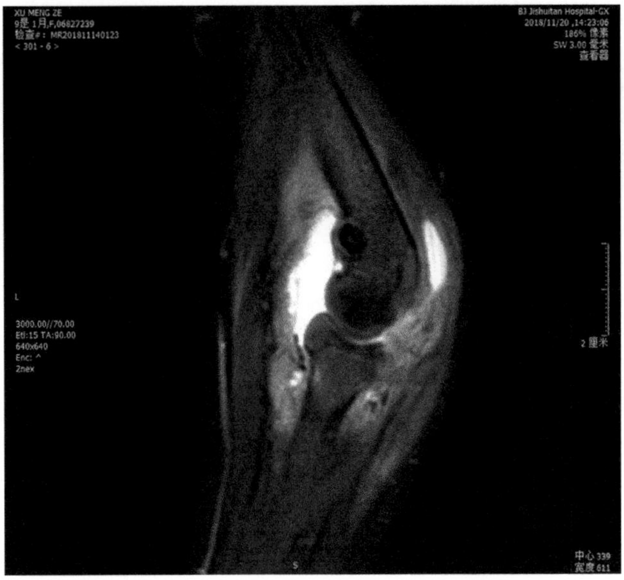

Fig. 43.11 Sagittal fat-suppressed T2-weighted MR image of the left elbow

MR images of the left elbow demonstrate low T1 and T2 signal at the distal lateral humeral epicondyle. Marrow edema is seen of the distal humerus. Moderate elbow joint effusion is present.

43.4 Description and Discussion from Residents

The patient is a 9-year-old girl with a history of symptoms for a year. Radiographs and CT images demonstrate the lesion at the distal lateral humeral epicondyle as a semicircular lytic lesion with internal high density and non-expansile. Peripheral sclerosis and periosteal reaction are noted. The joint effusion and hypertrophy of the synovium are reactive changes. Given the above findings, this is most likely an inflammatory process such as osteoid osteoma, Brodie's abscess, and eosinophilic granuloma. MR images show low T1 and T2 signals, not consistent with abscess or granuloma. Additionally, if there was an abscess, the peripheral cortex would be disrupted. Overall, the top consideration is osteoid osteoma.

43.5 Analysis and Comments from Professor Xiaoguang Cheng

The patient is a child. The circular lesion is at the distal lateral humeral epicondyle with internal nidus, clear margin, and peripheral osseous reactive changes. There is soft tissue swelling around the joint. The epiphysis is intact with preserved joint space. Infection can be excluded. In tuberculosis, the reactive changes in the adjacent bone would not be this significant and can be excluded. T2 signal tends to be high in cases of abscess or eosinophilic granuloma, not consistent with the current case. This is a relatively typical case of osteoid osteoma. Osteoid osteoma can incite inflammatory factors such as interleukin and cause extensive inflammatory changes.

43.6 Diagnosis

Osteoid osteoma.

Suggested Reading

Chai JW, Hong SH, Choi JY, et al. Radiologic diagnosis of osteoid osteoma: from simple to challenging findings. Radiographics. 2010;30(3):737–49.

Kransdorf MJ, Stull MA, Gilkey FW, et al. Osteoid osteoma. Radiographics. 1991;11(4):671–96.

44 Lipoma: Case 19

44.1 Medical History

The patient is a 60-year-old male. About 4 years ago, he incidentally noted a mass at his upper left arm, about the size of an egg and non-painful. However, he noticed an increase in size in the last 1 year.

44.2 Physical Examination

There is a palpable 26 cm × 15 cm × 10 cm mass along the medial aspect of the left upper arm.

44.3 Imaging Findings

44.3.1 Radiograph

X. Cheng et al., *Imaging of Bone Tumors in Shoulder and Elbow*,
https://doi.org/10.1007/978-981-33-6150-8_44

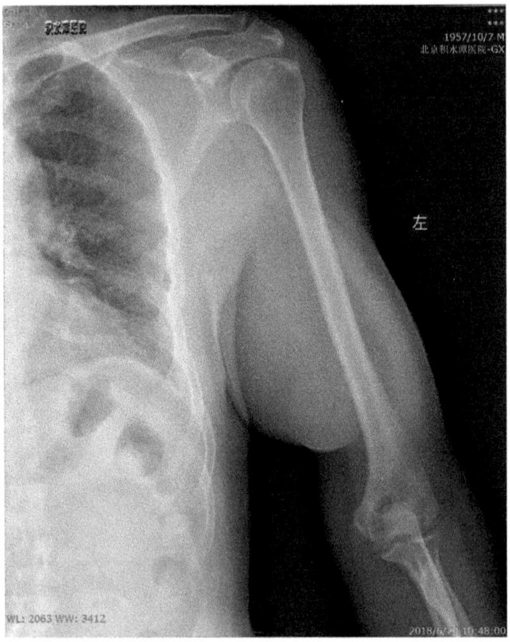

Fig. 44.1 Frontal view of the left humerus

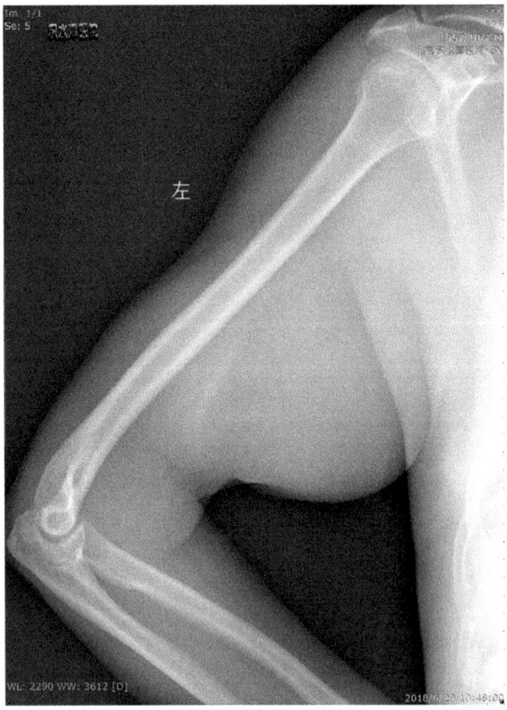

Fig. 44.2 Lateral view of the left humerus

Radiographs of the left humerus demonstrate a large low-density mass in the medial aspect of the left upper arm with a clear margin and normal adjacent bone.

44.3.2 CT Imaging

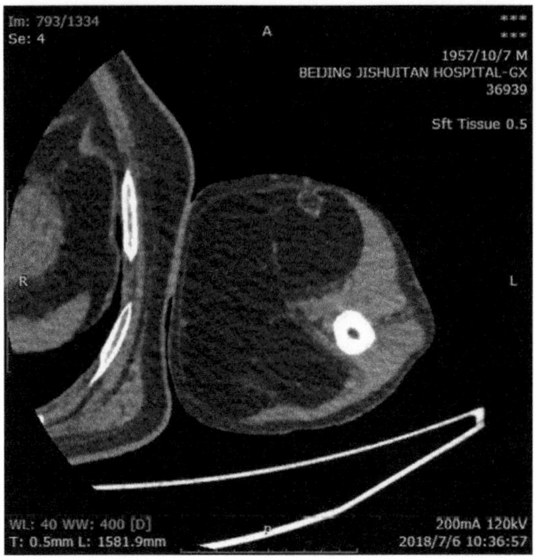

Fig. 44.3 Axial CT image of the left humerus in soft tissue window

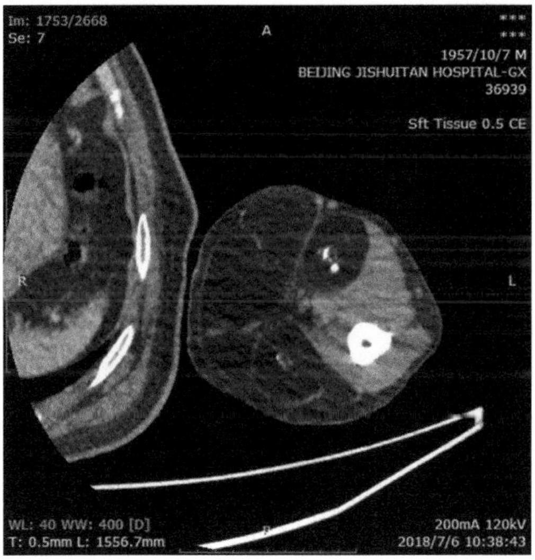

Fig. 44.4 Axial CT image of the left humerus in soft tissue window

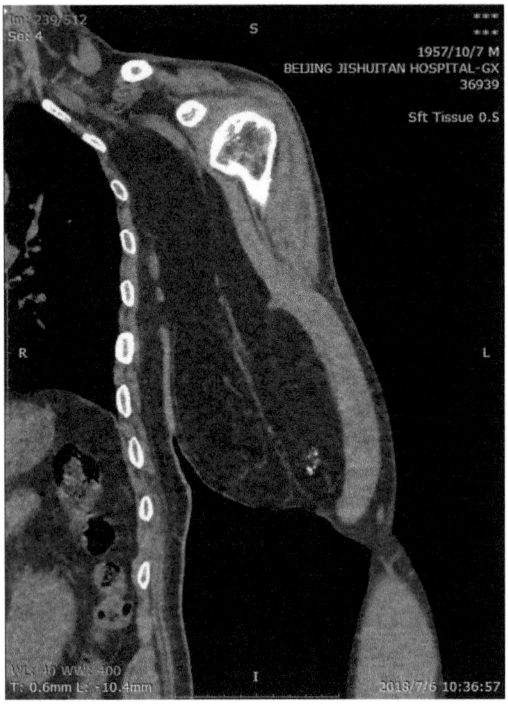

Fig. 44.5 Coronal CT image of the left humerus in soft tissue window

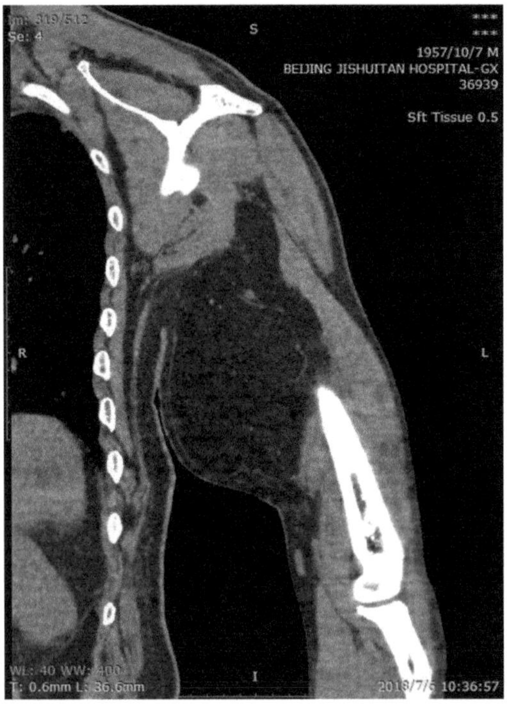

Fig. 44.6 Sagittal post-contrast CT image of the left humerus in soft tissue window

CT images of the left humerus demonstrate a large soft tissue mass in the medial aspect of the upper arm. The lesion measures of fat density with internal thin septations and some calcifications with clear margin. There is enhancement of the septations.

44.4 Description and Discussion from Residents

The patient is an older male. Radiographs demonstrate a large low-density soft tissue mass with clear margin but internal heterogeneous densities and septations, raising concern for malignant process. On the CT images, the lesion is well circumscribed with fat density and some internal thin septations and calcifications. The septations enhance but the majority of the lesion of fat does not enhance. Blood vessels are seen within the lesion. The adjacent humerus is normal. This is most consistent with a lipoma. However, with rapid growth in the past year, the possibility of liposarcoma is raised.

44.5 Analysis and Comments from Professor Xiaoguang Cheng

Fat density mass at the medial aspect of the left upper arm with some internal septations but no soft tissue nodule and only enhancement along the septations with clear margin is most likely a lipoma. When evaluating a fatty soft tissue mass, it is very important to make sure there is no soft tissue density or nodule within. If there is, the possibility of liposarcoma is raised

44.6 Diagnosis

Lipoma.

Suggested Reading

Burt AM, Huang BK. Imaging review of lipomatous musculoskeletal lesions. SICOT J. 2017;3:34.

Murphey MD, Carroll JF, Flemming DJ, et al. From the archives of the AFIP: benign musculoskeletal lipomatous lesions. Radiographics. 2004;24(5):1433–66.

45 Synovial Chondromatosis: Case 20

45.1 Medical History

The patient is a 37-year-old female. She presented with discomfort with restricted motion around the medial aspect of the right elbow for 5 years and worsening in the past 6 months. She has a history of biopsy.

45.2 Physical Examination

There was a palpable mass along the medial aspect of the right elbow, measuring about 3 cm × 3 cm × 2 cm without clear margin, smooth, rubbery, and nonmobile. There was point tenderness.

45.3 Imaging Findings

45.3.1 Radiograph

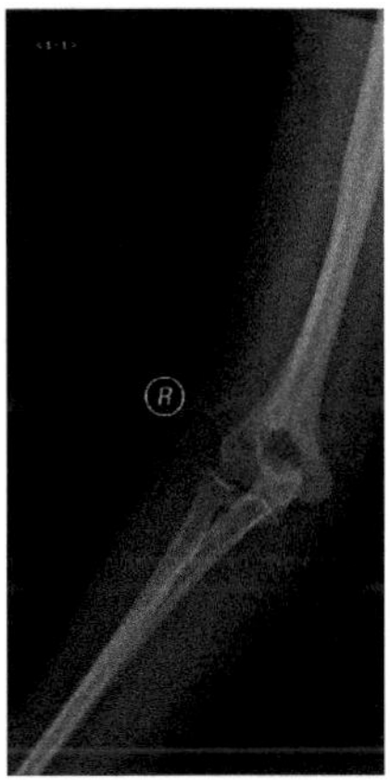

Fig. 45.1 Frontal view of the right elbow

X. Cheng et al., *Imaging of Bone Tumors in Shoulder and Elbow*,
https://doi.org/10.1007/978-981-33-6150-8_45

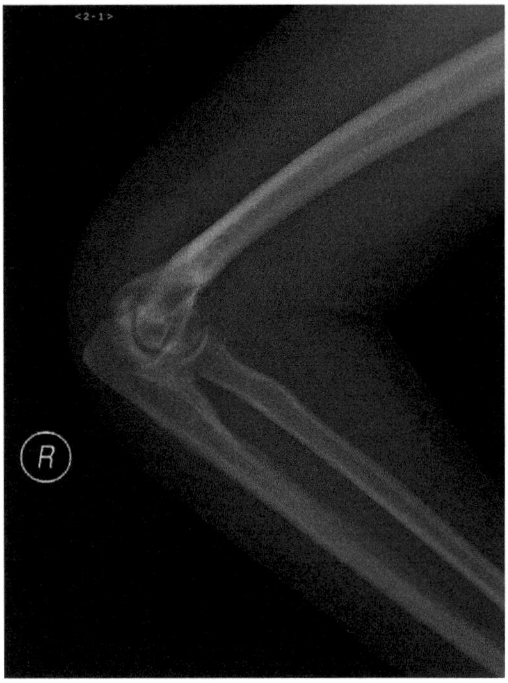

Fig. 45.2 Lateral view of the right elbow

Radiographs of the right elbow demonstrate enlargement of the olecranon fossa.

45.3.2 CT Imaging

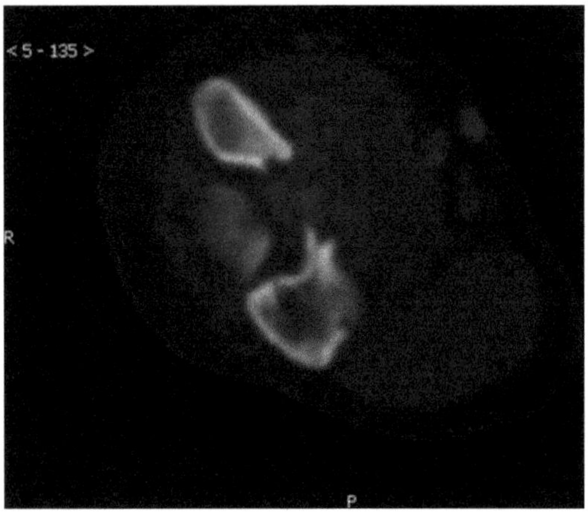

Fig. 45.3 Axial CT image of the right elbow in bone window

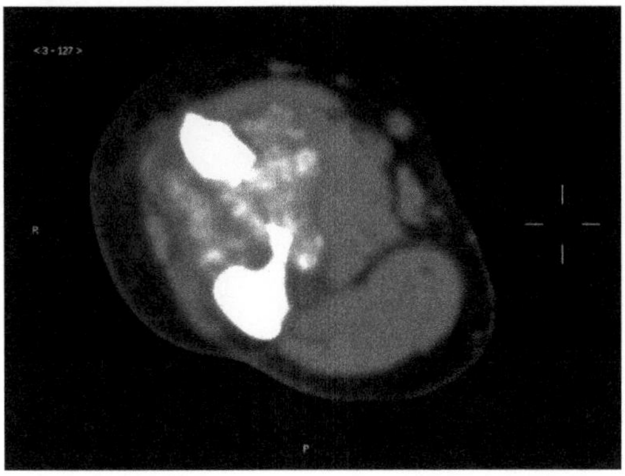

Fig. 45.4 Axial CT image of the right elbow in soft tissue window

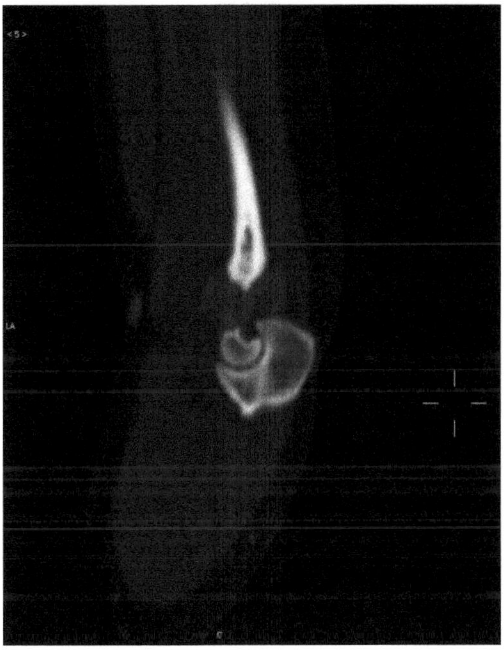

Fig. 45.5 Sagittal CT image of the right elbow in bone window

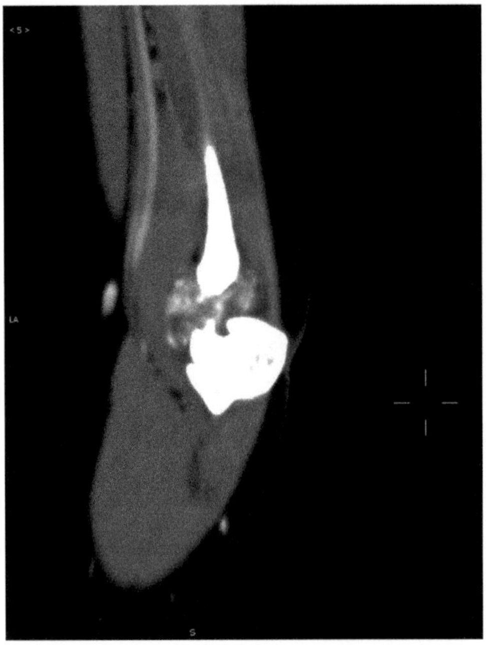

Fig. 45.6 Sagittal post-contrast CT image of the right elbow in soft tissue window

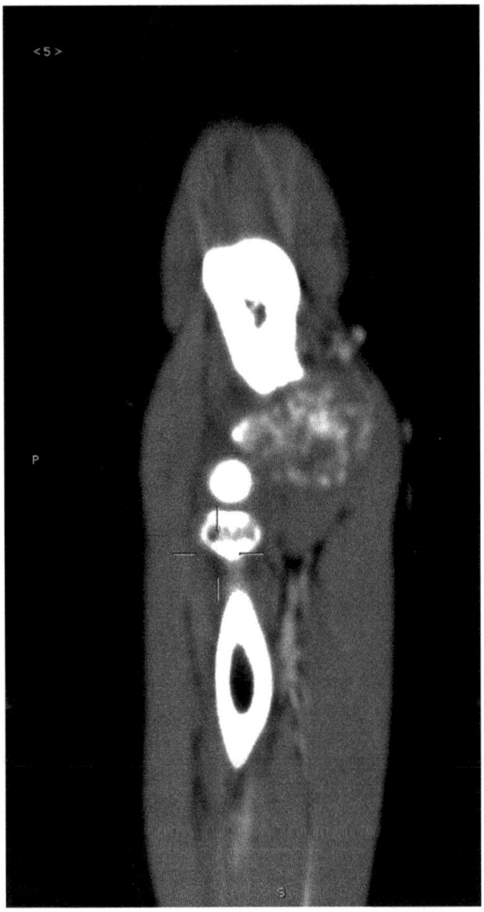

Fig. 45.7 Coronal post-contrast CT image of the right elbow in soft tissue window

CT images of the right elbow demonstrate intra-articular nodular and lobulated calcifications with clear margin and no enhancement. There is erosion into the distal humerus.

45.4 Description and Discussion from Residents

The patient is a young female with a prolonged history. Radiographs demonstrate enlargement of the olecranon fossa, focal bone resorption, and peripheral sclerosis, without soft tissue mass. CT scan images show a small amount of joint effusion with internal nodular and lobulated high densities and no enhancement. The overall findings are most suggestive of intra-articular benign process with top consideration of synovial chondromatosis. Differential diagnoses include pigmented villonodular synovitis (PVNS), synovial hemangioma, and tumor at the intercondylar region.

45.5 Analysis and Comments from Professor Xiaoguang Cheng

The patient is a young female with prolonged history. Radiographs show bone destruction around the right humeral olecranon fossa with clear margin and peripheral sclerosis. On the CT scan images, there is irregular shaped nodular and lobulated calcifications within the joint, without enhancement. This is most consistent with intra-articular pathology; the top consideration is synovial chondromatosis. However, on the sagittal images, there is cortical disruption of the distal humerus with focal soft tissue mass, favoring osseous pathology, such as osteoblastoma of the right distal humerus or osteoid osteoma. This should be differentiated from gouty arthropathy; however, that is rare in premenopausal women.

45.6 Diagnosis

Synovial chondromatosis.

Suggested Reading

Ho YY, Choueka J. Synovial chondromatosis of the upper extremity. J Hand Surg Am. 2013;38(4):804–10.

Murphey MD, Vidal JA, Fanburg-Smith JC, et al. Imaging of synovial chondromatosis with radiologic-pathologic correlation. Radiographics. 2007;27(5):1465–88.

46 Osteoblastoma: Case 21

46.1 Medical History

The patient is a 25-year-old male. He presented with on and off right elbow swelling with pain for 5 years.

46.2 Physical Examination

There was focal high temperature of the skin. No point tenderness but pain with percussion.

46.3 Imaging Findings

46.3.1 Radiograph

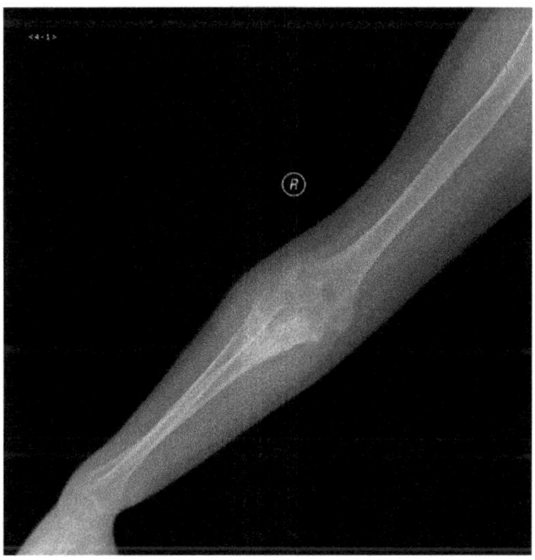

Fig. 46.1 Frontal view of the right elbow

X. Cheng et al., *Imaging of Bone Tumors in Shoulder and Elbow*,
https://doi.org/10.1007/978-981-33-6150-8_46

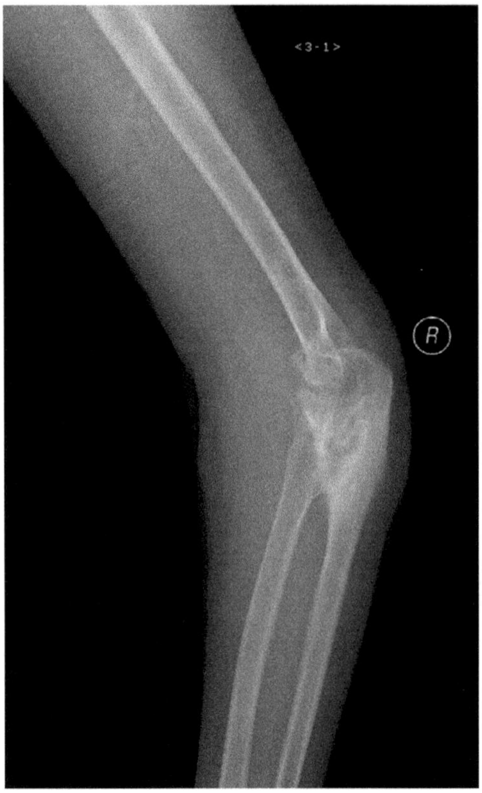

Fig. 46.2 Lateral view of the right elbow

Radiographs of the right elbow demonstrate sclerosis in the proximal right ulna with internal patchy low-density area and soft tissue swelling.

46.3.2 CT Imaging

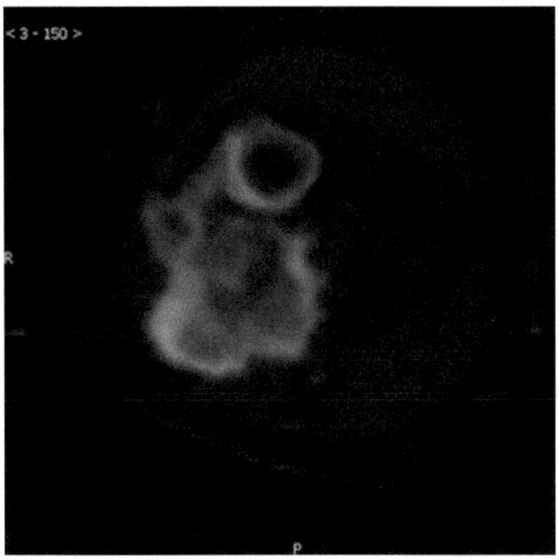

Fig. 46.3 Axial CT image of the right elbow in bone window

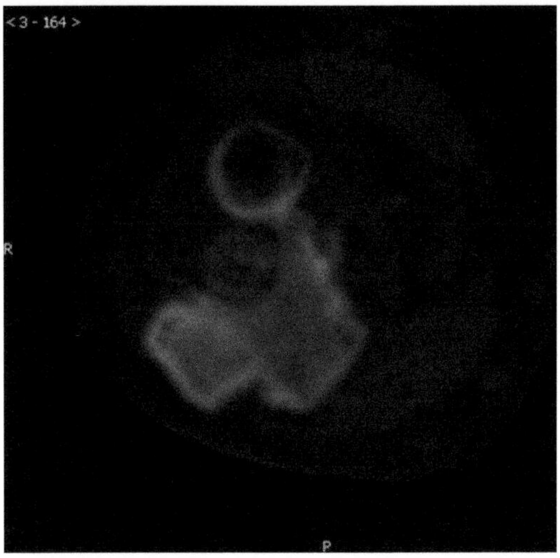

Fig. 46.4 Axial CT image of the right elbow in bone window

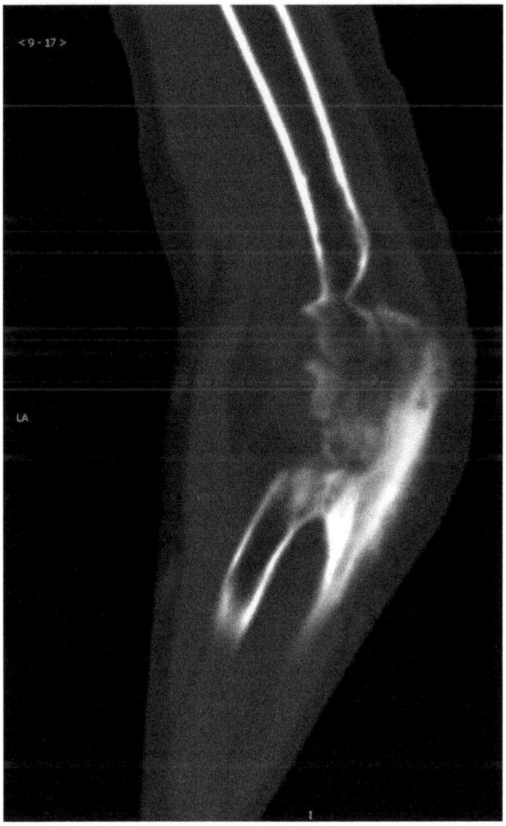

Fig. 46.5 Sagittal CT image of the right elbow in bone window

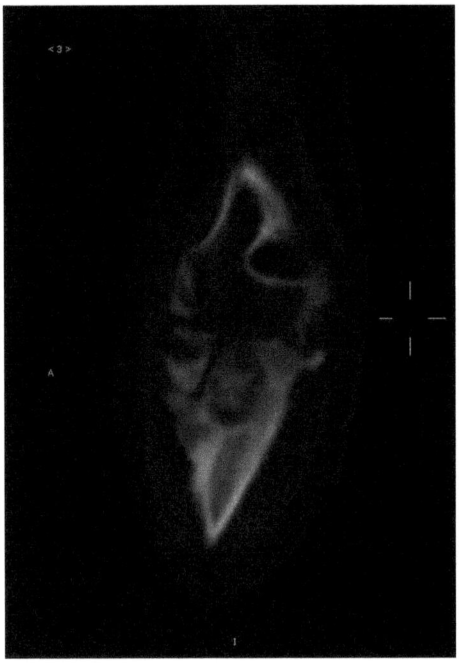

Fig. 46.6 Coronal CT image of the right elbow in bone window

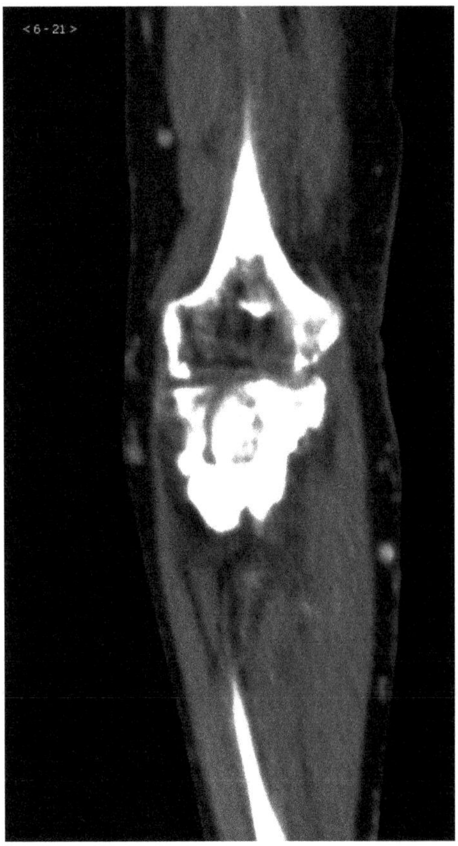

Fig. 46.7 Coronal post-contrast CT image of the right elbow in soft tissue window

CT images of the right elbow demonstrate low-density lesion in the proximal ulna with internal irregular shaped high density. There is peripheral sclerosis and soft tissue swelling. Mild heterogeneous soft tissue enhancement is noted.

46.4 Description and Discussion from Residents

The patient is 25 years old with 5 years of symptoms. Radiographs demonstrate deformity of the proximal ulna with sclerosis and internal patchy low-density area. The lesion demonstrates a clear margin with internal high density within the low-density lesion, consistent with osseous pathology, such as osteoblastoma or osteoid osteoma. On the CT scan, there is a low-density lesion at the proximal ulnar olecranon with a clear margin and internal irregular shaped high density. There is reactive sclerosis and soft tissue edema, but no soft tissue mass. Mild heterogeneous enhancement is noted in adjacent soft tissues. Overall, this is most consistent with osteoblastoma with chronic infection in the differential diagnosis.

46.5 Analysis and Comments from Professor Xiaoguang Cheng

The patient is a young male with 5 years of symptoms. Both radiographs and CT scan images demonstrate low-density lesion at the right olecranon with clear margin and internal irregular shaped high density, of the nidus and surrounding reactive sclerosis and soft tissue edema, most consistent with osteoblastoma. The high density within the lesion is plenty and not consistent with sequestrum, thus, chronic infection can be excluded.

46.6 Diagnosis

Osteoblastoma (Epithelioid osteoblastoma).

Suggested Reading

Kroon HM, Schurmans J. Osteoblastoma: clinical and radiologic findings in 98 new cases. Radiology. 1990;175(3):783–90.

Sonnylal L, Peterson JR, Decilveo AP, et al. Giant periosteal aggressive epithelioid osteoblastoma: 21-year-old male presents case in the midshaft of his femur. Skelet Radiol. 2018;47(10):1443–8.

47 Giant Cell Tumor of Bone: Case 22

47.1 Medical History

The patient is a 13-year-old boy. He presented with right elbow pain and swelling after trauma about 6 months ago. He underwent resection of the right distal humeral aneurysmal bone cyst about 4 months ago and recently experienced recurrent discomfort and swelling for about 1 month.

47.2 Physical Examination

There was swelling around the right elbow with a restricted range of motion.

47.3 Imaging Findings

47.3.1 Radiograph

X. Cheng et al., *Imaging of Bone Tumors in Shoulder and Elbow*,
https://doi.org/10.1007/978-981-33-6150-8_47

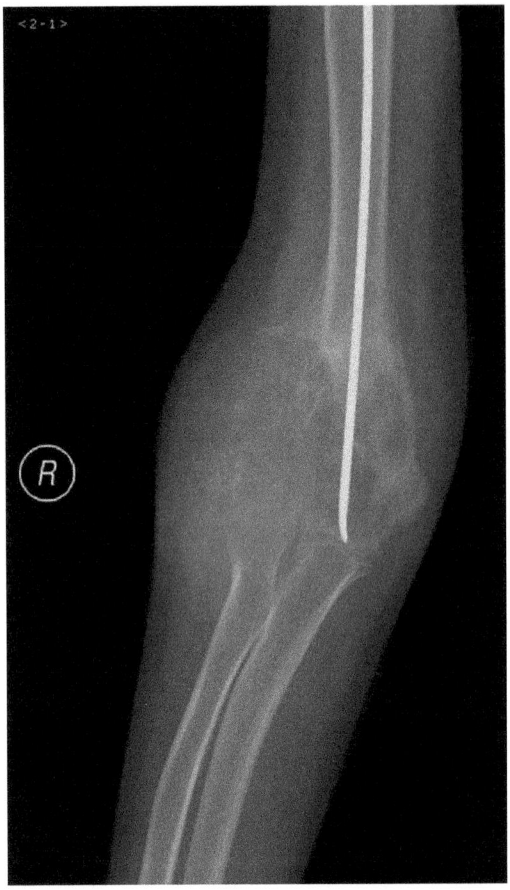

Fig. 47.1 Frontal view of the right elbow

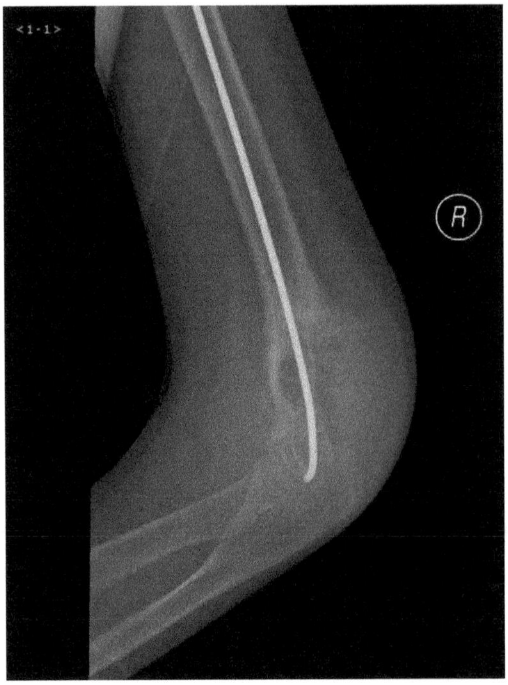

Fig. 47.2 Lateral view of the right elbow

Radiographs of the right elbow demonstrate post-surgical changes of the distal humerus and expansile osseous destruction with periosteal reaction and adjacent soft tissue swelling. An intramedullary nail is noted transfixing the right humerus.

47.3.2 CT Imaging

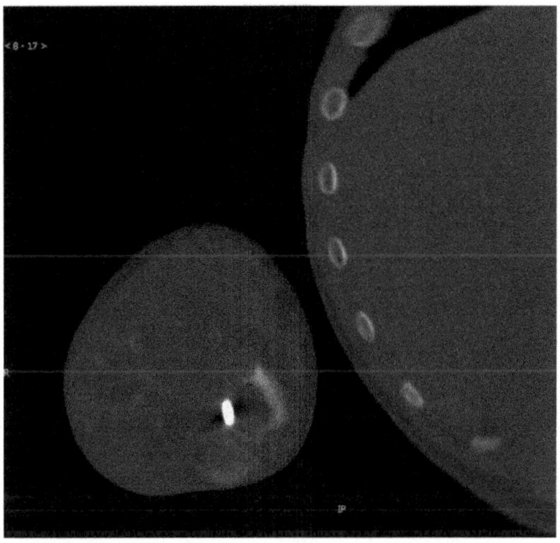

Fig. 47.3 Axial CT image of the right elbow in bone window

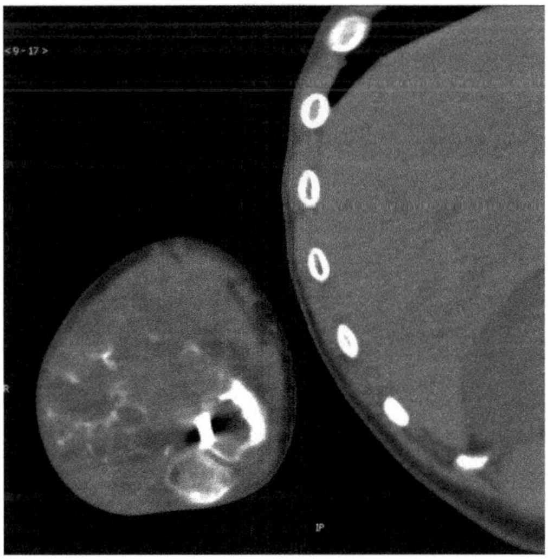

Fig. 47.4 Axial CT image of the right elbow in soft tissue window

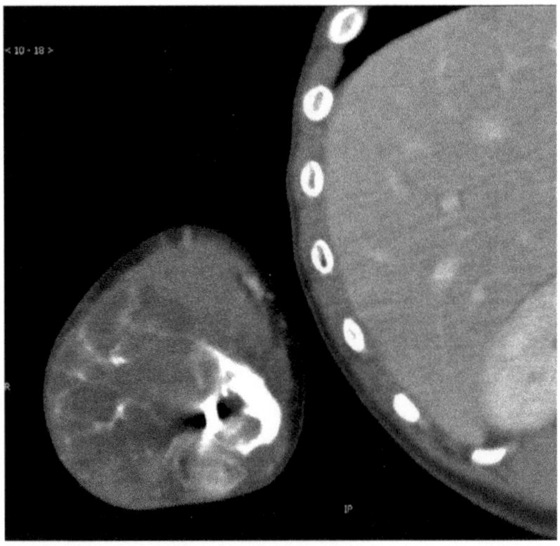

Fig. 47.5 Axial post-contrast CT image of the right elbow in soft tissue window

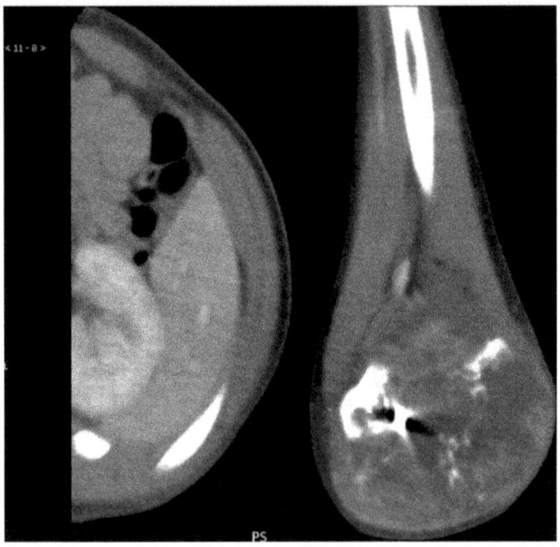

Fig. 47.6 Coronal post-contrast CT image of the right elbow in soft tissue window

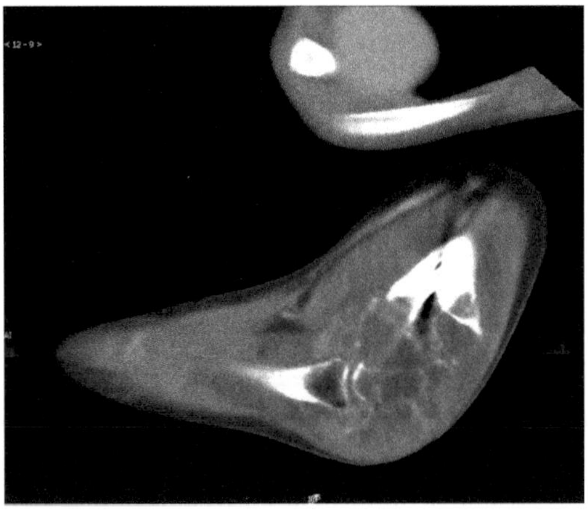

Fig. 47.7 Sagittal post-contrast CT image of the right elbow in soft tissue window

CT images of the right elbow demonstrate postsurgical changes at the distal humerus. There is expansile osseous destruction with the internal residual cortex. Heterogeneous enhancement is noted.

47.4 Description and Discussion from Residents

The patient is a 13-year-old boy with a history of resection of right distal humeral aneurysmal bone cyst. Radiographs demonstrate osseous postsurgical changes of osteopenia and expansile osseous destruction extending to the articular surface with irregular margin. There is focal reactive sclerosis and periosteal reaction. Destruction around the periosteal reaction is noted with adjacent soft tissue swelling. On the CT scan images, there is a residual osseous ridge in the lesion and internal heterogeneous enhancement with small fluid–fluid levels. Overall, the consideration is recurrence of aneurysmal bone cyst and telangiectatic osteosarcoma cannot be excluded.

47.5 Analysis and Comments from Professor Xiaoguang Cheng

The patient is a 13-year-old boy with a history of surgery at the right humerus. Images demonstrate the distal humeral osseous destruction with expansile appearance and internal residual osseous ridge and focal reactive peripheral sclerosis and periosteal reaction and preservation of the articular surface. There is heterogeneous enhancement with more avid enhancement at the solid portion of the lesion. Given the patient's age, history, and imaging findings, the top consideration is telangiectatic osteosarcoma.

47.6 Diagnosis

Giant cell tumor of bone with aneurysmal bone cyst.

Suggested Reading

Chakarun CJ, Forrester DM, Gottsegen CJ, et al. Giant cell tumor of bone: review, mimics, and new developments in treatment. Radiographics. 2013;33(1):197–211.

Kransdorf MJ, Sweet DE, Buetow PC, et al. Giant cell tumor in skeletally immature patients. Radiology. 1992;184(1):233–7.

Murphey MD, Nomikos GC, Flemming DJ, et al. Imaging of giant cell tumor and giant cell reparative granuloma of bone: radiologic-pathologic correlation. Radiographics. 2001;21(5):1283–309.

48 Hemangioma: Case 23

48.1 Medical History

A 46-year-old male with left elbow pain, swelling, and palpable mass for 2 months. No history of trauma.

48.2 Physical Examination

Mild swelling around proximal left elbow with palpable mass, no clear margin, hard with point tenderness. Restricted range of motion of the left elbow.

48.3 Imaging Findings

48.3.1 Radiograph

X. Cheng et al., *Imaging of Bone Tumors in Shoulder and Elbow*,
https://doi.org/10.1007/978-981-33-6150-8_48

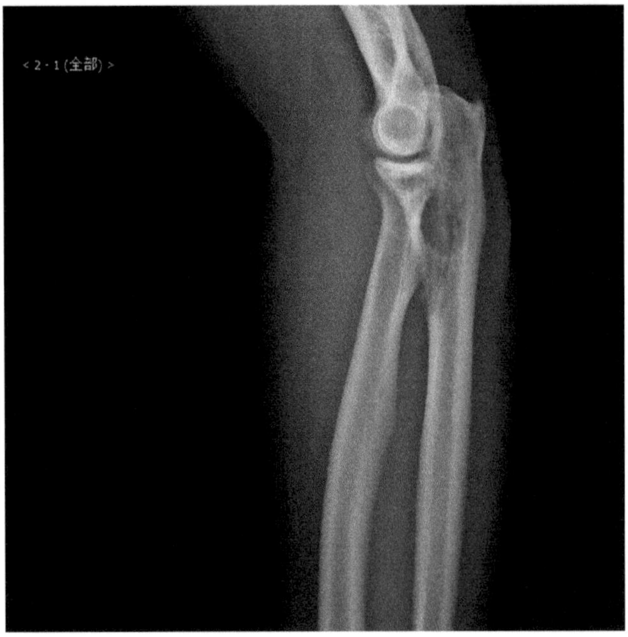

Fig. 48.1 Frontal view of the left forearm

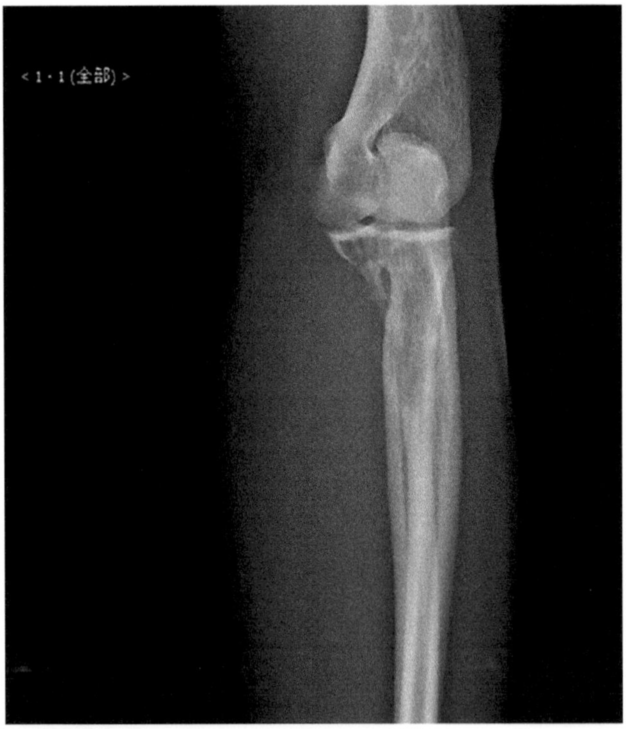

Fig. 48.2 Lateral view of the left forearm

Radiographs demonstrate focal osseous destruction around the left proximal ulna with peripheral sclerosis.

48.3.2 CT Imaging

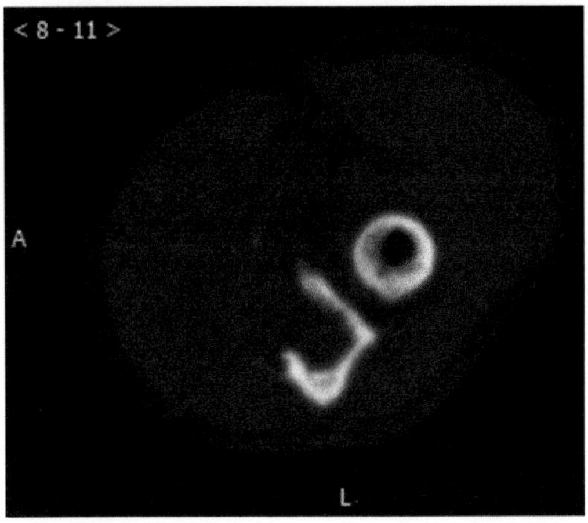

Fig. 48.3 Axial CT image of the left forearm in bone window

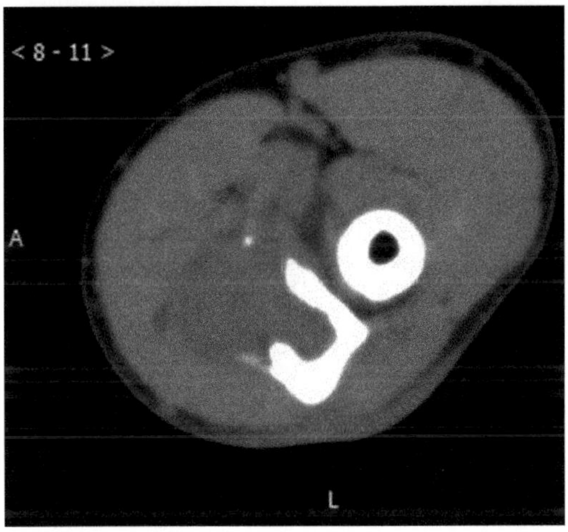

Fig. 48.4 Axial CT image of the left forearm in soft tissue window

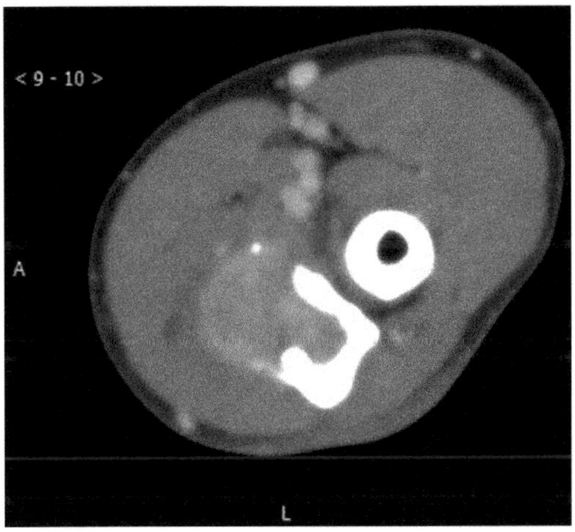

Fig. 48.5 Axial post-contrast CT image of the left forearm in soft tissue window

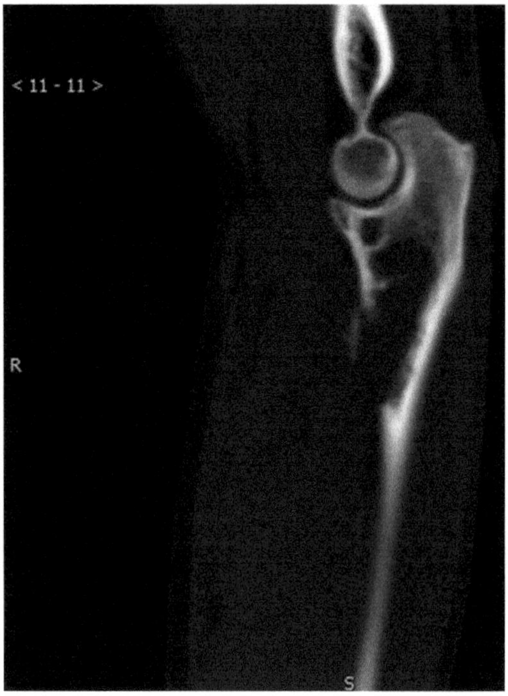

Fig. 48.6 Sagittal CT image of the left forearm in bone window

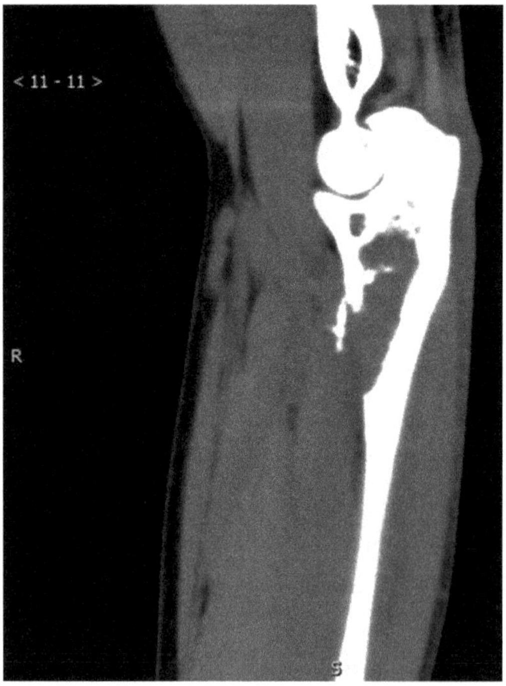

Fig. 48.7 Sagittal CT image of the left forearm in soft tissue window

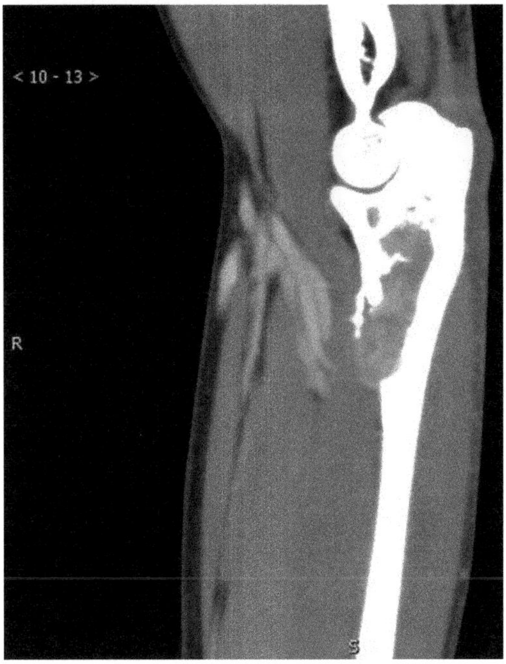

Fig. 48.8 Sagittal post-contrast CT image of the left forearm in soft tissue window

CT scan demonstrates focal osseous destruction of the left proximal ulna. There is related soft tissue mass with focal peripheral thin osseous shell. Avid enhancement is noted.

48.3.3 MR Imaging

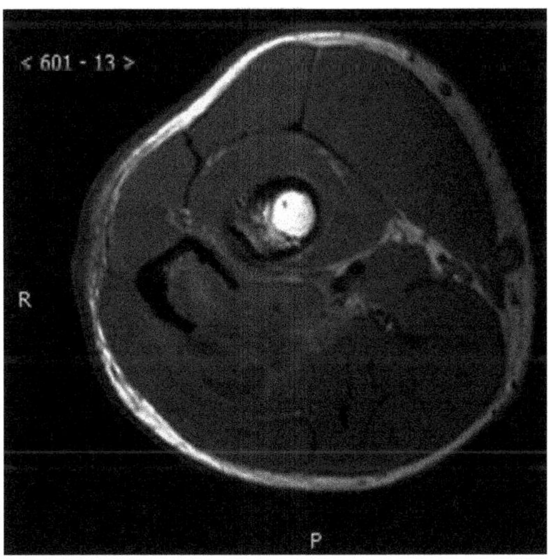

Fig. 48.9 Axial T1-weighted MR image of the left forearm

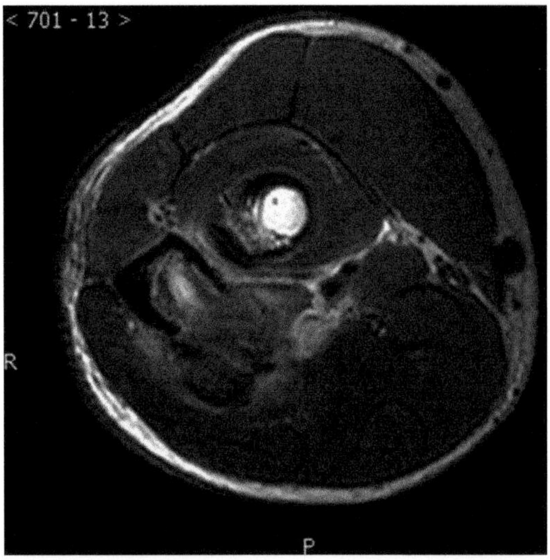

Fig. 48.10 Axial T2-weighted MR image of the left forearm

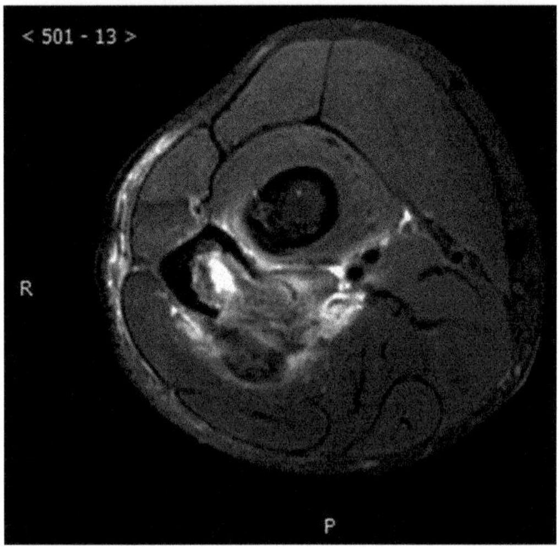

Fig. 48.11 Axial fat-suppressed T2-weighted MR image of the left forearm

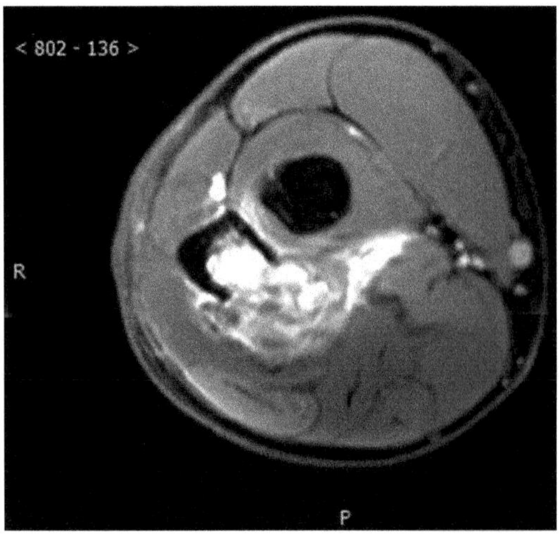

Fig. 48.12 Axial post-contrast fat-suppressed T1-weighted MR image of the left forearm

MRI scan demonstrates focal osseous destruction of the proximal ulna with related soft tissue mass. The mass demonstrates heterogeneous T1 signal and heterogeneous high T2 signal with inhomogeneous enhancement.

48.4 Description and Discussion from Residents

Radiographs demonstrate lytic osseous destruction of the proximal left ulna with internal homogeneous density and clear margin. There is a thinning of the cortex without periosteal reaction. Focal soft tissue mass is noted on CT scan with peripheral residual bone crest and shell and without internal osteoid matrix or calcification. Low signal is noted on both T1 and T2 weighted sequences, could be hemosiderin or fibrous tissue, nonspecific. There is heterogeneous enhancement. The findings favor aggressive neoplastic process, metastatic lesion should be included based on age.

48.5 Analysis and Comments from Professor Xiaoguang Cheng

There is osseous destruction around the proximal left ulna, mostly involved the cortex with expansion and invading into the medullary cavity. There is avid heterogeneous enhancement. Overall favors the malignant process and metastatic lesion is most common.

48.6 Diagnosis

Hemangioma.

Suggested Reading

Cohen EK, Kressel HY, Perosio T, et al. MR imaging of soft-tissue hemangiomas: correlation with pathologic findings. AJR Am J Roentgenol. 1988;150(5):1079–81.

Vermaat M, Vanel D, Kroon HM, et al. Vascular tumors of bone: imaging findings. Eur J Radiol. 2011;77(1):13–8.

49 Synovial Cyst: Case 24

49.1 Medical History

The patient is a 58-year-old female. She incidentally noted a mass at the anterior aspect of the left elbow about 1 month ago.

49.2 Physical Examination

There is a deep-seated mass at the midline of the front of the left elbow with a clear margin, rubbery, smooth, mobile with point tenderness.

49.3 Imaging Findings

49.3.1 Radiograph

X. Cheng et al., *Imaging of Bone Tumors in Shoulder and Elbow*,
https://doi.org/10.1007/978-981-33-6150-8_49

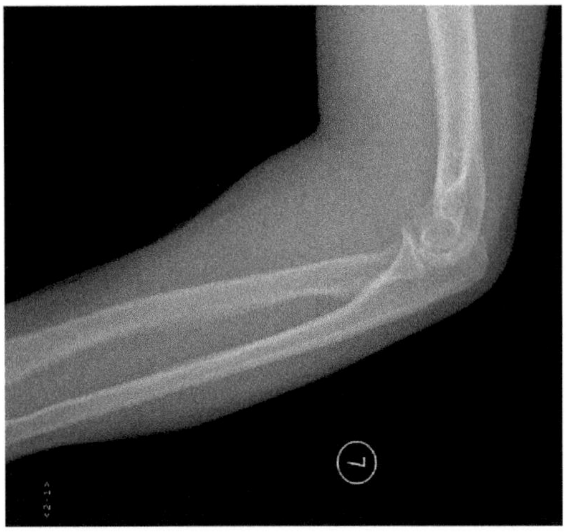

Fig. 49.1 Lateral view of the left elbow

The radiograph of the left elbow demonstrates compressive absorption of the left proximal ulna. The joint spaces are preserved. No soft tissue mass is noted.

49.3.2 CT Imaging

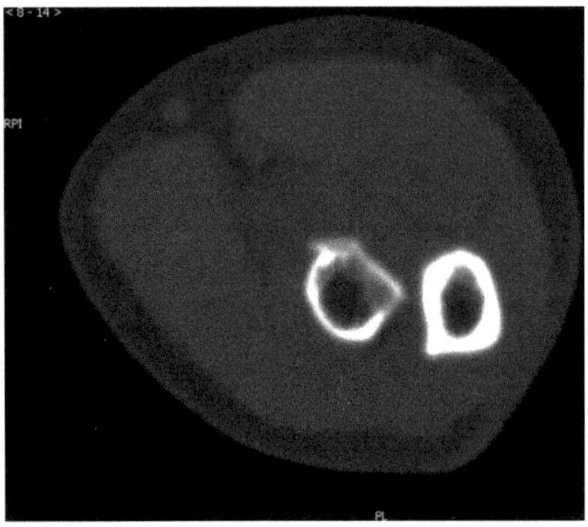

Fig. 49.2 Axial CT image of the left elbow in bone window

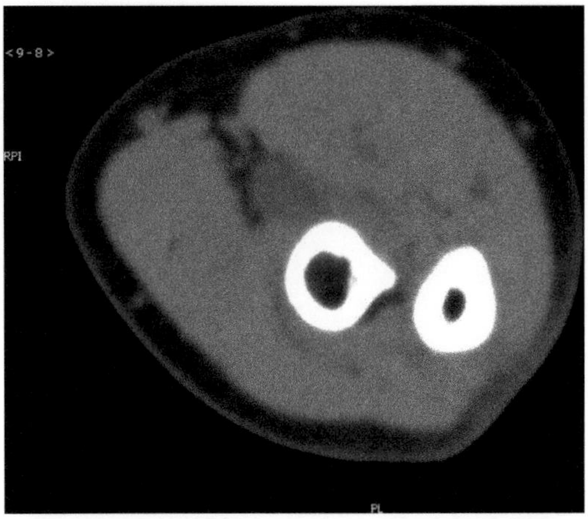

Fig. 49.3 Axial CT image of the left elbow in soft tissue window

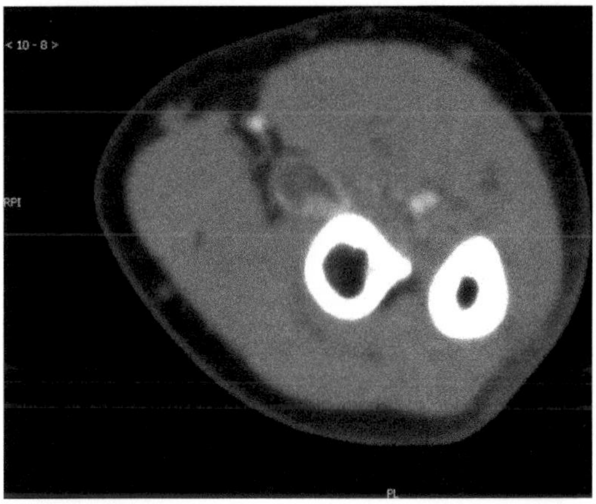

Fig. 49.4 Axial post-contrast CT image of the left elbow in soft tissue window

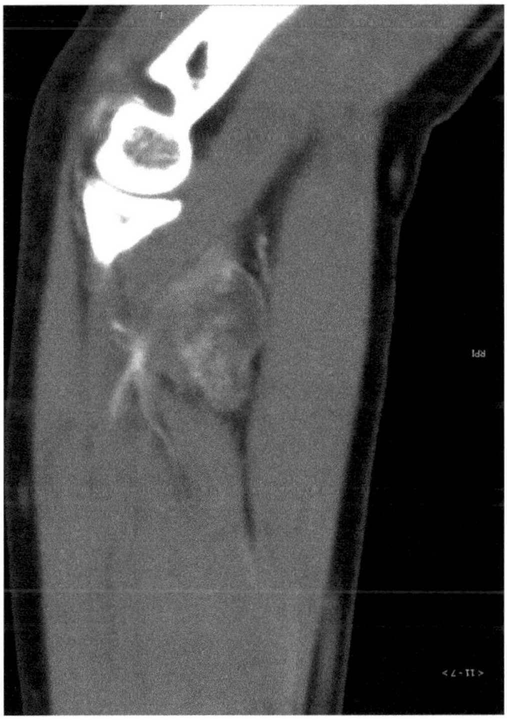

Fig. 49.5 Sagittal post-contrast CT image of the left elbow in soft tissue window

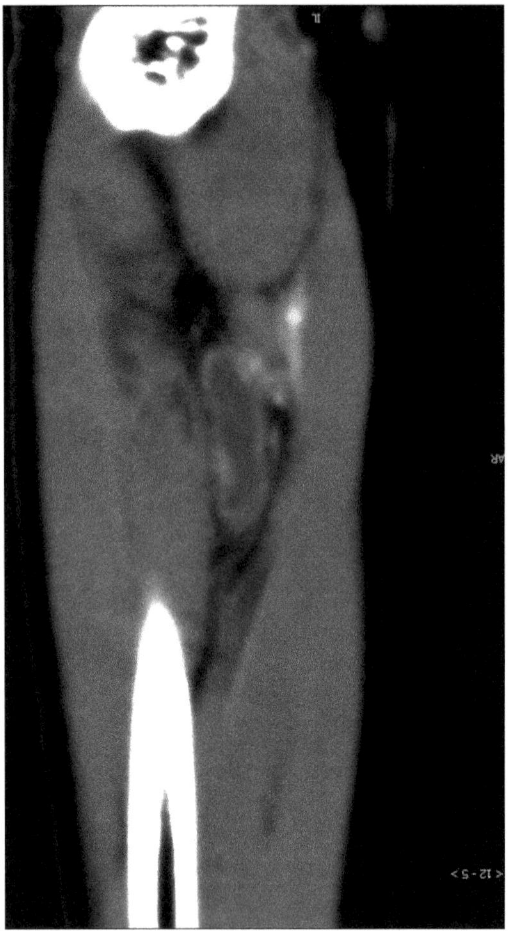

Fig. 49.6 Coronal post-contrast CT image of the left elbow in soft tissue window

CT images of the left elbow demonstrate a nodular lesion of low density around the intermuscular space of the proximal forearm with a clear margin. Peripheral circular enhancement is noted.

49.4 Description and Discussion from Residents

The radiograph demonstrates compressive change around the proximal left ulna without additional abnormality. On the CT scan, there is soft tissue mass noted along the intermuscular space of the left proximal forearm, around the neurovascular bundle. The lesion is well circumscribed with inhomogeneous density and circular peripheral enhancement. No enhancement is noted within the lesion of the area of low density. This is a benign process, likely of schwannoma.

49.5 Analysis and Comments from Professor Xiaoguang Cheng

Well-circumscribed, low-density soft tissue mass around the neurovascular bundle along the intermuscular space of the left proximal forearm demonstrates peripheral enhancement and no internal enhancement on CT scan. The above findings favor a benign process. The most common lesion in this location is schwannoma; however, with internal low density, not consistent.

49.6 Diagnosis

Synovial cyst.

Suggested Reading

Steiner E, Steinbach LS, Schnarkowski P, et al. Ganglia and cysts around joints. Radiol Clin N Am. 1996;34(2):395–425, xi–xii.

Treadwell EL. Synovial cysts and ganglia: the value of magnetic resonance imaging. Semin Arthritis Rheum. 1994;24(1):61–70.

50 Gout: Case 25

50.1 Medical History

A 59-year-old male patient presented with soft tissue nodules around multiple joints over the body for over 20 years.

50.2 Physical Examination

There are multiple hard nodules noted around feet and hands bilaterally and the right elbow, with swellings of both feet.

50.3 Imaging Findings

50.3.1 Radiograph

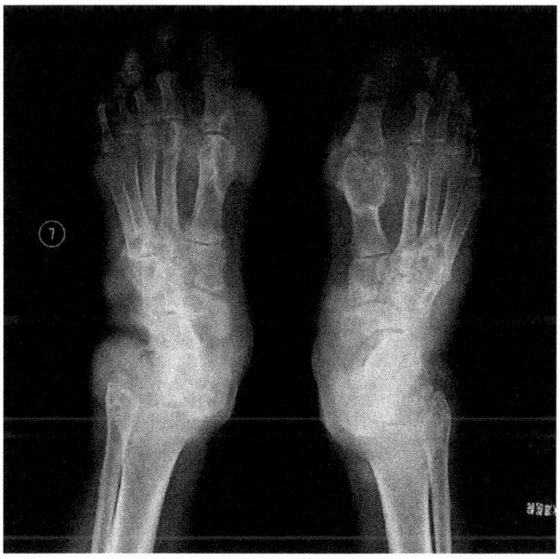

Fig. 50.1 Frontal view of both feet

X. Cheng et al., *Imaging of Bone Tumors in Shoulder and Elbow*,
https://doi.org/10.1007/978-981-33-6150-8_50

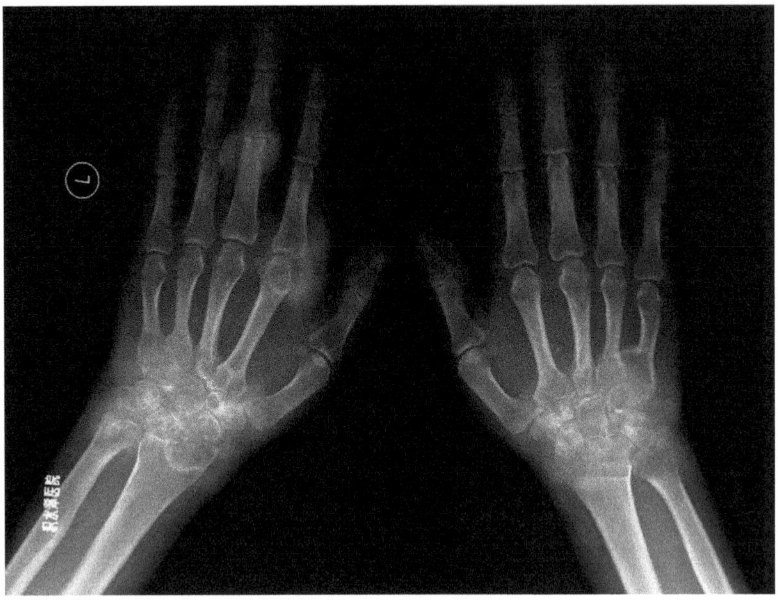

Fig. 50.2 Frontal view of both hands

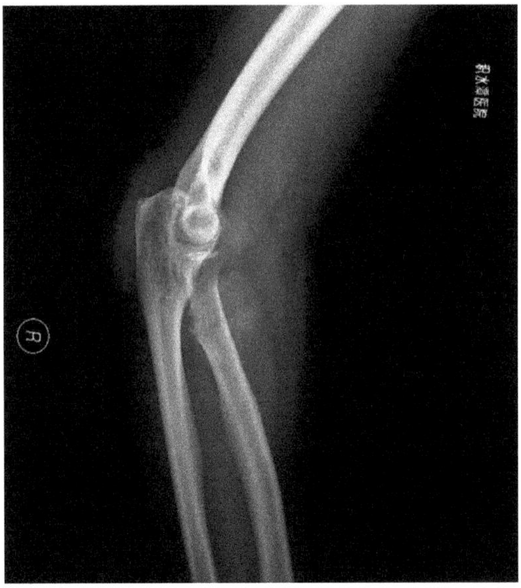

Fig. 50.3 Lateral view of the left elbow

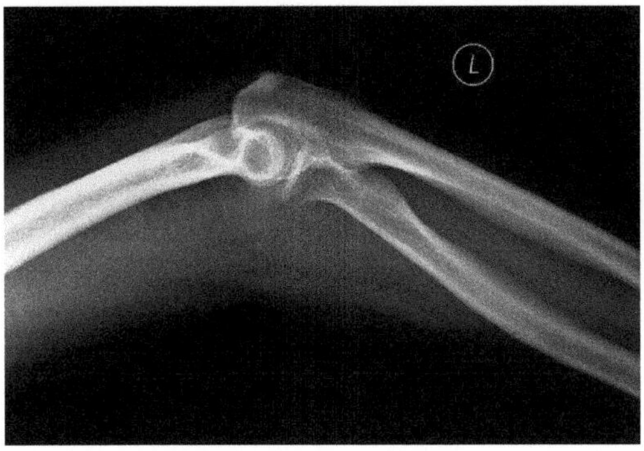

Fig. 50.4 Lateral view of the right elbow

Radiographs demonstrate multiple high-density soft tissue nodules around feet, elbows, hands, and wrists bilaterally. There are erosive changes around some of the articular surfaces.

50.3.2 CT Imaging

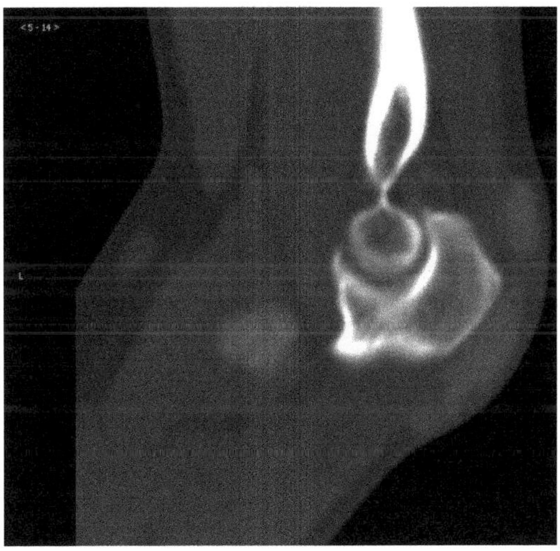

Fig. 50.5 Sagittal CT image of the right elbow in bone window

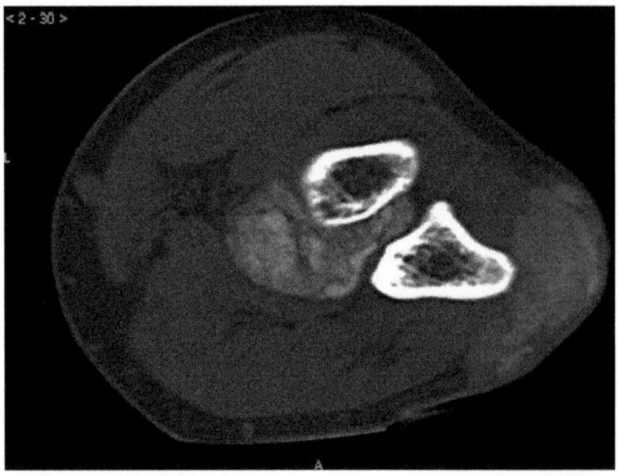

Fig. 50.6 Axial CT image of the right elbow in bone window

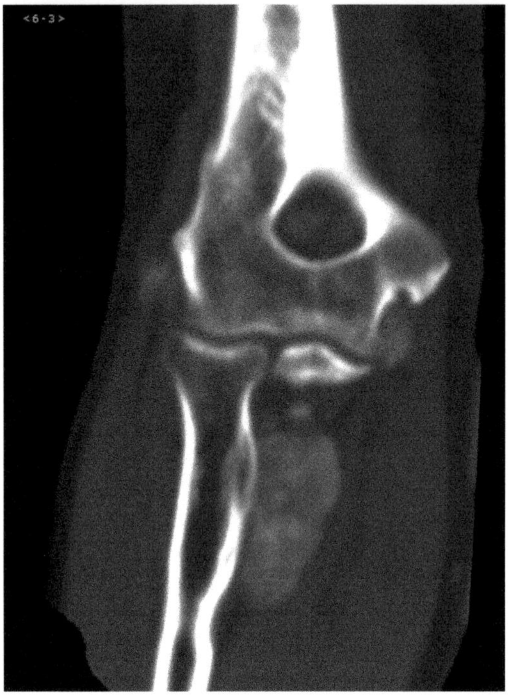

Fig. 50.7 Coronal CT image of the right elbow in bone window

CT images demonstrate multiple high-density patchy deposits around the tendon insertions and synovium of the right elbow. There are associated focal erosive changes with clear margin and peripheral sclerosis.

50.4 Description and Discussion from Residents

Images demonstrate multiple high-density soft tissue lesions around the feet, elbows, hands, and wrists bilaterally. There are focal erosive changes around the articular surface of the joints. On the CT scan images, there are multiple high-density soft tissue deposits around the tendon insertions of the elbow and focal osseous erosive changes with clear margin and peripheral sclerosis. The above constellation of findings is most consistent with gout.

50.5 Analysis and Comments from Professor Xiaoguang Cheng

There are multiple joints involved with multiple high-density soft tissue nodules around the joints with a clear margin. No obvious joint space loss or osteoporosis is noted and there is no deformity of the joint with alignment changes. On the CT scan images, the high-density soft tissue nodules are around the tendon insertions. The above findings are typical for gout. Even though multiple high-density nodules in the soft tissues can also be seen in tumoral calcinosis, the deposit pattern is different from gout.

50.6 Diagnosis

Gout.

Suggested Reading

Buckens CF, Terra MP, Maas M. Computed tomography and MR imaging in crystalline-induced arthropathies. Radiol Clin N Am. 2017;55(5):1023–34.

Omoumi P, Zufferey P, Malghem J, et al. Imaging in gout and other crystal-related arthropathies. Rheum Dis Clin N Am. 2016;42(4):621–44.